First International Conference on Rabies in Europe

Developments in Biologicals

Vol. 125

This series «Developments in Biologicals» begins with Vol. 102 and is the continuation of IABs symposia series «Progress in Immunobiological Standardization», Vols 1-5, «Immunobiological Standardization», Vols 1-22 and «Developments in Biological Standardization», Vols 23-101.

Organized and published by the International Association for Biologicals (IABs)

KARGER

Basel · Freiburg · Paris · London · New York ·
Bangalore · Bangkok · Singapore · Tokyo · Sydney

First International Conference on Rabies in Europe

Kiev, Ukraine
15-18 June, 2005

Volume editors

Betty Dodet
Dodet Biosciences
Lyon, France

Alejandro Schudel
World Organisation for Animal Health – OIE
Paris, France

Paul-Pierre Pastoret
Biotechnology and Biological Sciences Research Council (BBSRC)
Fontin, Belgium

Michel Lombard
International Association for Biologicals (IABs)
Geneva, Switzerland

Proceedings of a conference organized by the
World Organisation for Animal Health – OIE

62 figures and 28 tables, 2006

KARGER

Basel · Freiburg · Paris · London · New York ·
Bangalore · Bangkok · Singapore · Tokyo · Sydney

•••••••••••••••••

Developments in Biologicals

Library of Congress Cataloging-in-Publication Data

International Conference on Rabies in Europe (1st : 2005 : Kiev, Ukraine)
First International Conference on Rabies in Europe : Kiev, Ukraine, 15-18 June, 2005 / volume editors, Betty Dodet ... [et al.] ; proceedings of a conference organized by the World Organization for Animal Health -- OIE.
p. ; cm. -- (Developments in biologicals ; v. 125)
Includes bibliographical references.
ISBN 3-8055-8115-7 (pbk. : alk. paper)
1. Rabies--Europe--Congresses. 2. Rabies--Europe--Prevention--Congresses. I. Dodet, Betty. II. International Office of Epizootics. III. Title. IV. Series.
[DNLM: 1. Rabies--prevention & control--Europe--Congresses. 2. Disease Vectors--Europe--Congresses. 3. Rabies--epidemiology--Europe--Congresses. 4. Rabies Vaccines--immunology--Europe--Congresses. W1 DE997VKF v.125 2006 / WC 550 I616f 2006]
RA644.R3I38 2005
614.5'63094--dc22

2006017091

Bibliographic Indices. This publication is listed in bibliographic services, including Current Contents® and Index Medicus.

Drug dosage. The authors and the publisher have exerted every effort to ensure that drug selection and dosage set forth in this text are in accord with current recommendations and practice at the time of publication. However, in view of ongoing research, changes in government regulations, and the constant flow of information relating to drug therapy and drug reactions, the reader is urged to check the package insert for each drug for any change in indications and dosage and for added warnings and precautions. This is particularly important when the recommended agent is a new and/or infrequently employed drug.

Worldwide distribution by S. Karger AG, Basel (Switzerland).
Printed in Switzerland by Médecine et Hygiène, Genève.
ISBN-10: 3-8055-8115-7
ISBN-13: 978-3-8055-8115-8

Steering Committee

Dr N. Belev (OIE)
Dr F. Cliquet (AFSSA, France)
Dr J. Fevrier (EC)
Dr A. Fooks (VLA, United Kingdom)
Dr F. Meslin (WHO)
Dr T. Müller (FLI, Germany)
Dr C. Rogy (AFSSA, France)

Scientific Committee

Dr F. Cliquet (AFSSA, France)
Dr S. Edwards (VLA, United Kingdom)
Dr A. Fooks (VLA, United Kingdom)
Dr K. Gruzdev (FGI, Russia)
Dr P. Hostnik (University of Ljubljana, Slovenia)
Dr I. Kuzmin (CDC, United States of America)
Dr F. Meslin (WHO)
Dr T. Müller (FLI, Germany)
Dr P.-P. Pastoret (BBSRC, Belgium)
Dr Y. Rotivel (Institut Pasteur, France)
Dr A. Schudel (OIE)
Dr N. Tordo (Institut Pasteur, France)
Dr M. Warrell (CTM, United Kingdom)
Dr J. Zmudzinski (NVRI, Poland)

Preface

The First International Conference on Rabies in Europe was held at the President Hotel "Kyivsky", Kiev, Ukraine. The conference was opened by Dr Nikola Belev, President of the OIE Regional Commission for Europe, and Dr Alexander Wandeler, Director of the Collaborating Centre on Rabies. Dr Wandeler welcomed the participants and, on behalf of WHO, expressed gratitude to the Ukrainian Authorities for hosting the Conference. Dr Wandeler also thanked the co-sponsoring organisations and the World Organisation for Animal Health (OIE), for providing the general secretarial assistance.

Dr Wandeler stated that he wished to highlight the important role of WHO in the "European oral vaccination saga" and referred to the last major European rabies event, the Symposium on Wildlife Rabies Control held in Geneva, Switzerland, from 2 to 5 July 1990 (Wells Medical).

Dr Wandeler gave a personal account of the role of WHO in rabies control efforts in Europe, describing how he had joined the world of rabies research as a young Swiss wildlife biologist in 1966, when Switzerland was free of rabies, but invasion was imminent. Although rabies, seen predominantly in foxes, had been advancing from East to West in Europe since the end of World War II, it was around this time that international organisations began to recognise the problem at hand in Europe, and WHO organised the first European conference to address the problem in 1968. One of the recommendations of this conference was that epidemiological research should be intensified, and that wildlife biology should be included as a research topic. Also at that time, a challenging notion came from the East that rabies was not, as had been believed, a disease of foxes, but was a rodent epizootic with wild predators being sentinels only, and the isolation of rabies virus from rodents in the former Czechoslovakia and in Germany appeared to confirm this hypothesis. WHO invested considerable energy and resources into resolving this issue. With respect to rabies control, it had begun to be realised that even the most rigorous fox culling regimes only prevented the progress of the epizootic under extraordinary circumstances; and some researchers had experimented, with poor success, with trap – vaccinate – release schedules. At one of the early conferences on rabies, Dr W.G. Winkler from Centers for Disease Control (CDC), Atlanta, USA, had described George Baer's experiments with oral immunisation. The message had electrified the audience; oral immunisation of wildlife had appeared to be the solution to the rabies problem. Cooperation between several laboratories in Europe and the USA had then been facilitated by WHO. CDC had provided the ERA seed virus for laboratory studies that had eventually led to the first small-scale field trial on an island, to determine whether attenuated virus with a high residual pathogenicity could establish itself in rodent populations; no evidence for this had been found. In 1978, the late Franz Steck had then decided that the time was ripe to test the concept "real-time" on a wider scale and the ensuing success of these trials had led to new vaccines, better vaccines, safer vaccines, better baits, better baiting technologies, and more field applications.

Finally, Dr Wandeler described how the participation of WHO in the field of rabies control in the late 1960s and early 1970s had inspired and facilitated a number of national developments in Europe and North America, the most important of these being the creation of the Laboratoire d'études sur la rage et la pathologie des animaux sauvages, Centre national d'études vétérinaires et alimentaires (CNEVA) in Nancy, France.

The introduction to the conference was continued by Dr Florence Cliquet, Head of the French Food Safety Agency (AFSSA) in Nancy.

Dr Cliquet indicates that AFSSA was a key element in the system by which food safety, including the protection of animal health, is organised in France. By the provision of risk assessment and scientific and technical support, AFSSA enabled the authorities responsible for risk management, namely the Ministries of Agriculture, Health and Consumer Protection, to take actions based on sound science. The speaker explained that the activities of AFSSA covered the whole food chain, from primary production to final consumer, and concerned all kinds of food products of animal and vegetal origin (whether intended for human or animal consumption), and also drinking-water. Dr Cliquet said that AFSSA possessed 12 laboratories, which carried out research on food hygiene as well as on the health and welfare of different animal species, including fish. The work of the AFSSA laboratory located in Nancy, eastern France, is focused on rabies. It provides scientific and technical support to the French authorities, to OIE, WHO and the European Commission, and its activities mainly concern the surveillance and epidemiology of rabies and research programmes related to rabies. AFSSA also includes the National Agency for Veterinary Medicine Products, which delivers market authorisations for all veterinary products, controls the producing establishments and carries out pharmacovigilance.

Dr Cliquet declared that the rabies situation in Europe was a cause for concern. As with many other zoonoses, rabies does not respect borders, and national strategies are thus not sufficient. Dr Cliquet stated that strong international coordination was needed to determine and implement methods of prevention and control of the disease in a consistent way.

Dr Cliquet also explained that oral vaccination of rabies reservoirs was a key element of the French rabies control strategy. The determination of oral vaccination strategies required consideration of several parameters that would be discussed during the conference. It was emphasised that it was essential that options be based on strong scientific evidence and reliable epidemiological data.

Dr Cliquet suggested that the conference would provide an opportunity to share experience, and expressed her confidence that practical recommendations relevant to the situation prevailing in Europe would be elaborated. Dr Cliquet also assured the participants that AFSSA was ready to provide scientific support and to fully participate in international collaboration on rabies control.

The Conference was closed by Professor Nikola Belev, President of OIE Regional Commission for Europe, on behalf of the Director General of OIE, Dr Bernard Vallat.

Professor Belev stated that the most important aim of the conference had been achieved, that is, the bringing together of veterinarians, scientists, clinicians and public health officials to share their experience in modern rabies control, to agree strategies for the prevention and control of this fatal disease in reservoir animal species, and to examine the threat that classical rabies virus strains and new emerging strains of rabies virus, including bat rabies, may pose.

During the conference, 43 reports on the prevention and elimination of rabies had been presented by scientists of international renown, who also contributed greatly to the adoption of the conference recommendations. A total of 150 specialists, including young scientists, from 36 countries had participated in the conference.

Professor Belev indicated that now we are obliged:

- to provide the funds for national programmes in each European country, and for a programme for Europe in general;
- to coordinate the activities of reference laboratories and collaborating centres concerning rabies;
- to clearly develop measures for the prevention and elimination of rabies in domestic animals. These measures would involve the mass media, which would distribute information under the control of a Steering Committee to be created in Europe. Professor Belev thanked the Government, Parliament, Prime Minister and President of Ukraine for their invitation and support.

Professor Belev also thanked to:

- the Conference Steering Committee in Paris (which included representatives of OIE, WHO, the European Union [EU], and AFSSA), headed by Dr A. Schudel, Head of the OIE Scientific and Technical Department;
- the Conference Steering Committee in Ukraine, headed by Petro Verbitskiy, Chief Veterinary Officer of Ukraine, Secretary General of OIE Regional Commission for Europe;
- the Scientific Committee responsible for the preparation of the excellent conference programme;
- all the participants;
- the Ukrainian Mass Media for covering the conference in editorials and programmes following the press conference;
- the interpreters, who facilitated communication among the participants;
- staff of the company "Gestalt", which organised the logistical arrangements for the Conference.

Professor Belev informed the participants that all the conference materials would be published shortly in Russian and English by OIE Regional Commission for Europe and sent to the pertinent government representatives of all European countries.

Foreword

In 1885, Louis Pasteur produced the world's first rabies vaccine. Since then, significant advances have been made in reducing the burden of one of the best known and most feared zoonotic diseases in the world. Nevertheless, despite major advances in the past century, rabies control is still overlooked and rabies remains endemic in many parts of the world, including some parts of Europe, largely as a result of financial limitations and poor infrastructures. The control of animal rabies remains one of the major goals of Veterinary Services world-wide.

Experience shows that vaccination of rabies reservoirs – whether domestic or wildlife animals – offers a new and promising perspective in the global control of rabies. One particular example is the oral vaccination of wildlife, such as foxes, which led to the eradication of terrestrial rabies from large areas of Europe and to a reduction in the human burden of disease.

Each year, however, many unvaccinated people living in regions where rabies is endemic become anxious following contact with an animal suspected of harbouring the virus. Hence, great challenges remain in the 21st century to eliminate this zoonosis on a global scale. With this in mind, a jointly organised OIE/WHO/EU European Conference "Rabies in Europe" will be held in Kiev, Ukraine.

The most important aim of the conference will be to bring together veterinarians, scientists, clinicians and public health officials to share their experience in modern rabies control, to agree strategies for the prevention and control of this fatal disease in reservoir animal species, and to examine the threat that classical rabies virus strains and new emerging strains of rabies virus may pose, including bat rabies.

The result of a recent survey carried out by the OIE among its 167 Member Countries, supports the premise that a strong partnership among veterinary and public health authorities is needed in order to succeed in the control of zoonotic diseases.

I am convinced that the tools are available to successfully combat rabies. Now it is up to us to take the final steps toward a rabies-free Europe.

Dr. Bernard Vallat
OIE Director General

Organisation of the Meeting

Session I	Epidemiology Chairperson : *I.V. Kuzmin* (CDC, USA) Rapporteur : *F. Cliquet* (AFSSA, France)
Session II	Rabies Diagnosis Chairperson : *S. Edwards* (VLA, United Kingdom) Rapporteur : *P. Hostnik* (University of Ljubljana, Slovenia)
Session III	Animal Rabies Control Chairperson : *J. Zmudzinsky* (NVRI, Poland) Rapporteur : *F. Cliquet* (AFSSA, France)
Session IV	Human Rabies Prevention Chairperson : *Y. Rotivel* (Institut Pasteur, France) Rapporteur : *M. Warrel* (CTM, United Kingdom)
Session V	Vaccinology and Immunology Chairperson : *K. Gruzdev* (FGI, Russia) Rapporteur : *P.P. Pastoret* (BBSRC, Belgium)
Session VI	Bat Rabies Chairperson : *T. Müller* (FLI, Germany) Rapporteur : *A. Fooks* (VLA, United Kingdom)

Conclusions and Recommendations

Poster Session

Contents

Dodet B, Schudel A, Pastoret PP, Lombard M (eds): Rabies in Europe.
Dev Biol (Basel). Basel, Karger, 2006, vol 125, p 1.

SESSION I

Epidemiology

Chairperson: *I.V. Kuzmin* (CDC, USA)
Rapporteur: *F. Cliquet* (AFSSA, France)

Dodet B, Schudel A, Pastoret PP, Lombard M (eds): Rabies in Europe.
Dev Biol (Basel). Basel, Karger, 2006, vol 125, pp 3-13.

Rabies: Epidemiological Tendencies and Control Tools

N. Tordo[1], C. Bahloul[3], Y. Jacob[2], C. Jallet[1], P. Perrin[1], H. Badrane[4]

[1] Unit " Antiviral Strategies ", Virology Department, Institut Pasteur, Paris, France

[2] Unit " Papillomavirus and Human Cancer ", Virology Department, Institut Pasteur, Paris, France

[3] Institut Pasteur de Tunis, Tunisia

[4] University of Florida, Department of Molecular Genetics & Microbiology, Gainesville, GA, USA

Key words: Lyssavirus, rabies.

Abstract: Rabies encephalitis still generates 50,000 human deaths/year. It is due to neuron infection by lyssaviruses. Seven genotypes (GT) are currently distinguished within the *Lyssavirus* genus which segregate in two phylogroups (PG). This classification is constantly evolving due to isolation of new lyssaviruses within bat populations. Functional differences exist between GTs in term of neurotropism, pathogenesis, induction of apoptosis, immunogenicity, and their molecular basis are starting to be elucidated. Lyssavirus vectors are mammals, preferentially from the *Carnivora* and *Chiroptera* orders. Phylogenetic reconstruction strongly supports that lyssaviruses evolved in chiropters long before the emergence of carnivoran rabies which very likely occurred through host-switchings from bats to carnivores. If dog rabies control is possible by vaccination and population control, if oral vaccination demonstrated its potential to eliminate rabies from a terrestrial wildlife reservoir (fox in Western Europe), it is unrealistic today to clear lyssaviruses from bats, while bat rabies is a growing concern for both public and animal health. As bat transmit divergent lyssavirus GTs which are not well prevented by available vaccine strains, there is a need to increase the protection spectrum of vaccines. DNA-based immunization with plasmids expressing chimeric G proteins (fusion of two halves from different GTs) was shown to be effective in inducing a complete immune response and to broaden the spectrum of rabies vaccines toward lyssavirus vaccines. Further, the lyssavirus G protein can carry foreign epitopes/antigens in the perspective of multivalent vaccines against various zoonoses of carnivores.

Introduction

According to a recent re-evaluation of both public health and economic burden, rabies encephalitis remains responsible annually for 55,000 human deaths corresponding to 1.74 million disability-adjusted life years (DALYs) [1]. If Asia still pays the heaviest tribute (31,000 deaths), the death toll in Africa is also alarming (24,000 deaths). On the other hand, under the impulsion of PAHO over the last 15 years, Latin American governments have implemented strict control measures (mass vaccination of dogs and treatment of exposed people) resulting in a stringent reduction of canine rabies, followed by an immediate benefit for human health (< 50 cases/year) [2]. This success clearly demonstrates that, with political will and financial support, efficient tools are available today to reduce human and animal rabies incidence. In humans, safe and potent vaccines produced in cell culture, recommended by WHO, are progressively replacing old vaccines prepared from animal nervous tissue that are less immunogenic and occasionally suspected of adverse effects; in animals, classical vaccines in use under domestic conditions are complemented by a panel of recombinant and attenuated vaccines administrable by the oral route to vaccinate non-accessible dogs or wildlife.

Rabies and the Lyssavirus Infectious Cycle

The etiologic agents of rabies encephalitis belong to the order *Mononegavirales*, family *Rhabdoviridae*, genus *Lyssavirus* [3]. Lyssaviruses are most generally transmitted by the bite of an infected animal although transmission through aerosols could play a role in bat colonies. Even if inoculation generally occurs in non-nervous tissues, such as muscles, lyssaviruses are naturally neurotropic and propagate through the neuronal network up to the central nervous system (CNS). The incubation period, which corresponds to transfer up to the CNS, varies from 2 weeks to several years (average: 2 months) depending on the place of inoculation and the virulence of the variant. The symptomatic period, which results from neuronal dysfunctions still poorly understood, is shorter (1 week on average). It leads invariably to death although there are growing efforts to develop efficient therapies [4]. In the late stages, non-neuronal tissues such as the salivary glands are infected, allowing for virus transmission through biting.

The molecular bases for lyssavirus neurotropism are not fully understood but certainly implicate neuro-specific receptor recognition, first at the neuromuscular junction, then at inter-neuronal connexions. Three cellular proteins have been proposed to play some role in lyssavirus attachment [5]: the nicotinic acetylcholine receptor (nAChR), the neuronal cell adhesion molecule (NCAM) and the low affinity neurotrophin receptor (p75NTR). These receptors are bound by the viral transmembrane glycoprotein (G) which forms spike-like projections out of the lipid envelope of the bullet-shaped virion [6]. Then, the particule is internalized in an endosome, acidification provokes G mediated fusion of viral and endosomal envelopes and the internal helical ribonucleocapsid (or RNP) is delivered into the cytoplasm. The RNP is composed of the genomic RNA (12 kilobases, non-segmented, negative polarity) intimately associated with the nucleoprotein (N) and with a polymerase complex comprising the RNA-dependent RNA polymerase (L) and its cofactor the phosphoprotein (P, formally named M1). This RNP complex mediates viral transcription and replication in the cytoplasm [7]. The fifth viral structural protein, the matrix protein (M, formally named M2) is notably responsible for virus budding and bullet-shaped morphology. It occupies an intermediate position between the RNP and the envelope and interferes in both structures. In the neuron, between entry at the synapse and transcription/replication in the perinuclear space, the virus is actively transported along the axon and dendrites via retrograde or anterograde transport. It is unclear whether the RNP (upon release at the synapse) or the endosome vesicule is transported. A strong interaction between the P protein and the dynein light chain 8 (DLC8, a key element of the retrograde axonal motors) could play for the first hypothesis [8,9].

Natural History and Evolution of Lyssaviruses

Because the majority of human rabies infections worldwide are consecutive to dog bites in developing countries, rabies transmission has long been attributed to dogs only. Remnants of this profound dog/rabies association have integrated into common language, such as with the French word "canicule" designating the hot summer periods when dogs were presumed more effective at transmitting rabies due to the bad influence of Sirius, the dog constellation. However, with the progressive control of rabies in dogs and increased activity in field isolation, it has becoming clear that lyssaviruses are preferentially transmitted by wildlife vectors from two mammalian orders, *Carnivora* and *Chiroptera* (Fig. 1). Carnivoran vectors are members of the families *Canidae* (dog, fox, and raccoon dog), *Procyonidae* (raccoon), *Mustelidae* (skunk), and *Herpestidae* (mongoose). Chiropteran vectors have been found in more than 150 species of 50 genera including both megachiropters and microchiropters, frugivorous, insectivorous and hematophageous. The development of both antigenic and molecular methods for virus identification have progressively allowed for lyssavirus classification. Cross-reactivity between antisera against internal antigens (RNP in which N is highly conserved) first served to

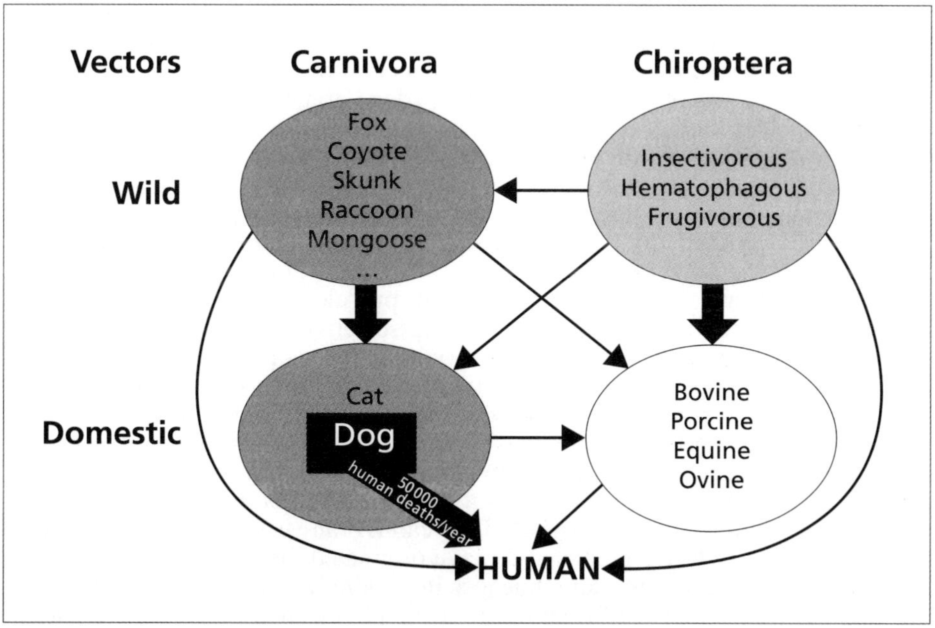

Fig. 1 : Dynamics of transmission of lyssaviruses from *Carnivora* and *Chiroptera* vectors to humans.

distinguish the *Lyssavirus* genus from the *Vesiculovirus* genus (VSV) within the *Rhabdoviridae* family. Virus-neutralising antibodies (VNAbs), which mainly recognized the G protein (less conserved), subdivided the *Lyssavirus* genus into three serotypes, and MAb studies further refined the classification into four serotypes: 1 (Rabies virus, RABV), 2 (Lagos bat virus, LBV), 3 (Mokola virus, MOKV) and 4 (Duvenhage virus, DUVV). Finally phylogenetic comparison of the N, G and P genes have delineated seven genotypes [10-12] (Table 1): the first four matched the four serotypes, and three additional genotypes were created for European bat lyssavirus type 1 (EBLV-1), type 2 (EBLV-2) and Australian bat lyssavirus (ABLV). The seven genotypes are distributed into two phylogroups [11]: phylogroup I includes genotypes 1 and 4 to 7; phylogroup II comprises genotypes 2 and 3 (Fig. 2). This current classification is bound to constantly evolve, particularly as surveillance of bat lyssaviruses is reinforced. Already, four additional divergent lyssaviruses have been isolated in bats of Central Asia, East Siberia and the Black Sea region and are proposed as new genotypes [13,14]: Aravan virus (ARAV), Khujand virus (KHUV), Irkut virus (IRKV) and West-Caucasian bat virus (WCBV). ARAV, KHUV and IRKV are more closely related to viruses of genotypes 4 (DUVV), 5 (EBLV-1) and 6 (EBLV-2) which altogether could form a distinct lineage of Old World (Africa-Europe-Asia) bat lyssaviruses. Although WCBV would appear phylogenetically closer to phylogroup II (LBV and MOKV) it is one of the most divergent lyssavirus isolated so far. It is predictable that increased surveillance of bat lyssaviruses in Asia will soon suggest a more complex classification [15-17].

Each genotype encompasses variants with distinct genetic patterns typical of the geographical area and/or the species of isolation. Each variant is primarily maintained in a single species under specific ecological conditions, but is also able to infect a variety of other species. These regular transmissions across the species barrier are more frequently dead-end infections, but may exceptionally result in variant adaptation and emergence of a new vector. In genotype 1 (classical rabies), a cosmopolitan lineage illustrates human influence in rabies epidemiology through the worldwide spread of the ancient European dog variant during colonization periods [11,18]. This variant has undergone successful adaptation to wildlife species (skunk, coyote, fox in North-America, etc.). With the increasing amount of genetic data on viral field isolates, the evolution mechanisms of the lyssavirus genome and their epidemiological consequences in nature have been analyzed [19-21]. Evolution primarily proceeds by point mutations (limited insertion/deletion, no visible role for recombination) at a low rate for an RNA virus estimated at about 4.10^{-4} synonymous mutations/site/year. There is a high prevalence of synonymous versus non-synonymous mutations suggesting strong selective constraints and purifying selection. It is, however, possible to identify limited regions or residues that seem subjected to some positive selection, particularly in G but also in N or P proteins. Although this local positive selection could result from virus/vector adaptation, no precise residue has been unambiguously pointed out as a signature of the variant adaptation to a specific vector. At the evolutionary level, phylogenetic reconstruction strongly supports an ancient evolution of lyssaviruses in chiropteran vectors with regular spillover and host-switching to carnivoran vectors [19]. Such bat/carnivore spillover is clearly predicted to have originated the raccoon lineage in the Eastern USA as well as the skunk lineages in South-Central USA and North-Central Mexico [22]. As a confirmation of these phylogenetic predictions, natural bat/carnivore host-switchings are regularly observed in nature. In most cases, they

Table 1 : Toxonomy classification of the *Lyssavirus* genus using phylogenetic and serologic characteristics.

Phylogroup	Geno-sero types	Species Tentative species	Abrev. (ICTV)	Geographical origin	Potential vector(s)
I	1-1	Rabies virus	RABV	World (except several islands)	Carnivores (world) Bats (Americas)
I	4-4	Duvenhage virus	DUVV	Southern-Africa	Insectivorous bats
I	5-?	European bat lyssavirus type 1	EBLV-1	Europe	Insectivorous bats *Eptesicus serotinus*
I	6-?	European bat lyssavirus type 2	EBLV-2	Europe	Insectivorous bats *Myotis sp*
I	7-?	Australian bat lyssavirus	ABLV	Australia (Philippines ?)	Frugivorous/insectivorous bats *Pteropus sp./Microchiroptera*
II	2-2	Lagos bat virus	LBV	Sub-Saharian Africa	Frugivorous bats *Megachiroptera*
II	3-3	Mokola virus	MOKV	Sub-Saharian Africa	**Unknown** (isolated from shrews)
?	?-?	*Aravan virus*	ARAV	Central Asia	Insectivorous bats (isolated from *Myotis blythi*)
?	?-?	*Khujand virus*	KHUV	Central Asia	Insectivorous bats (isolated from *Myotis mystacinus*)
?	?-?	*Irkut virus*	IRKV	East Siberia	Insectivorous bats (isolated from *Murina leucogaster*)
?	?-?	*West Caucasian bat virus*	WCBV	Caucasus region	Insectivorous bats (isolated from *Miniopterus schreibersi*)

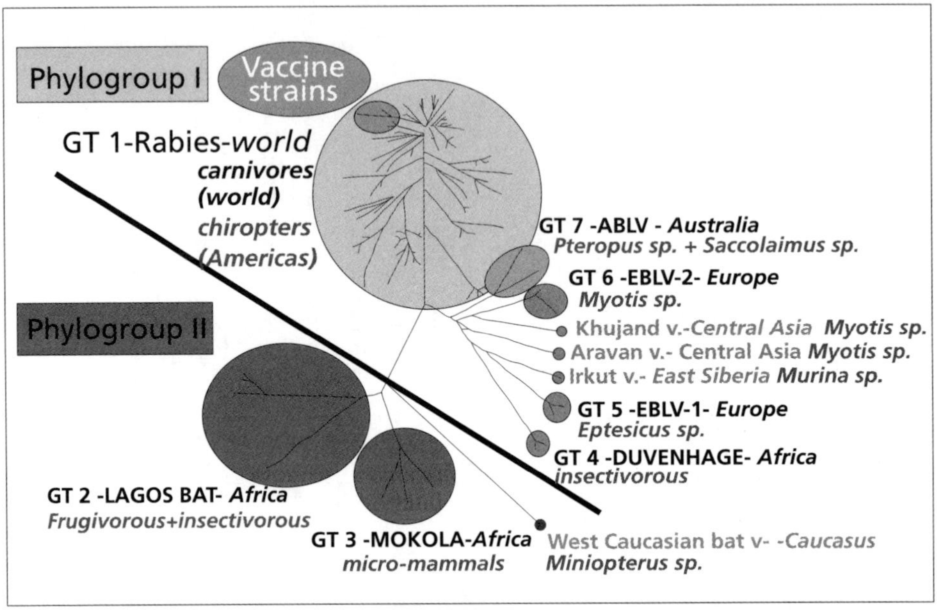

Fig. 2: **Diversity of the *Lyssavirus* genus:** A radial phylogenetic tree has been obtained by comparing partial nucleotide sequences of the G protein ectodomain using the Neighbour Joining Method (CLUSTAL-W; PHYLIP). The transversal bold line distinguishes phylogroups I and II. Circles illustrate the current genetic dispersion for each genotype (GT) which geographical location and principal vector species are indicated (bats in light, carnivores in dark). The vaccine strain position is indicated at the top of GT1.

only lead to dead-end infections like for EBLV1 transmission to sheep in Denmark [23] or to a stone-marten in Germany (24). More rarely, their adaptation is successful like for a RABV *Myotis* variant which circulated for a while among foxes in the Prince Edward Island, Canada [25] or more recently for a RABV *Eptesicus* variant which has been circulating among skunks since 2001 in Arizona [26].

Pathogenesis and Perspectives of Control

Efforts are currently underway worldwide to experimentally evaluate the pathogenicity of lyssaviruses, and particularly the transmissibility of bat lyssaviruses to terrestrial mammals including potential carnivore vectors. Lyssaviruses from different genotypes have been inoculated to various animal models such as the bat, dog, cat, red fox, sheep, ferret, hamster, and mouse [11,27-29]. Although the relevance of the rodent model for rabies infection can be discussed, it is the only one in which infection by a limited number of isolates from all genotypes of lyssaviruses has been tested. Globally, lyssaviruses of phylogroup I are pathogenic for mice when injected by the intracerebral or intramuscular routes, while lyssaviruses of phylogroup II are less pathogenic by the intramuscular route [11,29]. In non-rodent mammals, the pathogenicity is more variable depending on the species and the lyssavirus genotype. The molecular bases for these differences have been studied in vitro and in mice. Pathogenicity by the peripheral route results in the loss of responsivness of T-cells specific for lyssavirus antigens [30]. Apoptosis is also thought to play a key role in pathogenicity [31,32]. In vitro, it is more intensively induced in mouse neuroblastoma cells infected with lyssaviruses of phylogroup II [33]. By provoking more cell death, viral spread and pathogenesis in vivo is reduced. Coherently, a strong induction of apoptosis is also observed during human neuroblastoma cell infection with non-pathogenic mutants of phylogroup I [34,35]. Lyssaviral induction of apoptosis is probably multigenic and involves at least M and G proteins [33,35]. Concerning viral markers of pathogenicity, all lyssaviruses of phylogroup II sequenced so far, including the recently isolated WCBV, possess an acid residue (D or E) in position 333 of the G protein [11,14], while the maintenance of a basic residue (mostly R, sometimes K) at this position is an absolute prerequisite to maintain pathogenicity of phylogroup I laboratory strains [36,37]. R333D mutation could impair receptor recognition and penetration into neurons [38]. In this context, it is of note that G proteins from phylogroup II lyssaviruses (as well as from genotypes 4 (DUVV) and 5 (EBLV-1) in phylogroup I) are unable to specifically bind p75NTR, one potential receptor for rabies virus [39]. Other differences between G proteins from rabies virus (phylogroup I) and Mokola virus (phylogroup II) may also contribute to their different pathogenicity: RABV G protein trimers show greater stability and induce fusion at a lower pH than MOKV G protein trimers [40].

The constant potential of bat lyssavirus variants to spill-over and invade new carnivore vectors is currently impairing any perspective of global rabies eradication. It is clear that canine rabies can be controlled by systematic vaccination and population control, as has been demonstrated over the last century in many European countries, and as it is today successfully performed in Latin America [2]. In addition, it has also been beautifully demonstrated in Western Europe that the rational use of oral vaccination is a powerful tool to eliminate rabies from a terrestrial wildlife reservoir like the red fox [41]. Once adapted to each specific ecological context, a similar approach could be reasonably applied to many regions in the world still faced with terrestrial rabies: in Central, Eastern, and Northern Europe for fox rabies as well as for the emergent raccoon dog rabies; in the Americas, for the multiple existing terrestrial vectors: skunk, raccoon, fox, coyote, and mongoose [42]. However, it still appears unrealistic, today, to clear lyssaviruses from bats. This will remain a constant concern for both public and animal health, with the added potential of the virus to acquire new carnivore vectors. In the USA, over the last decades, RABV bat variants have progressively become the principal cause of indigenous human rabies cases [43]. Even in countries fulfilling the OIE rabies-free status (no terrestrial case for two consecutive years with effective surveillance) bat rabies remains present. In France, 26 EBLV-1 positive bats have been diagnosed so far with an increasing number since vulpine rabies elimination in 1998. In UK and Australia, which have been considered as a rabies-free countries for one century, EBLV2 and ABLV have been responsible for one (Scottland, 2002) and two human cases (since 1995), respectively [44]. Facing this situation, it is of note that all the current rabies vaccine strains belong to genotype 1 and were isolated a long time ago [45]. They are clearly protecting against RABV and ABLV, and they are more or less efficient against other genotypes in phylogroup I (EBLVs, DUVV), but they are unable to protect against lyssaviruses from phylogroup II (MOKV, LBV, WCBL) [11,29,46-48]. This absence of cross-neutralisation is globally inversely related to the genetic distance between each genotype and the vaccinal strain used

[11,29]. Assuming continued emergence in rabies epidemiology, especially in bats hosting divergent lyssaviruses, there is a need for a broader spectrum of protection. Perspectives in this direction have been opened using novel strategies such as DNA-based immunization, which has been shown to induce a complete immune response and protection in the mouse as well as in other target species like the dog [46,47,49,50]. Plasmids expressing chimeric G proteins were constructed by fusing the COOH-half of one genotype with the NH2-half of another genotype (Fig. 3). Upon intramuscular injection in mice, protection was obtained against the two parental genotypes but also against other genotypes, demonstrating the possibility of increasing the spectrum from anti-rabies to anti-lyssavirus vaccines. In addition, the capability of the lyssavirus G protein to carry foreign epitopes/antigens was also demonstrated in the perspective of a future DNA multivalent vaccine against various zoonoses for carnivores [51].

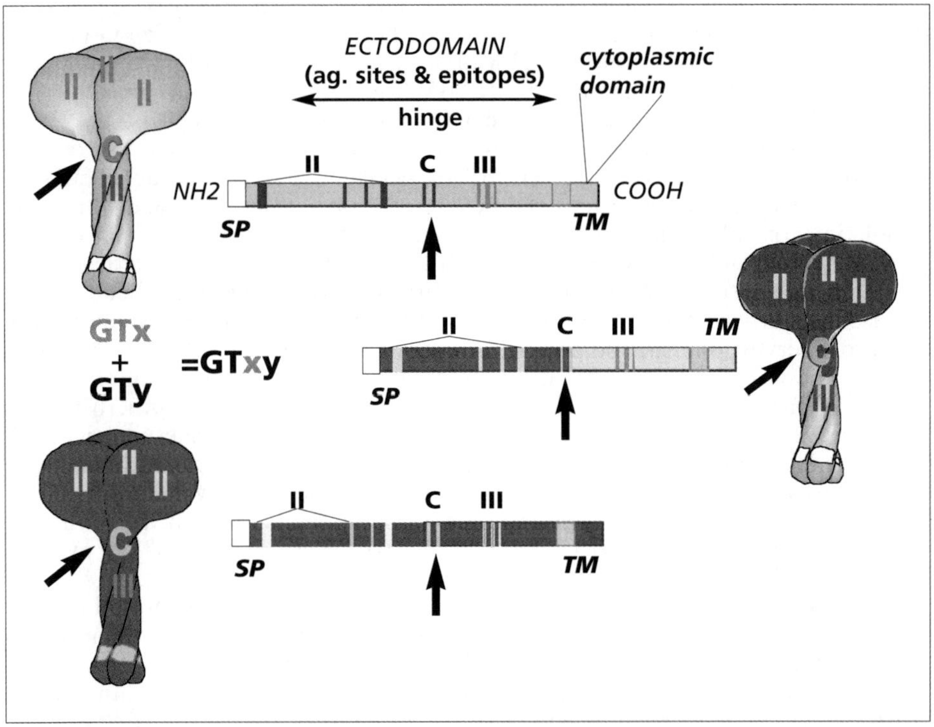

Fig. 3: **Chimerical Lyssavirus G proteins to increase the vaccine spectrum:** The transmembrane G protein comprises from the NH2 to the COOH extremity: a signal peptide (SP) removed from the mature protein; a glycosylated ectodomain carrying the antigenic sites and epitopes; a transmembrane peptide (TM); a cytoplasmic domain. There are 2 majors antigenic sites: site II is composed of epitopes dispersed along the NH2-half of the ectodomain that are put into contact by the protein folding (disulfide bridges); site III is more compact and limited in size (about 10 amino acids). Most G epitopes are conformational except one located between the 2 main antigenic sites and which constitutes a hinge region (region C). This region has been used to generate chimerical G proteins composed by the fusion of NH2- and COOH halves from divergent genotypes. The G protein structure proposed is purely hypothetical since the exact structure has not been solved so far.

References

1 Knobel D, Cleaveland S, Coleman PG, Fèvre EM, Meltzer MI, Miranda MEG, Shaw A, Zinsstag J, Meslin FX: Re-evaluating the burden of rabies in Africa and Asia. Bull WHO 2005; 83: 360-368.

2 Belotto A, Leanes LF, Schneider MC, Tamayo H, Correa E: Overview of rabies in the Americas. Virus Res 2005; 111: 5-12.

3 Tordo N, Benmansour A, Calisher C, Dietzgen RG, Fang R-X Jackson AO, Kurath G, Nadin-Davis S, Tesh RB, Walker, PJ: Rhabdoviridae, in Fauquet CM, Mayo MA, Maniloff J, Desselberger U, Ball A (eds): Virus Taxonomy, VIIIth Report of the ICTV. London, Elsevier/Academic Press, 2005, pp 623-644.

4 Willoughby RE, Tieves KS, Hoffman GM, Ghanayem NS, Amlie-Lefond CM, Schwabe MJ, Chusid MJ, Rupprecht CE: Survival after Treatment of Rabies with Induction of Coma. N Engl J Med 2005; 352: 2508-2514.

5 Lafon M: Rabies virus receptors. J Neurovirol 2005; 11: 82-87.

6 Tordo N, Ceccaldi PE, Gaudin Y, Wandeler A: Rhabdovirus: Rabies, in Collier L, Mahy B (eds): Topley & Wilson's Microbiology and Microbial Infections (10th ed). London, Hodder Arnold, 2005, pp 1102-1136.

7 Finke S, Conzelmann KK: Replication strategies of rabies virus. Virus Res 2005; 111: 120-131.

8 Raux H, Flamand A, Blondel D: Interaction of the rabies P protein with the LC8 dynein light chain. J Virol 2000; 74: 10212-10216.

9 Jacob Y, Badrane H, Ceccaldi PE, Tordo N: Cytoplasmic dynein LC8 interacts with lyssavirus phosphoprotein. J Virol 2000; 74: 10217-10222.

10 Bourhy H, Kissi B, Badrane H, Tordo N: Molecular diversity of the Lyssavirus genus. Virology 1993; 194: 70-81.

11 Badrane H. Bahloul C, Perrin P, Tordo N: Evidence of two lyssavirus phylogroups with distinct pathogenicity and immunogenicity. J Virol 2001; 75: 3268-3276.

12 Nadin-Davis SA, Abdel-Malik M, Armstrong J, Wandeler AI: Lyssavirus P gene characterisation provides insights into the phylogeny of the genus and identifies structural similarities and diversity within the encoded phosphoprotein. Virology 2002; 298: 286-305.

13 Kuzmin IV, Orciari LA, Arai YT, Smith JS, Hanlon CA, Kameoka Y, Rupprecht CE: Bat lyssaviruses (Aravan and Khujand) from Central Asia: phylogenetic relationships according to N, P and G gene sequences. Virus Res 2003; 97: 65-79.

14 Kuzmin IV, Hughes GJ, Botvinkin AD, Orciari LA, Rupprecht CE: Phylogenetic relationships of Irkut and West Caucasian bat viruses within the Lyssavirus genus and suggested quantitative criteria based on the N gene sequence for lyssavirus genotype definition. Virus Res 2005; 111: 28-43.

15 Arguin PM, Murray-Lillibridge K, Miranda MEG, Smith JS, Calaor AB, Rupprecht CE: Serologic evidence of Lyssavirus infections among bats, the Philippines. Emerg Infect Dis 2002; 8: 258-262.

16 Reynes J-M, Molia S, Audry L, Hout S, Ngin S, Walston J, Bourhy H: Serologic evidence of Lyssavirus infection in bats, Cambodia, Emerg Infect Dis 2004; 10: 2231-2234.

17 Lumlertdacha B, Boongird K, Wanghongsa S, Wacharapluesadee S, Chanhome L, Khawplod P, Hemachudha T, Kuzmin I, Rupprecht CE: Survey of bat lyssaviruess, Thailand. Emerg Infect Dis 2005; 11: 232-236.

18 Smith JS, Orciari LA, Yager PA, Seidel HD, Warner CK: Epidemiologic and historical relationships among 97 rabies virus isolates as determined by limited sequence analysis. J Infect Dis 1992; 166: 296-307.

19 Badrane H, Tordo N: Host-switching in lyssavirus history from chiroptera to carnivora orders. J Virol 2001; 75: 8096-8104.

20 Holmes EC, Woelk CH, Kassis R, Bourhy H: Genetic constraints and the adaptative evolution of rabies virus in nature. Virology 2002; 292: 247-257.

21 Hughes GJ, Orciari LA, Rupprecht CE: Evolutionary timescale of rabies virus adaptation to North American bats inferred from the substitution rate of the nucleoprotein gene. J Gen Virol 2005; 86: 1467-1474.

22 Velasco-Villa A, Orciari LA, Souza V, Juarez-Islas V, Gomez-Sierra M, Castillo A, Flisser A, Rupprecht CE: Molecular epizootiology of rabies associated with terrestrial carnivores in Mexico. Virus Res 2005; 111: 13-27.

23 Fooks AR, Brookes SM, Johnson N, McElhinney LM, Hutson AM: European bat lyssaviruses: an emerging zoonosis. Epidemiol Infect 2003; 131: 1029-1039.

24 Muller T, Cox J, Peter W, Schafer R, Johnson N, McElhinney LM, Geue JL, Tjornehoj K, Fooks AR: Spill-over of European bat lyssavirus type 1 into a stone marten (Martes foina) in Germany. J Vet Med B Infect Dis Vet Public Health 2004; 51: 49-54.

25 Daoust PY, Wandeler AI, Casey GA: Cluster of rabies cases of probable bat origin among red foxes in Prince Edward Island, Canada. J Wildl Dis 1996; 32: 403-406.

26 Smith J et al, 12th RITA Conference, Peterborough, Canada: 47.

27 Vos A, Muller T, Neubert L, Zurbriggen A, Botteron C, Pohle D, Schoon H, Haas L, Jackson AC: Rabies in red foxes (Vulpes vulpes) experimentally infected with European bat lyssavirus type 1. J Vet Med B Infect Dis Vet Public Health 2004; 51: 327-332.

28 Vos A, Muller T, Cox J, Neubert L, Fooks AR: Susceptibility of ferrets (Mustela putorius furo) to experimentally induced rabies with European Bat Lyssaviruses (EBLV). J Vet Med B Infect Dis Vet Public Health 2004; 51: 55-60.

29 Hanlon CA, Kuzmin IV, Blanton JD, Weldon WC, Manangan JS, Rupprecht CE: Efficacy of rabies biologics against new lyssaviruses from Eurasia. Virus Res 2005; 111: 44-54.

30 Perrin P, De Franco M, Gontier-Jallet C, Fouque F, Morgeaux S, Tordo N, Colle JH: Antigen-specific cell-mediated immune response in mice is suppressed by infection with pathogenic Lyssaviruses. Res Virol 1996; 147: 289-299.

31 Thoulouze MI, Lafage M, Montano-Hirose JA, Lafon M: Rabies virus infects mouse and human lymphocytes and induces apoptosis. J Virol 1997; 71: 7372-7380.

32 Fu ZF, Jackson AC: Neuronal dysfunction and death in rabies virus infection. J Neurovirol 2005; 11: 101-106.

33 Kassis R, Larrous F, Estaquier J, Bourhy H: Lyssavirus matrix protein induces apoptosis by a TRAIL-dependent mechanism involving caspase-8 activation. J Virol 2004; 78: 6543-6555.

34 Morimoto K, Hooper DC, Spitsin S, Koprowski H, Dietzschold B: Pathogenicity of different rabies virus variants inversely correlates with apoptosis and rabies virus glycoprotein expression in infected primary neuron cultures. J Virol 1999; 73: 510-518.

35 Prehaud C, Lay S, Dietzschold B, Lafon M: Glycoprotein of nonpathogenic rabies viruses is a key determinant of human cell apoptosis. J Virol 2003; 77: 10537-10547.

36 Dietzschold B, Wunner WH, Wiktor TJ, Lopes AD, Lafon M, Smith CL, Koprowski H: Characterization of an antigenic determinant of the glycoprotein that correlates with pathogenicity of rabies virus. Proc Natl Acad Sci USA 1983; 80: 70-74.

37 Tuffereau C, Leblois H, Benejean J, Coulon P, Lafay F, Flamand A: Arginine or lysine in position 333 of ERA and CVS glycoprotein is necessary for rabies virulence in adult mice. Virology 1989; 172: 206-212.

38 Coulon P, Ternaux JP, Flamand A, Tuffereau C: An avirulent mutant of rabies virus is unable to infect motoneurons in vivo and in vitro. J Virol 1998; 72: 273-278.

39 Tuffereau, C, Desmézières E, Bénéjean J, Jallet C, Flamand A, Tordo N, Perrin P: Interaction of lyssaviruses with the low-affinity nerve-growth factor receptor p75 NTR. J Gen Virol 2001; 82: 2861-2867.

40 Desmézières E, Maillard A, Gaudin Y, Tordo N, Perrin P: Differential stability and fusion activity of Lyssavirus glycoprotein trimers. Virus Res 2003; 91: 181-187.

41 Pastoret PP, Brochier B: Epidemiology and control of fox rabies in Europe. Vaccine 1999; 17: 1750-1754.

42 Slate D, Rupprecht CE, Rooney JA, Donovan D, Lein DH, Chipman RB: Status of oral rabies vaccination in wild carnivores in the United States. Virus Res 2005; 111: 68-76.

43 Messenger SL, Smith JS, Orciari LA, Yager PA, Rupprecht CE: Emerging pattern of rabies deaths and increased viral infectivity. Emerg Infect Dis 2003; 9: 151-154.

44 Fooks AR, McElhinney LM, Pounder DJ, Finnegan CJ, Mansfield K, Johnson N, Brookes SM, Parsons G, White K, McIntyre PG, Nathwani D: Case report: isolation of a European bat lyssavirus type 2a from a fatal human case of rabies encephalitis. J Med Virol 2003; 71: 281-289.

45 Tordo N: Characteristic and molecular biology of the rabies virus, in Meslin FX, Bögel K (eds): Laboratory Techniques in Rabies: World Health Organization, Geneva, 1996, pp 28-51.

46 Bahloul C, Jacob Y, Tordo N, Perrin P: DNA-based immunisation for exploring the enlargement of immunological cross-reactivity against the lyssaviruses. Vaccine 1998; 16: 417-425.

47 Jallet C, Jacob Y, Bahloul C, Drings A, Desmezières E, Tordo N, Perrin P: Chimeric lyssavirus glycoproteins with increased immunological potential. J Virol 1999; 73: 225-233.

48 Brookes SM, Parsons G, Johnson N, McElhinney LM, Fooks AR. Rabies human diploid cell vaccine elicits cross-neutralising and cross-protecting immune responses against European and Australian bat lyssaviruses. Vaccine 2005; 23: 4101-4109.

49 Nel LH, Niezgoda M, Hanlon CA, Morril PA, Yager PA, Rupprecht CE: A comparison of DNA vaccines for the rabies-related virus, Mokola. Vaccine 2003; 21: 2598-2606.

50 Perrin P, Jacob Y, Aguilar-Setien A, Loza-Rubio E, Jallet C, Desmezières E, Aubert M, Cliquet F, Tordo N: Immunization of dogs with a DNA vaccine induces protection against rabies virus. Vaccine 2000; 18: 479-486.

51 Desmezières E, Jacob Y, Saron MF, Delpeyroux F, Tordo N, Perrin P: Lyssavirus glycoproteins expressing immunologically potent B cell and cytotoxic T lymphocyte epitopes as prototypes for multivalent vaccines. J Gen Virol 1999; 80: 2343-2351.

Dr. N. Tordo, Unit Antiviral Strategies, Département de Virologie, Institut Pasteur, 25 rue du Docteur Roux, FR-75724 Paris Cedex 15, France.
E-mail: ntordo@pasteur.fr

Dodet B, Schudel A, Pastoret PP, Lombard M (eds): Rabies in Europe.
Dev Biol (Basel). Basel, Karger, 2006, vol 125, p 15.

Key Challenges Facing Oral Rabies Vaccination in the United States

D. Slate[1], *C. Rupprecht*[2]

[1] USDA, APHIS, Wildlife Services, Concord, NH, USA

[2] Centers for Disease Control and Prevention, Atlanta, GA, USA

Abstract: Containment and elimination of terrestrial rabies in wildlife is a daunting, multifaceted task. The challenges to achieving these rabies control goals can be broadly compartmentalized as ecological, technical, surveillance, economic and administrative. In the US, variants of the rabies virus are adapted to the raccoon, skunks (3 distinct variants), arctic fox (spillover into red fox), grey fox (2 variants) and coyote (spillover from domestic dogs south of the US border with Mexico). The ecological, physical and behavioural differences among these species profoundly impact oral rabies vaccination (ORV) strategies. Variable and generally high population densities for species like the raccoon require adaptive strategies to ensure appropriate spatial distribution of baits and bait density to effectively vaccinate target species. The ability of skunks, which are sympatric with all rabies reservoir species in the US, to " help maintain " rabies virus variants not unique to skunks further confounds control objectives. This obstacle can only be addressed on a broad geographical scale through the development and licensure of oral vaccines that are sufficiently immunogenic in skunks as well as all other terrestrial reservoir species. The need for real-time, enhanced rabies surveillance to bolster in-place public health surveillance is critical to delineating strategic areas for treatment as well as determining programmatic success. Garnering and maintaining state and federal support for ORV programmes represents a formidable challenge, given that the financial benefits to those governments are largely indirect under the health care system in the US, which is primarily insurance-based. Administratively, the key to successful programmes in the US requires that a coalition of federal, state and university expertise work together efficiently with available funding toward common research and management goals. In presenting these challenges and steps taken to address them, we emphasize similarities and differences between wildlife rabies control in the US and Europe to promote an understanding and dialogue that leads to enhanced, science-based ORV.

Dodet B, Schudel A, Pastoret PP, Lombard M (eds): Rabies in Europe.
Dev Biol (Basel). Basel, Karger, 2006, vol 125, pp 17-28.

Molecular Epidemiology of Rabies Viruses in Europe

L.M. McElhinney[1], D. Marston[1], N. Johnson[1], C. Black[1], O. Matouch[2], D. Lalosevic[3], S. Stankov[3], K. Must[4], M. Smreczak[5], J.F. Zmudzinski[5], A. Botvinkin[6], O. Aylan[7], E. Vanek[8], F. Cliquet[9], T. Muller[10], A.R. Fooks[1]

1 Veterinary Laboratories Agency (Weybridge), WHO Collaborating Centre for the Characterisation of Rabies and Rabies Related Viruses, Surrey, United Kingdom
2 State Veterinary Institute, Liberec, Czech Republic
3 Pasteur Institute Novi Sad, Serbia
4 Estonian Veterinary and Food Laboratory, Tartu, Estonia
5 Panstwowy Instytut Weterynaryjny, Pulawy, Poland
6 Plague Control Research Institute of Siberia and Far East, Irkutsk, Siberia, Russia
7 Etlik Central Veterinary Control and Research Institute, Etlik-Ankara, Turkey
8 Austrian Agency for Health and Food Safety Vet. Med. Mödling, Modling, Austria
9 Agence Française de Sécurité Sanitaire des Aliments, Malzeville, France
10 Friedrich-Loeffler-Institute, Wusterhausen, Germany

Abstract: Several different strains of classical rabies virus co-circulate in Europe. In order to investigate the roles of the host species and topography on the molecular epidemiology of these viruses, a 400 bp region of the nucleoprotein gene was sequenced and compared with more than 500 European virus isolates. Viruses from 21 European countries were represented including some unique panels of archived isolates from the former Republic of Yugoslavia, Estonia, the Czech Republic, Poland and Austria. Phylogenetic analysis of 198 unique sequences demonstrated numerous groups of viruses clustered at both geographical and host-species levels.

INTRODUCTION

The Lyssavirus genus, a member of the *Rhabdoviridae* family, consists of seven related viruses (genotypes 1-7). Rabies cases in Europe are principally attributed to three of these genotypes, namely genotype 1 (RABV, classical rabies) and to a lesser extent genotypes 5 and 6 (European bat lyssaviruses type-1 and -2). In 2004, the number of reported rabies cases in Europe [1], was approximately half that reported for 2003. The substantial reduction of rabies in large parts of Europe is attributed to the successful implementation of oral vaccination campaigns targeted at the principal reservoir, the red fox (*Vulpes vulpes*). Despite the fact that the majority of live attenuated or sub-unit rabies vaccines are derived from viruses obtained between 50-100 years ago [2], vaccine failures are rare. However, under specific circumstances they do occur [3,4] and differences between 'street' and vaccine ('fixed') strains may be a factor in these failures. An earlier study of rabies viruses circulating in France in 1989-1990 showed a marked divergence (13.3 %-16.5 %) of street strains from vaccine seed strains (PV, CVS, ERA, SAD_{B19}, PM, HEP, PAS) [2]. Hence, it is essential to conduct molecular epidemiological surveillance to assess and monitor the levels of genetic divergence between the viral strains currently circulating in animals and the oral vaccine seed strains that are employed throughout Europe (principally SAD_{B19}, SAD_{Bern}, SAD P5/88, SAG-1, SAG-2 and VRG).

Advances in molecular epidemiological methods over the past 15 years have resulted in an increase in genetic data on rabies viruses (RABV) circulating in a range of host species worldwide. The main focus of molecular epidemiology studies of lyssaviruses is the nucleoprotein (N) gene. It was chosen for several reasons including the effectiveness of this region for genotyping and evolutionary analysis [5]. More recently, the large number of partial N gene sequences available in various databases have facilitated detailed virus, host, geographical and temporal comparisons [6-11].

Temporal changes with respect to both reservoir species and geographical distribution are well documented for rabies in Europe. For reasons which are not fully understood, large areas of central Europe were apparently free of rabies in the early decades of the 20th century [12]. Reductions in wolf and stray dog populations, two ancestral reservoirs for rabies, in combination with quarantine and movement restrictions, may have been partially responsible. However during the Second World War, a new epizootic of rabies began on the Russian-Polish border and in Northern Poland and was spread to the rest of Europe by red foxes, moving west and south, reaching France by 1968 and northern Italy in the early 1980s [12]. The main reservoir host species of sylvatic RABV in Europe are the red fox and the raccoon dog (*Nyctereutes procyonoides*). In 2004, the red fox accounted for 46.2 % of 5,452 reported cases, while the raccoon dog accounted for 9.2 % [1]. However, in some countries the raccoon dog is increasingly replacing the red fox as the main reservoir species, for example, in the final quarter of 2004, Estonia reported 30.6 % of its cases were in red foxes, whereas 51.4 % of cases were associated with raccoon dogs. Rabies in companion animals (domestic dogs and cats) has largely been controlled in Europe, but cases are still reported in Eastern Europe and the Russian Federation.

The molecular diversity of lyssaviruses within genotype 1 has been studied at the global level and reference has been made to the existence of a number of European strains in a range of mammalian species [5,7]. They are believed to be clustered within a "Cosmopolitan Lineage" having ancestral roots in Europe in the 17th century before its widespread dispersal to Asia, Africa and the Americas as a result of European exploration and colonisation [13,14].

A previous study analysed 245 RABV isolates by sequencing or RFLP [6]. The European isolates were collected from 15 different countries between 1972 and 1996 and included 51 red fox, 13 raccoon dog and 22 other mammalian isolates. Phylogenetic analyses indicated that there was a gradual dispersal of rabies from the north-east to the south-west across Europe, matching the epidemiological data. Surveillance and phylogenetic evidence suggests that two spillover events occurred in Europe, resulting in host adaptation. The first was a spillover from dogs to red foxes in Eastern Europe/Western Russia during the first half of the 20th century. The second host change appears to have occurred in north-east Europe when fox RABV colonised raccoon dogs [6]. Obstacles, such as mountains, lakes and wide rivers are believed to have disrupted the fluidity of virus transmission in Europe, resulting in virus variants correlated strongly with geographical isolation and/or host species [15,16].

Three phylogenetic groups of RABV have been associated with red foxes in Northern Europe (NE), Central Europe (CE) and Eastern Europe (EE). A red fox-raccoon dog variant has also been demonstrated in North East Europe (NEE) [6,16]. Furthermore, two virus isolates from the former Republic of Yugoslavia and Hungary were proposed as possible "intermediates" between the dog and fox viruses. A single isolate from cattle in the former Republic of Yugoslavia was reported as the most divergent of the European isolates. Understanding the importance of these divergent viruses was difficult due to the low numbers analysed. In an attempt to extend previously published studies and to examine the potential existence of "dog-fox" or "fox-raccoon dog" intermediate virus isolates in Eastern Europe, we obtained and analysed extensive panels of genotype 1 rabies isolates from Europe, including the former Republic of Yugoslavia, Estonia, the Czech Republic, Turkey and Poland, originating from a range of hosts.

Materials and Methods

Viral isolates

A summary of the European RABV isolates, usually original brain material or first passage mouse brain, held in the virus archive at the Veterinary Laboratories Agency, Weybridge, are provided in Table 1. RNA was extracted from all isolates submitted ($n = 718$) and tested by RT-PCR. Amplified material was subjected to purification and genetic sequencing. In addition, sequence data previously published for European isolates [5,6,8] was obtained from Genbank and included in the phylogenetic analysis. After the removal of identical sequences, 198 partial N gene sequences (400 nucleotides) were available for analysis. In total, isolates from 21 European countries are represented in this review (Table 1).

RNA extraction, reverse transcription – PCR

The protocols used followed previously published methods [17]. Briefly, total RNA was extracted using the Trizol (Gibco BRL) method following the manufacturers' instructions and resuspended in HPLC purified water (Aldrich). Each sample was quantified and the RNA concentration adjusted to 1 µg/µl. Samples were then reverse transcribed using the primer JW12 (5-ATGTAACACC [C/T] CTACAATG-3) which anneals to genomic positions 55–73 at the start of the nucleoprotein coding sequence. Following incubation for one hour at 42° C, cDNAs were diluted to 100 µl with water and 5 µl used in a PCR reaction with primer JW12 and a combination of primers JW6 (DPL) (5-CAATTCGCACACATTTTGTG-3), JW6(E) (5-CAGTTGGCACACATCTTGTG-3) and JW6(M) (5-CAGTTAGCGCACATCTTATG-3). Positive PCR reactions produced a fragment of 606 base pairs (bp) in size. PCR products (5 µl) were visualised by agarose gel electrophoresis (1.8 % agarose). The remaining 45 µl product was purified using the QIAquick™ PCR purification kit (Qiagen) following the manufacturer's instructions.

Sequencing

300-500 ng of purified PCR product was sequenced directly using 3.2 pmol of the PCR primers JW12 and JW6DPL. Either the Big Dye sequencing kit (Applied Biosystems) or the Quickstart Kit (Beckman) was used to sequence the products which were subsequently run on either ABI 3100, or the Beckman CEQ8800 respectively. Sequences were edited using the DNAstar programme (DNAstar Inc., Madison, USA).

Phylogenetic analysis

After the removal of identical sequences, 198 unique nucleoprotein sequences coding for the first 400 bp were aligned using the Clustal W programme (1.83) and transition/transversion ratios calculated using the Puzzle 4.0.2 programme of the PHYLIP package (version 3.5). Phylogenetic analysis was performed to generate consensus trees and bootstrap values as previously described [9]. Phylogenetic trees were visualised using Treeview (Version 3.2).

Table 1 : European RABV isolates.

Country	No of isolates	Host species	Chronology
Austria	24*	Red fox, dog, sheep, cattle, horse	1990-2002
Bosnia & Herzegovina	3*	Red fox, dog	1986, 1999
Czech Republic	71*	Red fox, deer, cat, cattle	1995-1999
Estonia	78*	Raccoon dog, red fox, dog, cattle, cat, badger	1989-2000
Finland	2*	Fox, dog	1988
France	250*	Red fox, cattle, sheep, dog, cat, badger	1988
Georgia	4*	Dog, cattle, human	1989
Germany	10*	Red fox	1990
Kazakhstan	2*	Fox	1988
Montenegro	2*	Cattle, horse	1978, 2000
Poland	28*	Red fox, Raccoon dog, rodent, dog, badger	1985-2002
Russia	64*	Fox sp, Raccoon dog, dog, cat, wolf, rodent, badger, reindeer, horse	1983-2002
Serbia	142*	Red fox, dog, cat, deer, horse	1972-2000
Turkey	38*	Dog, red fox, cattle	1989-2001
Total (VLA archive)	**718***		
Belgium	Kissi et al 1995 Bourhy et al 1999	Country represented only by Genbank sequences	
Hungary			
Lithuania			
Slovak Republic			
Slovenia			
Switzerland			
Latvia	Vanaga et al 2003	Country represented only by Genbank sequences	

* Held at VLA Weybridge archive.

RESULTS

The four main European groups (NEE, EE, WE and CE) were resolved on our tree despite the inclusion of larger numbers of viruses (Fig. 1). As previously observed for the 400 bp analysis, bootstrap support for these groups was poor. In addition to the four main European groups, a number of divergent variants were represented from Russia, Serbia and Turkey.

North East Europe (NEE)

The North East Europe group was represented on the tree by 45 RABV isolates from Western Russia, Finland, Estonia, Latvia, Lithuania, Poland and Slovakia. The majority of isolates within NEE originated from both raccoon dogs and red foxes. However, isolates from badgers, dogs, cats, polecats, rodents and cows were also represented. All raccoon dog isolates clustered in the NEE group with the exception of three within the CE group. This indicates that this variant is equally well supported by both reservoir species or that it represents an emergent biotype for raccoon dogs. As previously reported [8], all the Latvian isolates clustered within this group. Without exception, all the Estonian isolates analysed were also included within the NEE group, despite testing a large panel ($n = 78$) from a range of species collected between 1989 and 2000. No conclusions can be drawn for Finland, Lithuania and Slovakia as the sequence data for only one or two isolates were available for comparison.

The NEE group was referred to as Russian Group E in a recent molecular epidemiological review of Russian isolates [18].

Eastern Europe (EE)

The EE variant was represented on the tree by 38 RABV isolates. The geographical distribution of this group has now been extended and includes Austria, Bosnia, the Czech Republic, Hungary, Montenegro, Poland and Serbia. The large majority of Serbian isolates fell within this group ($n = 20$). The associated host species is mainly the red fox ; however, there were a number of isolates originating from dogs, cats, horses and deer.

Western Europe (WE)

The vast majority of isolates analysed were in the WE group, including all 250 French isolates submitted for diagnosis in 1988. Large numbers of the isolates had identical sequences and the group was consequently represented on the tree by 45 unique sequences, mainly associated with red foxes or their spill-over hosts. The Western Europe group, therefore, reflects the variant responsible for the epizootic which spread from East to West across Europe during the latter half of the 20th century and which has been successfully controlled in many countries by large-scale oral vaccination campaigns. As expected, the WE group was widely dispersed and formed a band from Serbia in the east to France and Belgium in the west. On the radial tree (Fig. 1), the WE group appears to be split into two clades by the projection of the Central Europe (CE) group on a long branch. This topology has been previously described for the 400 bp tree but not when the complete N gene is analysed and it is thought to be of little significance.

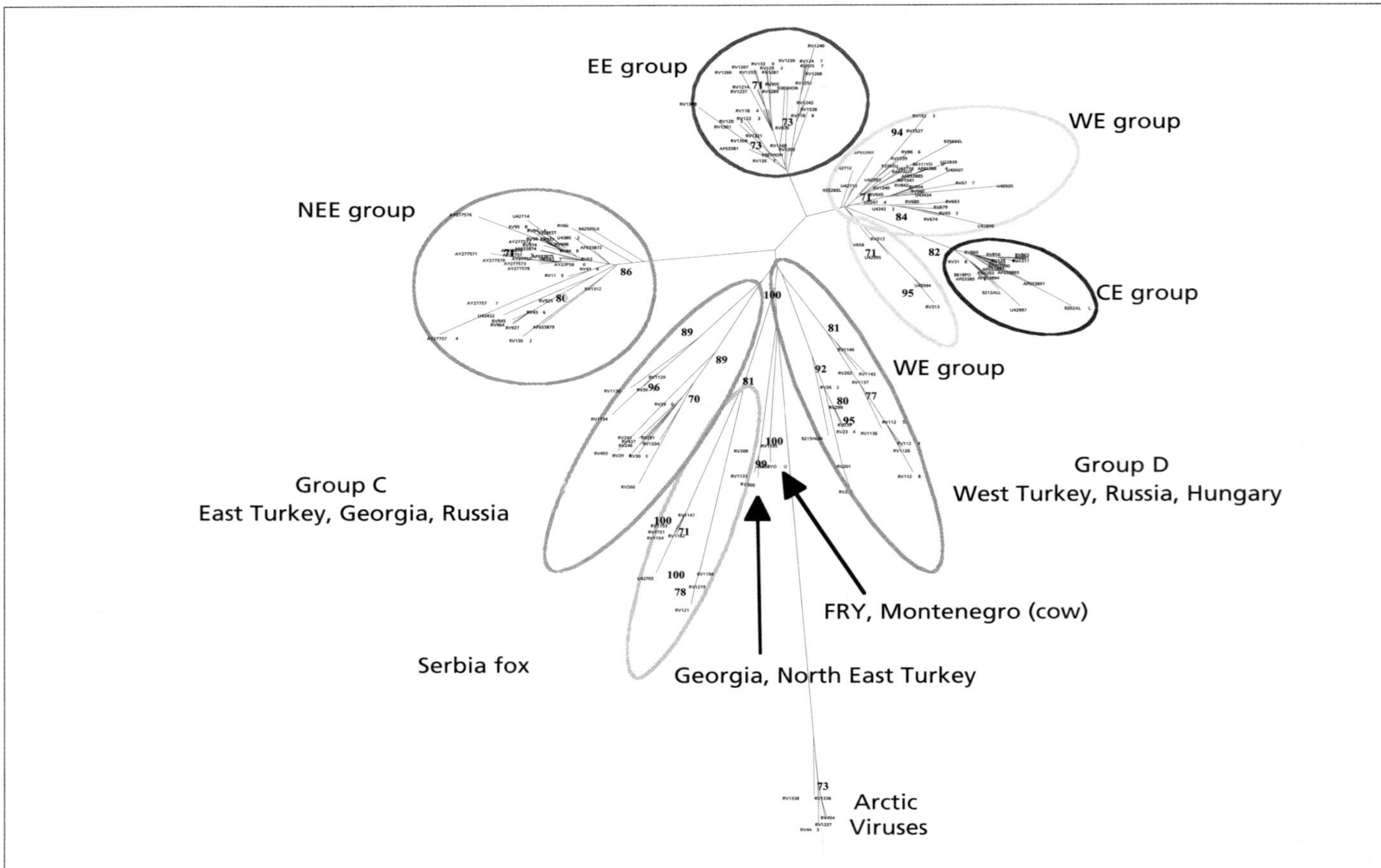

Fig. 1: Phylogenetic relationship between 198 European RABV isolates based on partial N gene sequence (400 nucleotides). Significant bootstrap values (> 70%) are marked on the tree. Arctic isolates from Russia are included as an outgroup.

Within this group of viruses, clusters can be observed at the geographical level. For example, all of the German isolates analysed tended towards small sub-lineages within WE, as did the French, Belgian and Austrian isolates.

Central Europe (CE)

The Central Europe variant was represented by 24 unique sequences on the tree (19 fox, three raccoon dog, one water rat and one marten). As previously reported, this group is restricted in distribution to Poland, the Czech Republic and Germany [6]. Two sub-lineages are supported by a good bootstrap value (82 %). With the exception of a single divergent isolate from Germany (9202ALL), the first sub-lineage contains isolates from Poland and the Czech Republic. The second sub-lineage contains only isolates from Germany and Poland. Geographical obstacles such as rivers may have played a role in defining these subsets. The small number of raccoon dog isolates within this group may reflect dead-end spillover events.

Russian Group A – Arctic Russia

Group A consisted of five isolates originating from the Arctic zone of Eurasia and was used as an outgroup.

Russia Group C – East Turkey, Georgia, Kazakhstan & South West Russia

A group of divergent viruses was derived from locations throughout East Turkey, Georgia, Kazakhstan and South West Russia (including Tula, Orenburg, Krasnodar, Bryansk and Omsk). The group was represented by 12 unique sequences derived from red foxes ($n = 4$), dogs ($n = 2$), cats ($n = 2$), cows ($n = 2$), a human ($n = 1$) and a wolf ($n = 1$). This group is believed to represent a red fox variant dispersed throughout the vast steppe regions of South West Russia and South East Europe, previously reported as Russia Group C viruses [18]. Its dispersion has perhaps been impeded by topographical barriers such as the Caucasian Mountains. In previous studies, this group has been shown to be related to viruses circulating in Iran and, to a lesser extent, Israel [10].

Russia Group D – West Turkey, Hungary and West Russia

A cluster of isolates (eight dog, six fox and two human), previously designated as Russian Group D viruses [10], originated from the west of the European part of Russia at the borders of Russia, Ukraine and Belarus. This group included a second set of Turkish viruses derived from dogs and red foxes in the west of Turkey, including the major cities of Istanbul, Bursa, and Izmir. Isolates within this lineage grouped together depending on the place of origin with good bootstrap support. Two viruses isolates from Turkish dogs (RV202 and RV203), isolated in the Samsun region in 1989, aligned with the Turkish isolates collected in North West Turkey over a decade later. A human isolate from Hungary in 1991 (9215HON) was also included in this group. This group may represent an intermediate variant between the dog and fox viruses.

Molecular epidemiological data from Bulgaria, Romania, Ukraine and Belarus is required to confirm that this variant is widespread throughout East Europe and West Russia.

Group G – Georgia and North East Turkey

As previously reported [10], a single isolate from the Ardahan region of North East Turkey (RV1133) did not segregate with either of the two groups which contained Turkish isolates including a second isolate from Ardahan. Instead, it was most closely related to two divergent isolates from Georgia (human and dog isolates).

The segregation of this cluster from all other European lineages was supported by significant bootstrap values (100 %).

Group SF – Serbia Fox

The majority of Serbian isolates clustered within the EE group (*n = 20*). However, a distant lineage, represented by nine unique sequences (eight fox and one cat), was evident on the tree. Only isolates from North and North East Serbia were included in this group, which was divided into two lineages with good bootstrap support (81 %). For the first time in this study a clear chronological association was observed between sub-lineages. The first sub-lineage was represented by three unique sequences from foxes collected in 1986 (*n = 1*) and 1997 (*n = 2*). The second sub-lineage was represented by fox isolates collected between 1972 and 1977. A single cat isolate was included in the latter group.

Former Republic of Yugoslavia Cattle

Two closely related isolates from cattle obtained in 1978 (RV1185 Cow, Montenegro) and 1981 (8658YOU, cattle, former Republic of Yugoslavia) were shown to be more closely related to the Georgian and North East Turkey isolates than the other variants identified in the former Republic of Yugoslavia (EE, WE and Serbia fox). The isolate, 8658YOU, was previously shown to be more closely related to dog and jackal variants from the Middle East and Africa than to other European isolates, and was proposed as a spillover with a virus from a lineage which was established in the earlier part of the 20th century, before the epizootic in red foxes [6].

Discussion

Molecular typing methods are playing an increasingly important role in the understanding of RABV epidemiology and control. In this study, we have extended previously published findings with regards to the range of variants circulating in Europe and Western Russia over the past 30 years. To this end, we collected panels of isolates from countries not fully represented in previous reviews of European RABV e.g. the former Republic of Yugoslavia, Austria, Estonia, the Czech Republic and Turkey. Twenty-one countries are represented in this review, although some, e.g. Lithuania, Slovenia and Slovakia, have only a single representative isolate.

Reviews of this kind are dependent on the quality and quantity of the data available. It should be viewed as a starting point and continually updated as further information becomes available. For example, rabies molecular epidemiology remains uninvestigated in large areas of Europe and the Middle East, making it difficult to understand the dynamics of viral dispersion and adaptation fully. Even when large panels of isolates are obtained, they may only reflect part of the existing rabies epidemiology in that country due to inherent biases in surveillance techniques and sample selection. For example, when we analysed 78 isolates from Estonia, we observed that all virus isolates were included in the NEE group, despite the range of host species and time intervals between isolation (1989 to 2000). In a recent study [19], two antigenic variants (I and II) were reported to occur in Estonia. The profile for variant II was only reported for two isolates and the authors suggested that this variant was rare. It is difficult to make firm conclusions on whether a particularly rare virus is capable of maintaining rabies cycles, represents an intermediate variant or indeed if it has been eliminated in a region, unless typing is performed on all submitted specimens over a number of years. Similarly, 250 isolates collected in France from a range of species in 1988, yielded only a handful of unique sequences, all falling in the WE group. The latter was not surprising, as this variant is well documented to be associated with the epizootic that swept from East to West Europe in the second half of the last century. However, 2,223 rabies cases were reported in France in 1988 and so we do not know whether the 250 isolates which were typed were representative of the situation as a whole.

Despite these limitations, the data provide clear evidence that a number of well established RABV variants cocirculate in Europe (Fig. 2). The large majority are associated with red foxes, although there is substantial evidence to support the continued presence of dog-associated rabies, particularly in Turkey and Russia and the increasing role of raccoon dogs in maintaining RABV in the Baltic countries. With the possible exception of the dog and raccoon dog variants, the lineages are defined by the geographical derivation of the virus. For example, the CE group only contains isolates from localised regions of the Czech Republic, Germany and Poland, and sub-lineages are further defined geographically. Similarly, despite the widespread dispersion of the WE variant, isolates were observed to cluster based on the country of isolation. The NEE group is represented by both raccoon dogs and red foxes, and its distribution is limited to the countries of North East Europe and North West Russia. As for the CE, EE, Russia Group C and Russia Group D variants, topographical obstacles have been implicated in halting the spread of NEE and facilitating localised evolution [18]. In Poland, the Vistula River forms a well-established barrier impeding the dispersal of NEE to the West. However, there is no clear geographical definition of the isolates within this group, for example, Estonian, Polish and Latvian isolates are well distributed throughout the branches. The raccoon dog has been reported as far west as France [20], albeit intermittently, so it is vital that wildlife rabies cases are monitored throughout Europe, to determine whether the NEE variant will follow the westward distribution of its reservoir species.

Surveillance is also essential for detecting potential host adaptations which may result in the emergence of new biotypes and reservoir species, posing a significant threat to areas in which rabies has been controlled or eliminated in a particular niche. A biotype is a virus strain adapted to a particular reservoir host species and is typified by high pathogenicity for that species with high levels of virus excretion and a low infectious dose. This optimises transmission between members of the same species without generating substantial herd immunity. Conversely, for a spillover infection to a different species to occur, a very large infectious dose is usually required and infection may not give rise to excretion of virus in the new host or, if it does, excretion may be at a low level.

Spillover events of bat lyssaviruses, including European bat lyssavirus type 1 [21-23] to a terrestrial species, have been reported but there is little evidence that the virus is maintained by an enzootic transmission within the new species. However,

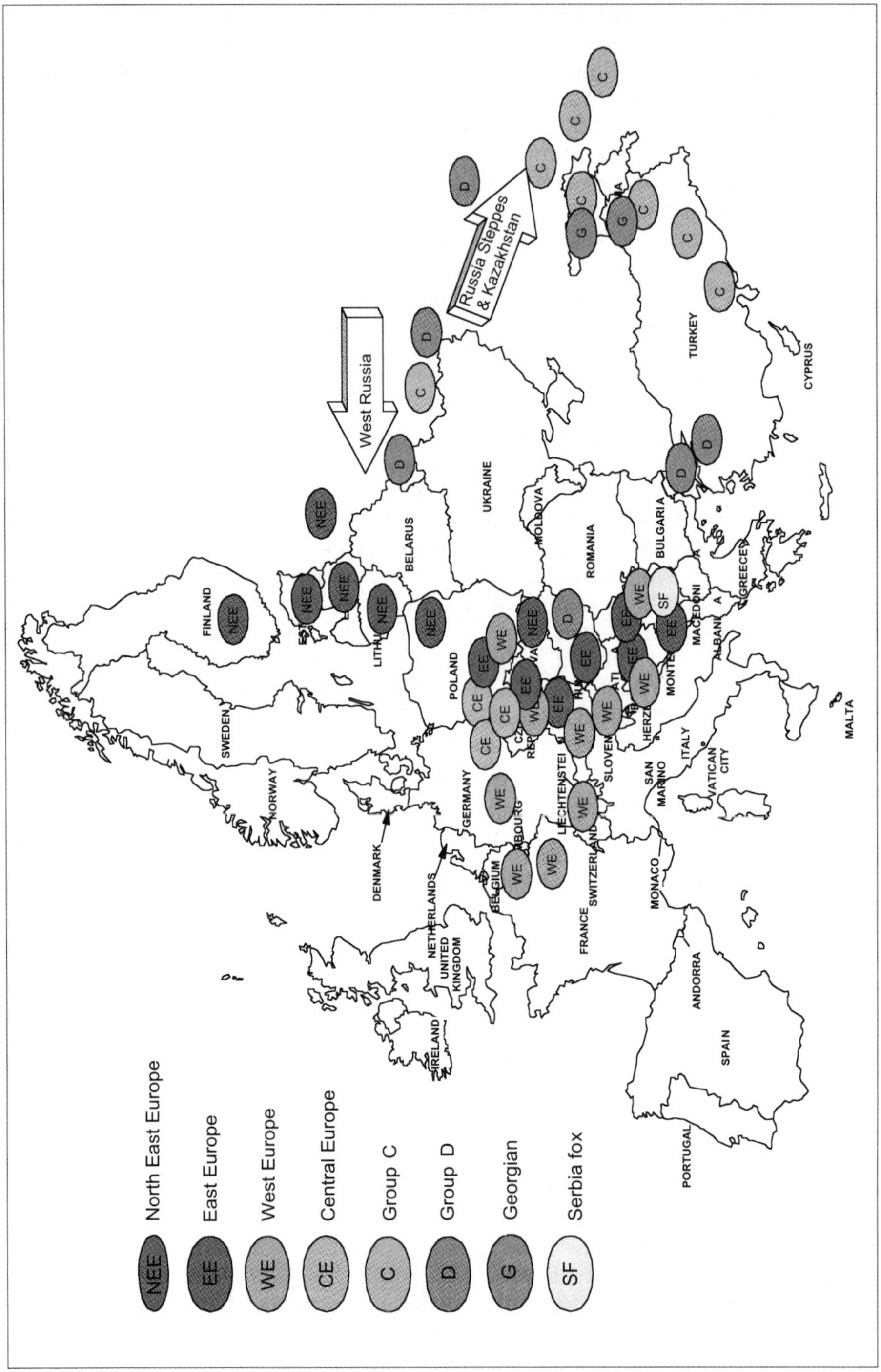

Fig. 2: Distribution of Genetic Variants of RABV in Europe.

exceptions have been documented. The epizootic of fox rabies in Europe in the latter half of the last century and the possible maintenance of rabies in raccoon dogs in North East Europe, provide examples of the impact of virus adaptation on previously rabies-free areas [24]. Of equal concern is the adaptation of bat variants to terrestrial species as seen in 2001, when a rabies outbreak in skunks in the Flagstaff area of Arizona in North America was attributed to a spillover infection of a bat variant (RABV, genotype 1), followed by a rare host adaptation and maintenance within the skunk population [25]. Typing the viruses responsible for such events is essential to determine the origins of sporadic cases in previously rabies-free regions and to allow specific targeting of the subsequent control programmes. With the aid of molecular epidemiological data, it is not unreasonable to expect a successful conclusion to the concerted efforts to control rabies in Eastern Europe

Further analysis of the divergent variants from Turkey, Serbia, Georgia and Hungary, particularly at the amino acid level and within other genomic regions, is necessary to determine whether they represent intermediate dog-fox viruses. The two divergent viruses isolated from cattle in the former Republic of Yugoslavia may represent an early ancestor of the 'Cosmopolitan Lineage', so representative viruses will be studied in greater detail at the global level. In addition, further detailed analysis of the available data is necessary in countries of Eastern Europe and the Middle East, such as Poland, Turkey, Serbia and Israel [26], where several variants are known to co-circulate. Studies of this kind may help us understand the role of host ecology and the effects of topography in the maintenance and evolution of RABV in Europe.

Acknowledgements

This work was supported by a grant from the Department for Environment, Food and Rural Affairs (Defra), UK (ROAME SE0417).

References

1 Rabies Bulletin Europe 28: 4/2004.

2 Sacramento D, Badrane H, Bourhy H, Tordo N: Molecular epidemiology of rabies virus in France: comparison with vaccine strains. J Gen Virol 1992; 73: 1149-1158.

3 Selimov MA, Mikhailovskii EM, Gribencha SV: Epidemiology of rabies in the USSR between 1964 and 1971. Simpozium Po Beshenstvu (Symposium on Rabies). 1972: 79-82.

4 Larghi OP, Diaz AM: Cross protection of mice against different rabies virus isolates Zentralbt Bakteriol, Mikrobiol Hygiene 1985; 259: 268-274.

5 Kissi B, Tordo N, Bourhy H: Genetic polymorphism in the rabies virus nucleoprotein gene. Virology 1995; 209: 526-537.

6 Bourhy H, Kissi B, Audry L, Smreczak M, Sadkowska-Todys M, Kulonen K, Tordo N, Zmudzinski JF, Holmes EC: Ecology and evolution of rabies virus in Europe. J Gen Virol 1999; 80: 2545-2557.

7 McElhinney LM, Johnson N, Mansfield KM, Finnegan CJ, Smith J, Lowings JP, Fooks AR: Molecular Characterisation of rabies and rabies related viruses, in Dodet B, Meslin FX (eds): Rabies Control in Asia. Paris, John Libbey Eurotext, 2001, pp 178-184.

8 Vanaga S, van der Heide R, Joffe R, van der Poel WH: Rabies in Wildlife in Latvia. Vector Borne Zoonotic Dis 2003; 3,3: 117-124.

9 Johnson N, McElhinney LM, Smith J, Lowings P, Fooks AR: Phylogenetic comparison of the genus Lyssavirus using distal coding sequences of the glycoprotein and nucleoprotein genes. Arch Virol 2002; 147: 2111-2123.

10 Johnson N, Black C, Smith J, Un H, McElhinney LM, Aylan O, Fooks AR: Rabies emergence among foxes in Turkey. J Wildl Dis 2003; 39 (2): 262-270.

11 Johnson N, McElhinney LM, Ali YH, Saeed IK, Fooks AR: Molecular Epidemiology of Canid Rabies in Sudan: Evidence for a common origin of rabies with Ethiopia. Virus Res 2004; 104 (2): 201-205.

12 Wandeler A: Epidemiology and Ecology of Fox Rabies in Europe, in King AA, Fooks AR, Wandeler A, Aubert MA (eds): Perspectives of Rabies in Europe and the Mediterranean Basin. OIE 2004, pp 201-214.

13 Smith JS, Orciari LA, Yager PA, Seidel HD, Warner CK: Epidemiologic and historical relationships among 87 rabies virus isolates as determined by limited sequence analysis. J Infect Dis 1992; 166: 296-307.

14 Nadin-Davis SA, Bingham J: Europe as a Source of Rabies for the Rest of the World, in King AA, Fooks AR, Wandeler A, Aubert MA (eds): Perspectives of Rabies in Europe and the Mediterranean Basin. OIE 2004, pp 259-280.

15 Sadkowska-Todys M: Phylogenetic relationship of street rabies virus strains and their antigenic reactivity with antibodies induced by vaccine strains. I. Analysis of phylogenetic relationship of street rabies virus strains isolated in Poland. Med Dosw Mikrobiol 2000; 52: 173-183.

16 Brookes S, McElhinney LM, Johnson N, Badrane H, Tordo N, Fooks AR: Rabies virus variants and molecular epidemiology in Europe, in King AA, Fooks AR, Wandeler A, Aubert MA (eds): Perspectives of Rabies in Europe and the Mediterranean Basin. OIE 2004, pp 243-258.

17 Heaton PR, Johnstone P, McElhinney LM, Cowley R, O'Sullivan E, Whitby JE: A hemi-nested PCR assay for the detection of six genotypes of rabies and rabies-related viruses. J Clin Microbiol 1997; 35: 2762-2766.

18 Kuzmin IV, Botvinkin AD, McElhinney LM, Smith JS, Orciari LA, Clark J, Hughes GJ, Fooks AR, Rupprecht CE: Molecular Epidemiology of Terrestrial Rabies in the former Soviet Union. J Wildl Dis 2004; 40 (4): 617-631.

19 Metlin AE, Cox J, Rybakov SS, Huovilainen A, Grouzdev KN, Neuvonen E: Monoclonal antibody characterization of rabies virus isolates from Russia, Finland and Estonia. J Vet Med B. 2004; 51 (2): 94-96.

20 Sillero-Zubiri C, Hoffmann M: Nyctereutes procyonoides, in IUCN 2004. 2004 IUCN Red List of Threatened Species. <www.redlist.org>.

21 Muller T, Cox J, Peter W, Schafer R, Johnson N, McElhinney LM, Geue JL, Tjornehoj K, Fooks AR: Spill-over of European bat lyssavirus type 1 into a stone marten (Martes foina) in Germany. J Vet Med B 2004; 51 (2): 49-54.

22 Rønsholt L: A new case of European Bat Lyssavirus (EBL) infection in Danish sheep. Rabies Bulletin Europe 2002; 26 (2): 15.

23 Fooks AR, McElhinney LM, Pounder DJ, Finnegan CJ, Mansfield K, Johnson N, Brookes SM, Parsons G, White K, McIntyre PG, Nathwani D: Case Report: Isolation of a European bat lyssavirus type-2a from a fatal human case of rabies-encephalitis. J Med Virol 2003; 71: 281-289.

24 Johnson N, Fooks AR: Archival study of a Finnish isolate from the 1988/89 rabies outbreak. Arch Virol 2005; 150 (7): 1407-1414.

25 Krebs JW, Noll HR, Rupprecht CE, Childs JE: Rabies surveillance in the United States during 2001. JAMA 2002; 221 (12): 1690-1701.

26 David D, Yakobson B, Smith JS, Stram Y: Molecular epidemiology of rabies virus isolates from Israel and other middle- and Near-Eastern countries. J Clin Microbiol 2000; 38 (2): 755-762.

Dr. L.M. McElhinney, Rabies and Wildlife Zoonoses Group, Veterinary Laboratories Agency (Weybridge), WHO Collaborating Centre for the Characterisation of Rabies and Rabies Related Viruses, Surrey, Woodham Lane, New Haw, Surrey, KT15 3NB, United Kingdom.
E-mail: l.mcelhinney@vla.defra.gsi.gov.uk

Dodet B, Schudel A, Pastoret PP, Lombard M (eds): Rabies in Europe.
Dev Biol (Basel). Basel, Karger, 2006, vol 125, pp 29-32.

The Epidemiological Situation of Enzootic Rabies in the Republic of Lithuania over the Past Ten Years

P. Mačiulskis, K. Lukauskas, A. Dranseika, V. Kiudulas, A. Pockevičius

Lithuanian Veterinary Academy, Kaunas, Lithuania

Objective

Rabies is widespread across the Republic of Lithuania. While urban rabies has been eradicated, it remains enzootic in wildlife. Infected wild animals are the main reservoir of the disease and they cause sporadic cases of rabies in domestic animals. Since 1960, 11 people have died of rabies in Lithuania. The objective of this study was to analyse the development of the epidemiological situation of enzootic rabies, looking at associations between animals submitted for examination and reported cases, the incidence and trends of infection in certain species of domestic and wild animals, geographical distribution, monthly and seasonal variations, and the impact of rabies control activities on rabies cases in Lithuania over a ten-year period, between 1994 and 2003.

Materials and Methods

Rabies has been enzootic in Lithuania for many years and the reporting of cases is compulsory. The State Food and Veterinary Service carries out rabies prevention and control measures. Suspected cases are notified to the local State Food and Veterinary Services and samples are collected and submitted to veterinary laboratories for investigation by direct immunofluorescence and biological testing. Mouse inoculation is used to verify samples tested negative by immunofluorescence.

Data on rabies prevention and control measures along with rabies cases in domestic and wild animals were collected retrospectively from the records of the Animal Health Department of the State Food and Veterinary Service. The records of the hunters' organization were used to obtain data on the size of wildlife populations.

Descriptive epidemiology and time series data analyses were used to compile data on animals submitted for examination and reported cases. The incidence, monthly, seasonal and geographical variations, and the influence of applied control measures on rabies cases were also examined. Evaluation of the relationship between animal submissions and reported cases and correlations between the rabies incidence rates in certain species (foxes, raccoon dogs, cattle, dogs and cats), taking into account geographical location and forested areas, was performed using Prism 2.01 software. The correlation coefficient, r, and its 95 % confidence interval and P values were calculated.

RESULTS

In the ten years studied, the number of animal submissions increased more than six times; from 298 in 1994 to 1,989 in 2003. The greatest annual increases occurred during the last four years. During the 10-year period, 3,972 domestic animals and 5,294 wild animals were submitted for examination. There was a positive correlation between the number of submissions and the number of positive cases.

The number of reported rabies cases increased 16 times over the 10-year period: from 69 cases in 1994 to 1,108 cases in 2003. The incidence rate of rabies in domestic animals increased nearly seven fold from 44 cases in 1994 to 301 cases in 2003. In wildlife it increased 32 fold from 25 cases in 1994 to 807 cases in 2003. The number of animal rabies cases has greatly increased in the last four years: 850 cases in 2000, 677 cases in 2001, 933 cases in 2002 and 1108 cases in 2003.

From 1994 to1997, more rabies cases occurred in domestic animals than in wildlife. Since 1998, the reverse has been true. In 1998, 58.9 % of all rabies cases occurred in wildlife, 75.3 % in 1999, 66.5 % in 2000, 71.6 % in 2001, 73.1 % in 2002 and 72.8 % in 2003.

In 1994, most rabies cases were registered in the northern regions of Lithuania, with a prevalence of fox and raccoon dog rabies. Sporadic rabies cases were diagnosed in other parts of the country. In 1999 and 2003, domestic and wildlife rabies was more prevalent in the northern, southern and central regions of Lithuania.

Two seasonal peaks of wild animal rabies were found in spring and autumn. The first, moderate peak occurred from March to May and a second, higher peak was found from October to November. On an annual basis, 7.7 % of all cases occurred in March, 7.3 % in April, 7.2 % in May, 13.1 % in October and 12.5 % in November. Domestic animal rabies showed only one seasonal peak, in autumn: 12.5 % of cases were recorded in September, 16.2 % in October and 17.2 % in November.

The incidence rate of rabies in foxes increased nearly 1.5 times, from 23.5 % in 1994 to 34.1 % in 2003, with a peak of 35.4 % of all rabies cases recorded in 1999. A slight decrease in fox rabies cases occurred from 2000 to 2002. In 2000, 31.3 % of rabies cases diagnosed occurred in foxes, with 29.1 % in 2001 and 29.3 % in 2002.

The incidence rate of raccoon dog rabies increased nearly three fold from 11.8 % of all rabies cases in 1994 to 27 % in 2003, with a rise in the incidence rate to 35 % in 2001 and a slight decrease to 27 % in 2003. The incidence of cases of cattle rabies decreased 1.8 fold from 25 % in 1994 to 13.7 % in 2003, with an increase in the incidence rate to 42.6 % in 1996 and 43.8 % in 1997. The incidence rate of dog rabies decreased by more than three fold from 19.1 % in 1994 to 5.95 % in 2003 and the incidence rate of cat rabies decreased 2.4 fold from 17.6 % in 1994 to 7.3 % in 2003.

Of all diagnosed rabies cases, 28.8 % were foxes, 21.3 % were raccoon dogs, 22.9 % were cattle, 10.3 % were cats and 7.5 % were dogs, totalling 90.8 %. Of all wildlife rabies cases, fox rabies accounted for 52.8 %, raccoon dog rabies 34 %, martens 8.5 % and other wild animal species 4.6 %. Other wild animal cases involved polecats, badgers, hamsters, muskrats, rats, roe deer, otters, wolves, hedgehogs, beavers, mink, elk and lynxes. Of all diagnosed domestic animal rabies cases, dogs accounted for 17.1 %, cats 24.8 %, cattle 54.2 % and other species 3.8 %. Other domestic animals cases involved sheep and goats.

A significant correlation was found between the number of cases of fox and raccoon dog rabies and between wild animal rabies and dog rabies. There was a non-significant correlation between wild animal rabies and cat and cattle rabies, and also between the number of rabies cases and the number of vaccinated domestic animals, oral vaccination of wildlife and forested areas. A significant correlation was found between the number of rabies cases and the size of the fox and raccoon dog populations as well as the number of hunted foxes and raccoon dogs.

Discussion

This report analyses data from animal rabies records obtained from rabies surveillance, which plays an important part in the planning of rabies control. Domestic animals submitted for rabies examination had usually shown clinical signs of rabies or had bitten, scratched or attacked other domestic animals and sometimes humans. Wild animals, mostly foxes and raccoon dogs, with unusual behaviour were brought to the veterinary laboratories by the official veterinarians of the State Food and Veterinary Service. The total number of submissions for rabies diagnosis has increased more than six fold since 1994. This is probably related to the increased number of animals with suspected rabies and increased public awareness of the danger rabies poses to humans and animals. The records showed a significant correlation between submissions and recorded rabies cases. Geographical location did not prevent the submission of animals for examination. This is probably due to the availability of rabies diagnostic facilities in each county's veterinary laboratory.

The last four years have seen the highest number of registered rabies cases in wild animals, mainly in foxes and raccoon dogs. A similar epidemiological situation may exist across Europe. Since 1994, the number of reported cases in Europe has increased nearly 1.3 fold. In 1997 there was a reduction in rabies cases, and then the number of cases doubled in 2003. The available data cannot explain whether these developments were due to a change in rabies incidence or a change in case reporting in Europe. The political and economical developments in Eastern European countries during this period may have contributed to changes in both the epidemiological situation of rabies and disease surveillance.

Intensive control measures have been implemented in Lithuania and urban rabies has been eradicated. An estimated 70 % of the dog population and about 10 % of the cat population are vaccinated against rabies. Emergency vaccination of domestic animals is carried out in areas where confirmed cases of rabies are detected. Stray dogs are quarantined and most of them are put down. In our study, cattle, dogs and cats were the most commonly effected domestic animals. Other domestic animals accounted on average for less than 4 % of all rabies cases in domestic animals. More rabies cases occurred in domestic animals than in wildlife for the period 1994-1997. This could indicate that, during this period, the main focus of rabies surveillance was on domestic animals. Foxes and raccoon dogs were the main reservoir of this disease. Wild predators moved into areas of human settlements and animal holdings and close contact between wildlife and susceptible domestic animals increased, increasing the incidence rate of rabies in domestic animals. In Europe, the main groups of domestic animals affected with rabies between 1994 and 2003 were cattle, dogs, cats, sheep and goats.

For many years, foxes were the main wildlife reservoir of rabies in Lithuania. Recently, raccoon dogs have become the main wildlife species infected with rabies. In 2001 and 2002 there were more rabies cases in raccoon dogs than in foxes in Lithuania. In other Baltic States and in Poland in 1994-2003 most rabies cases occurred in raccoon dogs. This probably reflects the distribution and density of raccoon dog populations in parts of Europe. Martens play a local role in rabies epidemiology. They accounted for between 4.7 % and 13.2% of all rabies cases in wildlife in Lithuania between 1994 and 2003. Other wildlife species accounted for an average of less than 5 % of all wildlife rabies cases.

Rabies is endemic in Lithuania. Records show that in 1994 most sporadic rabies cases were registered in the northern part of Lithuania and later the disease became widespread across the country. Several factors may have effected the prevalence of the disease in different regions. From 1995-2000, a short-term, wildlife oral vaccination campaign against rabies was carried out in discrete areas of Lithuania. More rabies cases were subsequently registered in the regions where oral vaccination had taken place. It might therefore be considered that the campaign had a negative rather than a positive effect on the incidence rate of rabies in the fox and raccoon dog populations in the short-term. However, the increase could be explained by a significant increase in the overall populations of foxes and raccoon dogs at the time (attested to by the number of animals hunted), which would lead to a proportional increase in the number of rabies cases quite independently of the vaccination campaign.

The significant correlation between wild animal rabies and dog rabies suggests that rabid wild animals frequently approach animal holdings and commonly bite restrained dogs. Rabid animals also attack cattle at pasture. The occurrence of the disease in cattle kept in the cowshed indicates a long incubation period. Cats are probably infected after having been in contact with infected small animals.

We found seasonal variations in rabies in wild and domestic animals. The number of wild animal rabies cases increased during the spring, when foxes and raccoon dogs breed, and again during autumn, when they migrate to new habitats. During these seasons, contact and fighting among animals increase the likelihood of transmission of the rabies virus. In summer there is also an increase in the young fox population. The number of domestic animal rabies cases increased in autumn, when the number of infected wild animals is at its highest, and they encroach on animal holdings and attack the animals.

Conclusions

Rabies is a public health concern as well as a problem of wildlife and domestic animals in Lithuania. Foxes and raccoon dogs are the main species involved in rabies transmission.

A long-term wildlife rabies control programme coordinated with neighbouring countries will be the only means of solving the problem. The oral vaccination of foxes and raccoon dogs should be applied to control rabies in Lithuania.

Dr. P. Mačiulskis, Lithuanian Veterinary Academy, Tilzes str. 18, Kaunas, Lithuania.
E-mail: pmaciulskis@vet.lt

Dodet B, Schudel A, Pastoret PP, Lombard M (eds): Rabies in Europe.
Dev Biol (Basel). Basel, Karger, 2006, vol 125, pp 33-37.

Antigenic and Molecular Characterization of Field and Vaccine Rabies Virus Strains in the Russian Federation

A.E. Metlin[1], S.S. Rybakov[1], K.N. Gruzdev[1], E. Neuvonen[2], J. Cox[3], A. Huovilainen[2]

[1] Federal Centre for Animal Health, Yur'evets, Vladimir, Russia
[2] National Veterinary and Food Research Institute, Helsinki, Finland
[3] Federal Research Centre for Virus Diseases of Animals, Wusterhausen, Germany

Introduction

Different panels of monoclonal antibodies (mAbs) have been successfully used worldwide to study the antigenic characteristics of field rabies viruses and vaccine strains [1-6]. The combination of mAb studies and nucleotide sequencing of different viral genes (mainly nucleoprotein gene [N-gene]) has also successfully been used for this purpose [7,8]. In this case, the glycoprotein gene and the so-called ψ-region (hypervariable intergenic region) are significantly more variable than N-gene and therefore they are suitable targets for molecular epidemiological studies [9].

The study of nucleotide and amino acid sequences of attenuated rabies virus strains used for vaccine production is most important. Such investigations allow for the detection of conserved and variable genome regions and the development of reliable methods for the differentiation of vaccine strains and field isolates [10].

The main objective of this work is to characterize the antigenic and genetic properties of the field rabies viruses isolated recently in the Russian Federation. Attenuated vaccine strains were also studied and correlated with the field strains. Furthermore, a reverse transcriptase-polymerase chain reaction (RT-PCR) test suitable for the diagnostic and molecular epidemiological study of rabies virus was developed.

Materials and Methods

Brain samples from diagnosed or suspected rabid animals were obtained from regional veterinary laboratories in Russia. Both field and vaccine strains were isolated in MNA and/or BHK-21 cell culture using previously published methods [11]. Antigenic characteristics of 154 field viruses isolated in cell culture were studied by indirect immunofluorescence test (IFAT) using a panel of five mouse anti-nucleocapside mAbs: W-239.17, W-187.5, W-187.11.2, MW-187.6.1 and P-41 (J. Cox, Tübingen, Germany). In addition to the field strains, three Russian vaccine strains (PB-97, "ARRIAH" and "Sheep") were studied with this panel.

The total RNA for RT-PCR was isolated from cell culture suspension using "RNeasy Mini Kit" (QIAGEN®, GB). The cDNA synthesis with 5µl of purified total RNA as a template was carried out with MuLV-reverse transcriptase and 5 pmols of Random Hexamers primer (Applied Biosystems) at 37 °C for 90 minutes in a volume of 20 µl.

Two pairs of primers were designed: the first pair (N-primers) amplified an N-gene segment of 384 base pairs (bp) (nt 626-1010) and the second pair (G-primers) amplified 280 bp (nt 4835 – 5115) covering the end of the G-gene and a part of the pseudogene ψ region. The numbering of the nucleotides is according to the SAD B19 sequence [12].

All PCR reactions were carried out in a volume of 50 µl. Mixtures included 5 µl of 10-fold buffer for DNA polymerase, 5 pmol of each primer, 1 U Dynazyme II of DNA polymerase (Finnzymes) and 1 µl 10 mM of dNTP's. Thirty-five cycles of template denaturation at 94° C for one minute, primer annealing at 55° C for one minute and polymerization at 72° C for one minute were run. The products were run on 2 % agarose gel and the results were visualized by ethidium bromide staining under UV.

Before sequencing, the PCR products were purified using "MicroSpin S-400HR" columns (Amersham Pharmacia Biotech, USA). The sequencing was carried out in 16 channel automatic sequencer ABI 3100 (Applied Biosystems) at the Institute of Biotechnology, University of Helsinki. The nucleotide identities were calculated with the program WATER of the EMBOSS (The **E**uropean **M**olecular **B**iology **O**pen **S**ource **S**oftware **S**uite) Package, version 2.9.0.

Results and Discussion

Monoclonal antibody studies

On the basis of the mAb results (Table 1), antigenic variant I seems to correspond to the Arctic antigenic variant, while antigenic variants III and IV correspond to European fox and West European antigenic variants, respectively. Antigenic variants II and V do not correspond to any of the previously recovered variants.

It has been shown previously that antigenic variant I circulates mainly in the Northwestern regions of Russia, in Finland and in Estonia. Antigenic variant II has been isolated only in the Estonian islands [3], and antigenic variants III and IV in the Central and Southwest regions of Russia. Antigenic variant V was isolated in the Tver region [6]. In addition, antigenic variant III circulates in the Novosibirsk, Vladimir and Mordovia regions and variant IV in Nizhni Novgorod and Mordovia regions. The results of the determination of antigenic variants of field rabies virus isolates using mAbs are presented in Table 1.

Fixed rabies virus strains can be divided into two groups according to their reaction pattern with these five mAbs: SAD B19 belongs to antigenic group V and PB-97, and "ARRIAH", "Sheep" and CVS strains belong to the antigenic group III.

RT-PCR, sequencing and the sequence analysis

About 50 field rabies viruses and the vaccine strains PB-97, "Sheep" and "ARRIAH" were successfully amplified with N- and G-primer pairs producing bands of expected sizes. Examples are shown in Figure 1.

In addition to the "Sheep" and the PB-97 vaccine strains, over 20 Russian field rabies virus isolates originating in different geographical areas and isolated from different animal species were partially sequenced, covering the genome regions amplified by PCR. The two vaccine strains turned out to be identical at the G/pseudogene ψ region and shared 99.7 % nucleotide identity at the N-gene region. The

Table 1 : Determination of antigenic variants of rabies virus isolates using mAbs.

Antigenic variant/Region	Genotype	Reaction with mAb				
		W-239.17	W-187.5	W-187.11.2	MW-187.6.1	P-41
	Results of present investigation					
I. Finland[1], Estonia[1], Pskov[1], Kursk[1], Tver[1]	1	+	+	+	+	+
II. Estonia[1]	1	+	-	+	+	+
III. Belgorod[1], Kursk[1], N. Novgorod[1], Orel[1], Penza[1], Voronezh[1], Tver[1], Vladimir, Mordovia, Novosibirsk	1	+	+	+	+	-
IV. Tver[1], Tula[1], Ryazan[1], Vladimir[1], N. Novgorod, Mordovia	1	+	-	+	+	-
V. Tver[1]	1	+	-	+	-	-
	Results in the literature					
Arctic[2]	1	+	+	+	+	+
European fox[3]	1	+	+	+	+	-
West European[3]	1	+	-	+	+	-
Logos bat[4, 5]	2	+	-	-	+	-
Mocola[4, 5]	3	+	-	-	+	-
Duvenhage[4, 5]	4	+	-	-	+	-
EBL1[3]	5	+	-	-	-	-
EBL[2]	6	+	-	-	+	-

[1] Metlin et al [6]; [2]Schneider et al [13]; [3]Cox et al [2]; [4]Umoh et al [14]; [5]Mebatsion et al [15].

vaccine strains differed clearly from the field strains, sharing approximately 93 % and 84 % nucleotide identities with the field isolates on the N-gene and the G/pseudogene ψ region respectively.

Conclusion

Based on our mAb data, the majority of Russian rabies virus field isolates can be easily differentiated with this panel from the vaccine strain SAD B19. On the other hand, the strain PB-97 used widely for oral vaccination in Russia is impossible to distinguish from the field strains belonging to antigenic group III. For this purpose the extended panel of mAbs should be used.

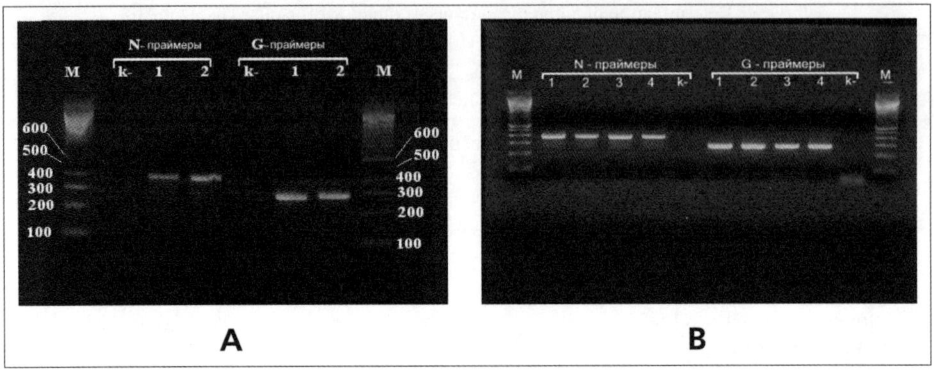

Fig. 1: **Amplification of vaccine and field rabies virus strains with RT-PCR. A.** Isolate n° 96 (tracks 1, N and G) and vaccine strain PB – 97 (tracks 2, N and G). M – marker. The numbers along the track indicate the size of PCR-product. k – negative control. **B.** Isolates n° 1 (tracks 1, N and G), 13 (tracks 2, N and G), 18 (tracks 3, N and G) and 85 (tracks 4, N and G).

The primary sequence analysis shows that the vaccine strain PB-97 included in the oral antirabic vaccine "Sinrab" in many regions (Tver, Novosibirsk, Belgorod and other Russian regions) differs considerably from the field strains. This makes the future development of reliable methods for the differentiation of Russian vaccine and field strains possible.

References

1 Botvinkin AD, Selimov MA, Kluyeva EV, et al: Antigenic characterization of rabies virus field isolates from different USSR regions using anti-nucleocapside monoclonal antibodies. J Microbiol Epidemiol Immunobiol 1990; 1: 50-54.

2 Cox JH, Schneider LG, Muller WW: Eine antigenvariante der fuchstollwut in Europa. Tierartztl. Umschau 1992; 47: 824-828.

3 Kulonen K, Boldina I: Differentiation of two rabies strains in Estonia with reference to recent finish isolates. J Wildl Dis 1993; 29 (2): 209-213.

4 Kuzmin IV: An Arctic fox rabies virus strain as the cause of human rabies in Russian Siberia. Arch Virol 1999; 144: 627-629.

5 Goto H, Minamoto N, Ito H, Ito N, et al: Mapping of epitopes and structural analysis of antigenic sites in the nucleoprotein of rabies virus. J Gen Virol 2000; 81: 119-127.

6 Metlin AE, Cox J, Rybakov SS, Huovilainen A, Grouzdev KN, Neuvonen E: Monoclonal antibody characterization of rabies virus isolates from Russia, Finland and Estonia. J Vet Med B Infect Dis Vet Public Health 2004; 51: 94-96.

7 Favoretto SR, Carrier ML, Cunha EMS, et al: Antigenic typing of Brazilian rabies virus samples isolated from animals and humans, 1989-2000. Rev Inst Med Trop Sao Paulo 2002; 44 (2): 91-95.

8 Nadin-Davis SA, Simani S, Armstrong J et al: Molecular and antigenic characterization of rabies viruses from Iran identifies variants with distinct epidemiological origins. Epidemiol Infect 2003; 131: 777-779.

9 Johnson N, McElhinney M, Smith J, et al: Phylogenetic comparison of the genus Lyssavirus using distal coding sequences of glycoprotein and nucleoprotein genes. Arch Virol 2002; 147: 2111-2123.

10 Fodor I, Grabko VI, Khozinski VV, Selimov MA: Nucleotide and deduced amino acid sequences of glycoprotein gene of rabies virus vaccine strain Vnucovo-32. Arch Virol 1994; 135: 451-459.

11 Manual of standards for diagnostic techniques, 2004, OIE, Geneva.

12 Conzelmann KK, Cox JH, Schneider LG, Thiel HJ: Molecular cloning and complete nucleotide sequence of the attenuated rabies virus SAD B19. Virology 1990; 175 (2): 485-499.

13 Schneider LG, Odegaard OA, Mueller J, Selimov M: Application of monoclonal antibodies for epidemiological investigations and oral vaccination studies, in Kuwert E, Merieux C, Koprowski H, Bogel K (eds): Rabies in the Tropics. Berlin, 1985, pp 47-59.

14 Umoh JU, Cox JH, Schneider LG: Antigenic characterization of street rabies virus isolates from Nigeria using monoclonal antibodies. Zentralbl Veterinarmed B 1990; 37: 222-228.

15 Mebatsion T, Cox JH, Frost JW: Isolation and Characterization of 115 street rabies virus isolates from Ethiopia by using monoclonal antibodies: identification of 2 isolates as Mokola and Logos bat viruses. J Infect Dis 1992; 166: 972-977.

Dr. A.E. Metlin, Federal Centre for Animal Health, RU-600901, Yur'evets, Vladimir, Russia.
E-mail: artem.metlin@inbox.ru

Dodet B, Schudel A, Pastoret PP, Lombard M (eds): Rabies in Europe.
Dev Biol (Basel). Basel, Karger, 2006, vol 125, p 39.

Epidemiological Characteristics of Rabies in the Republic of Srpska from 1995 to 2003

V. Santrac[1], J. Maric[1], S. Golubovic[2], R. Babic[1], D. Nedic[3], D. Kubelka[1]

[1] Veterinary Institute of Republic of Srpska " Dr Vaso Butozan ", Republic of Srpska, Bosnia and Herzegovina

[2] Department of Infectious Diseases, Banja Luka General Hospital, Republic of Srpska, Bosnia and Herzegovina

[3] Chief Veterinary Officer, Republic of Srpska, Bosnia and Herzegovina

Abstract: The authors studied epidemiological features of rabies over a 7-year period by analysing the collected data from protocols of the CVL of the Republic of Srpska (RS) and the protocols of the public health service and by interviewing field veterinarians. From 1995 to 2003, by passive surveillance using the fluorescent antibody test (FAT) and the mouse inoculation test (MIT), 284 positive cases were diagnosed by the CVL. The ratio between the number of positive samples to the number of submitted samples ranged from 14.29 % to 54.72 %. Rabies was present in 12 terrestrial animal species: foxes (79 %), cattle (7 %), dogs (5 %), small ruminants and cats (3 %). The remaining species were on average 1 % positive. The highest incidence of rabies was in October (12.68 %), and the lowest in July (2.93 %). There were no officially reported human rabies cases. The authors used data from only one unit for human antirabies treatment as a model to show whether rabies was a threat to human health. The unit received 2,636 patients within the period. Among them 14.6 % received specific antirabies treatment. The majority of reported attacks happened in May and August. Children between seven and 15 years of age were under the greatest risk. Males were more frequently exposed (61 %). Ninety-three per cent of injuries originated from dogs, 23 % from cats, 18 % from rodents, 14 % from cattle, 12 % from pigs and 1 % from foxes. Fifty-four percent of cases received post-exposure treatment within the first 24 hours after injury, 19 % after one day, 1.8 % after 7 days, and 4.1 % after 15 days. Only 10 % of interviewed veterinarians received pre-exposure treatment. According to the interviews, the greatest risk to the field veterinarians is contact with pasture animals. Rabies is present in RS as a sylvatic enzootic disease. This paper is intended to show the significance of the disease and should also serve as a warning to both the veterinary service and the public health service of RS.

Dodet B, Schudel A, Pastoret PP, Lombard M (eds): Rabies in Europe.
Dev Biol (Basel). Basel, Karger, 2006, vol 125, pp 41-49.

Epizootic Situation and Fox Rabies Prophylaxis in the Territory of Tatarstan

N.A. Khismatullina[1], A.N. Chernov[2], R.H. Yusupov[1], A.Z. Ravilov[1], A.V. Ivanov[1], M.S. Zaydullin[2]

[1] Federal State Scientific Establishment All-Russian Scientific Research Veterinary Institute, Kazan, Russia

[2] Council of Ministers of the Republic of Tatarstan, Kazan, Russia

Abstract: Data on the epizootic situation of rabies in the Republic of Tatarstan from 1970-2003 were obtained from epizootological and immunological monitoring. The districts in Tatarstan were divided into four groups according to the intensity of indices and a map of epizootics was developed. A three- to five-year cyclic recurrence of rabies, with peaks in the spring-winter-autumn seasons of the year was established. Foxes are the basic source and spreader of rabid infection in the Republic amounting to 96.5 % of rabies cases among wild animals. The present study gives the results of epizootological analysis of the efficacy of oral immunization of foxes in the republic since 1996.

INTRODUCTION

Rabies poses a constant threat to humanity in some parts of the world. In spite of significant scientific progress, the fight against this infection is complicated by the wide circulation of the virus in nature. The presence of natural foci and the increase in the population of wild animals has intensified the level of its spread. Since 1994, the World Health Organisation (WHO) has given much attention to the elaboration of national and inter-governmental programmes against rabies based on current epidemiological knowledge. However, according to several authors [1-4], scientifically well-grounded anti-epizootic and anti-epidemic measures should be based on the particularities of the regional epizootology of this zoo-anthroponosis. Oral immunization of wild animals is highly effective in the fight against rabies and is ecologically acceptable [5-11].

The aim of our investigation was to carry out an analysis of the epizootic situation regarding the number of rabies cases and the efficacy of oral immunization of wild fauna in the Republic of Tatarstan (RT).

Materials and Methods

We studied epizootic and statistical data from RT using the reported data from the Chief Veterinary Administration of the Council of Ministers of RT, the Kazan Municipal Animal Diseases Control Station, the Republic's Veterinary Laboratory, the Centre of Sanitary and Epidemiological control of RT, and the Administration for Regulations on the Protection, Control and Use of Hunting Animals. Regulations, guidelines, instructions, and recommendations were studied when available, as well as documents concerning programmes aimed at the control and elimination of animal rabies. The immunological monitoring of rabies cases in RT was carried out with diagnostic kits using enzyme immunoassay and fluorescence immunoassay, at the All-Russian Research Veterinary Institute (Kazan, Russia) and approved by the Ministry of Agriculture and Provision of the Russian Federation.

Results and Discussion

Efforts to decrease rabies morbidity in the Republic of Tatarstan over the past several years remain unsuccessful [3,9]. During the period 1970-2003, 1,306 cases of rabies in animals and humans were registered in 42 administrative districts and six towns. Foxes are the main source and transmitter of rabies in the republic and they account for 96,5 % of rabid wild animals (Fig. 1). We determined a three to five year periodicity in the rabies morbidity rate (Fig. 2) with maximal manifestation in the spring-winter-autumn periods (33.8 %, 31,3 %, 20,9 % respectively) (Fig. 3) connected with the fox's life-cycle. The first rise, which coincides with the mating season of foxes, can be observed in winter and early spring, and the second, connected with the dispersal and settling of young animals, is in autumn-winter. In summer when foxes are engaged in bringing up their litters, their mobility is limited and the number of rabies cases is minimal. In autumn, we have observed an increase in the sickness rate as a result of the increase in the population of young animals [3]. During rabies enzootics, 20-70 % of animals become infected and die. The year following enzootics, the number of rabid foxes decreases due to a decrease in the population. The population is usually restored in three to five years with the increase in population leading to a new rise in rabies cases among foxes [12].

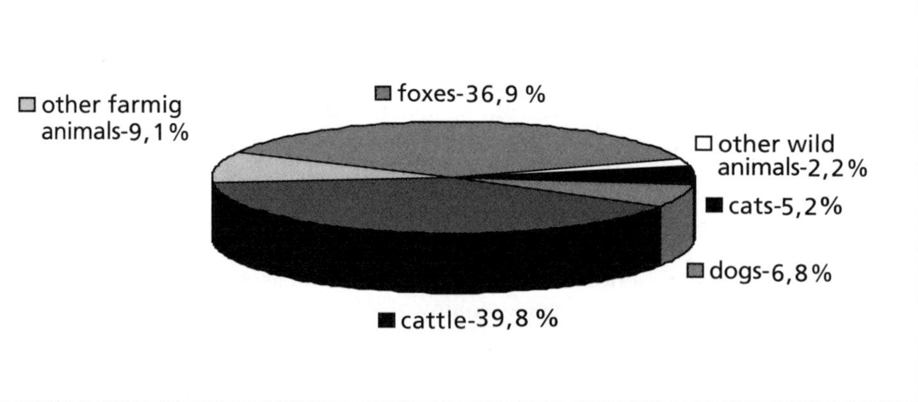

Fig. 1: Proportion of infection among different species of animals in the Republic of Tatarstan for the period 1970-2004.

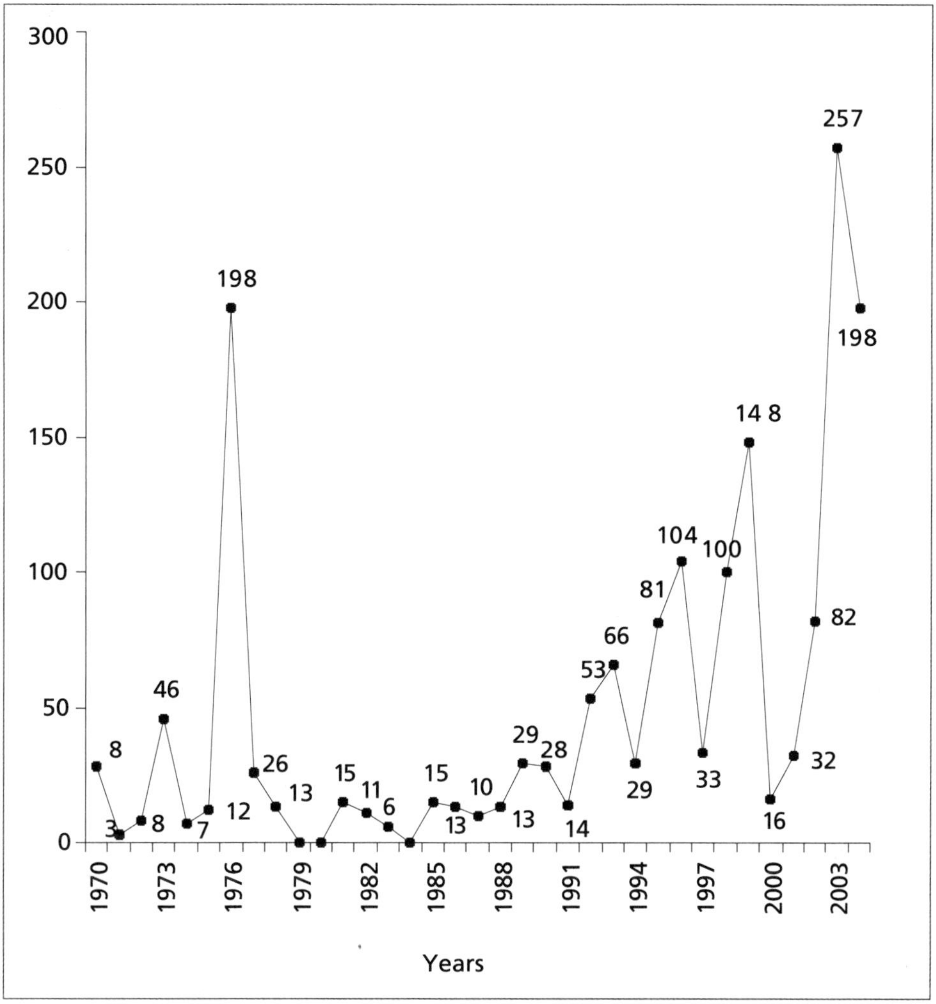

Fig. 2 : Dynamics of rabies infection found in animals in the Republic of Tatarstan for the period 1970-2004.

It was determined that the worst affected districts for rabies are situated in the eastern part of Zakamie, in the Bugulma-Belebey Hills which represent the epicentre of rabies in the republic.

The districts of RT were divided into four groups according to the intensity of the epizootic situation and a map showing affected districts was drawn up (Fig. 4). Cross-border transmission of the pathogen into RT cannot be ignored so official reports for the period of 2002-2004 (including eight months of 2004) were examined in bordering regions. In the Republic of Bashkortostan 969 rabies cases were registered; in the Orenburg region, 422 cases; in the Samara region, 267 cases; in the Ulyanovsk region, 74 cases; in the Chuvash Republic, 27; in the Republic of Mariy El, 13; in the Kirov region, 1 and in the Udmurt Republic, 2 cases.

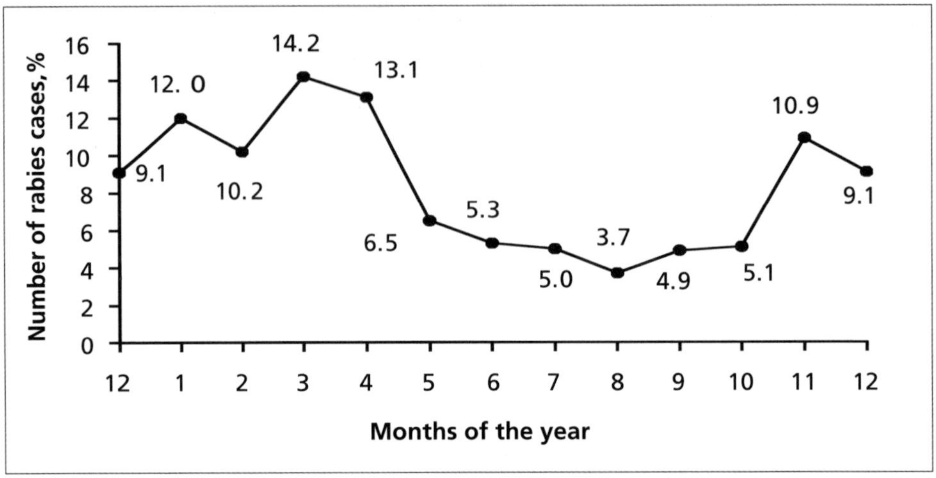

Fig. 3: Seasonality of rabies in the Republic of Tatarstan for the period 1970-2003.

Rabies control requires not only protective measures but also direct actions aimed at controlling epizootic process in natural disease reservoirs. Oral immunization of wild carnivores together with active measures to control their populations are effective and should be carried out where possible.

According to the decree No.403 of the Cabinet of Ministers of RT of 22.05.96, together with the Chief Veterinary Administration, we elaborated a "Plan of measures for Fox Rabies Prophylaxis" which was approved by the Chief Veterinary Administration on 25.02.1997 and determined the territory for the distribution of vaccine in the worst affected republican districts (Appendix).

Meetings were held in all districts to discuss the problems of anti-epizootic measurements, vaccination of wild carnivores and how to maximise coverage. Representatives of the Chief Veterinary Administration of the Cabinet of Ministers of RT, chief state veterinarian inspectors, the representatives of the Regional Centers of Sanitary and Epidemiologic Inspections, the heads of Administrations of all the regions of Tatarstan, the heads of hunters' societies, veterinarian specialists and chasseurs all participated. The peculiarities of recent rabies epizootics in the territory of the Russian Federation and Tatarstan and the danger of rabies to humans, were discussed.

Veterinarian specialists and chasseurs were acquainted with the manual on vaccine use and precautionary measures to be taken during the application of vaccine. The heads of the hunters' societies supplied information about the habitats of foxes. Teams including veterinarian specialists, chasseurs and representatives of village councils were organised to distribute bait containing oral vaccine with the aim of maximal immunization coverage of the fox population. Bait consumption was recorded at six, 10 and 18 days, and uneaten bait was recorded and eliminated.

A resolution was made to intensify the work on regulating the number of foxes and other wild predators and to inform the veterinary service immediately about unusual behaviour in wild animals and to send dead, wild animals to the veterinary laboratories to be examined for rabies. Municipal services were to intensify the catching and shooting of stray dogs and cats as well as monitoring registration and compliance with the rules for keeping domestic animals.

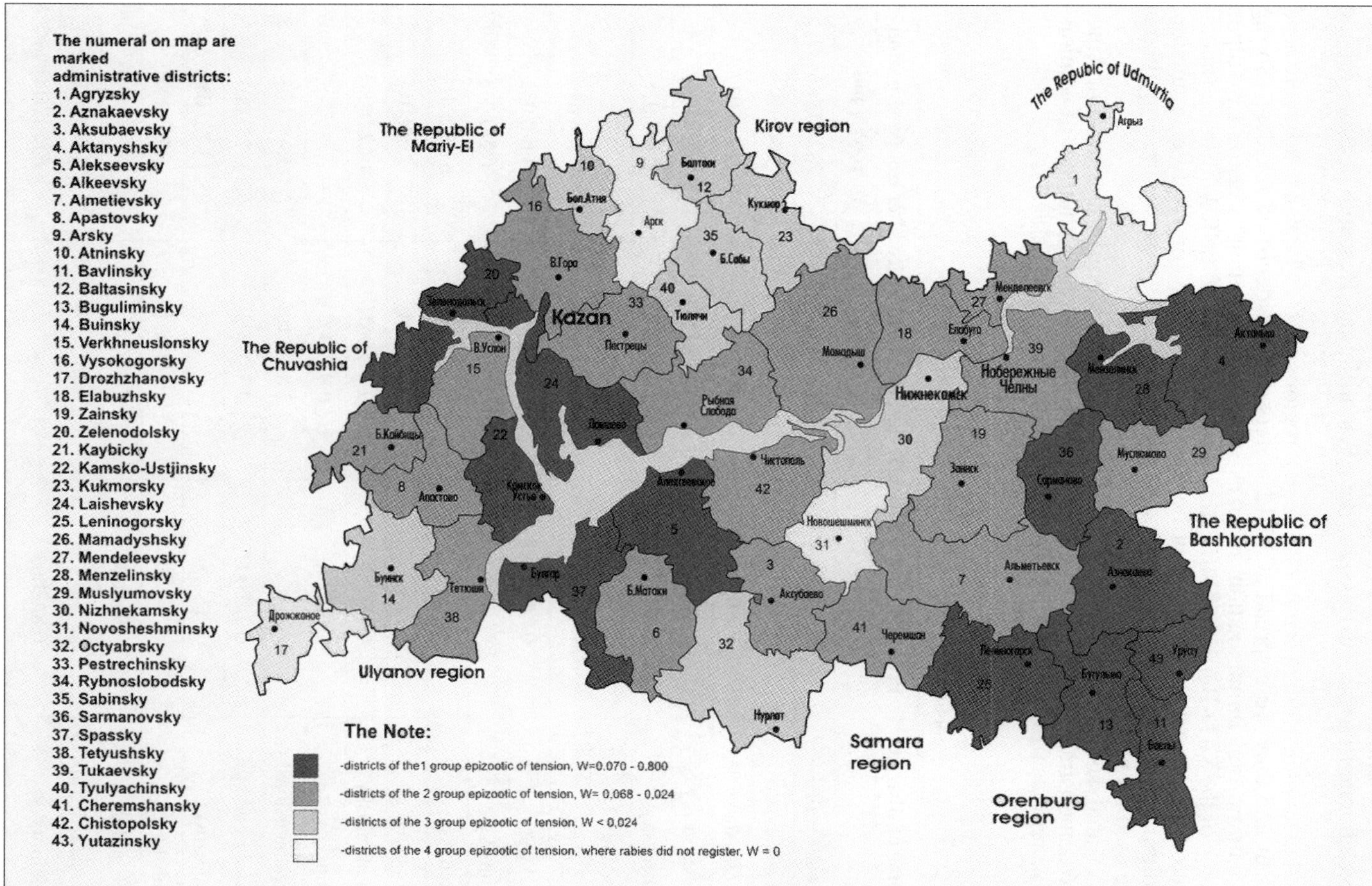

Fig. 4: Epizootic map of animal's rabies in the Republik of Tatarstan for the period from 2000 till 2004.

Oral immunization of wild carnivores (mainly foxes) with anti-rabic viral vaccine elaborated in the All-Russian State Scientific and Research Institute for the Control, Standardization and Certification of Veterinary Preparations (Moscow) began in autumn 1996 in six worst affected regions of RT. Chicken heads were used for bait and they were spread at 10-12 meters around identified fox-dens. Spring and autumn oral immunization of foxes was repeated annually using Lysvulpen vaccine of the SAD-Bern virus strain and Sinrab vaccine of the RB-71 strain (manufactured by the All-Russian Scientific Research Institute for Wildlife Protection, Vladimir). Briquettes containing tetracycline as an indicator of vaccine prophylaxis were used for bait.

An analysis of the efficacy of wildlife oral vaccination in the republic since 1996 demonstrated an improvement in the rabies situation in a number of administrative regions from 1997 to 1999 compared to 1994-1996 (Table 1).

Table 1 : The epizootic situation in rabies affected districts in the Republic of Tatarstan 1991-1999.

Name of district	Proportion of badly affected areas/intensity of epizootic situation		
	1991-1993	**1994-1996**	**1997-1999**
Aznakaevsky	35.1/0.351	45.5/0.303	28.6/0.286
Aksubaevsky	–	–	3.6/0.012
Aktanyshsky	1.2/0.004	11.5/0.115	11.5/0.077
Alekseevsky	–	11.7/0.117	1.7/0.006
Alkeevsky	1.4/0.005	9.6/0.096	2.6/0.018
Almetievsky	2.1/0.007	3.1/0.031	–
Apastovsky	1.3/0.004	1.3/0.004	2.6/0.017
Arsky	0.8/0.003	–	4.6/0.031
Atninsky	–	–	6.5/0.043
Bavlinsky	–	11.6/0.078	62.8/0.419
Baltasinsky	–	1.3/0.004	2.6/0.017
Bugulminsky	6.1/0.020	9.1/0.061	18.2/0.061
Buinski	–	0.9/0.003	–
Verkhneuslonsky	–	2.8/0.019	1.4/0.005
Vysokogorsky	0.7/0.003	0.7/0.003	0.7/0.003
Elabuzhsky	–	–	13.7/0.046
Zainsky	–	1.2/0.004	1.2/0.004
Zelenodolsky	0.9/0.003	–	–
Kamsko-Ustjinsky	–	5.9/0.039	5.9/0.039
Kukmorsky	0.8/0.003	–	6.6/0.044

Table 1: continued.

Name of district	Proportion of badly affected areas/intensity of epizootic situation		
	1991-1993	**1994-1996**	**1997-1999**
Laishevsky	–	13.0/0.087	5.8/0.039
Leninogorsky	12.5/0.042	6.3/0.021	26.6/0.177
Mamadyshsky	–	3.8/0.038	3.0/0.030
Mendeleevsky	–	–	2.8/0.009
Menzelinsky	1.5/0.005	18.8/0.188	2.9/0.019
Musliumovsky	7.1/0.024	22.9/0.229	4.3/0.043
Nizhnekamsky	–	–	1.5/0.005
Novosheshminsky	14.3/0.048	–	8.6/0.057
Oktybrsky	1.1/0.004	–	–
Pestrechinsky	1.3/0.004	1.3/0.004	1.3/0.004
Rybnoslobodsky	1.2/0.004	–	6.2/0.062
Sabinsky	4.5/0.029	1.5/0.005	32.8/0.328
Sarmanovsky	9.9/0.033	16.9/0.169	4.2/0.028
Spassky	8.5/0.057	2.1/0.007	–
Tetiushsky	1.3/0.004	2.6/0.018	1.3/0.004
Tukaevsky	1.1/0.004	4.5/0.045	1.1/0.004
Tiulyachinsky	1.8/0.006	–	23.6/0.157
Cheremshansky	–	2.0/0.007	2.0/0.007
Chistopolsky	18.8/0.125	10.9/0.073	1.6/0.005
Iutazinsky	–	10.5/0.105	65.8/0.658

As shown in Table 1, the decrease in the number of badly affected sites and tension of the epizootic situation for the Aznakayevskiy district are 1.6 and 1.1 times respectively, for the Alkeevskiy district, 3.7 and 5.3; for the Mendeleyevskiy district, 6.5 and 9.8; for the Muslumovskiy district, – 5.3 and 5.3; for Sarmanovskiy, 4.0 and 6.0; for Tetyushskiy, 6.0 and 4.5; Tukayevskiy district, 4.1 and 11.3 and others. In 2000, the incidence of rabies decreased to just 16 cases. Nevertheless, for the last three years (2001-2003) we have registered a deterioration in the rabies situation in the republic: in 2001, 32 rabies cases were registered, in 2002, 78, in 2003, 257 cases (including 35 administrative districts and two cases in the city of Kazan), and in 2004, 198 (an improvement in the situation of 1.3 times compared to 2003).

Conclusion

Rabies is transmitted by a very mobile carrier which does not take account of administrative or state boundaries. Permanent information exchange between all the administrative regions in the Republic of Tatarstan and neighbouring regions is required. To decrease rabies enzootics a programme of simultaneous, large-scale, wildlife oral immunization operations in the Mid-Volga region should be elaborated in combination with population control of host species.

References

1 Avilov VS, Sedov VA, Kolomytsev SA, Vedernikov VA, Pytalev PN, Guljukin AM, Khakin GV: The count of new features of an epizootology of a rabies. Veterinary.1998; 6: 3-6. (In Russian).

2 Bakulov IA: New problems of epizootology. Mater. international scientific-practikal. conference, devoted to 40-anniversary VNIIVVM. Pokrov 1998: 135-138. (In Russian).

3 Ravilov AZ, Khismatullina NA, Jusupov RH et al: The Epizootologo-epidemiological characteristics of a rabies in the Republic of Tatarstan and modification of measures to control this infection. Newslett Kazan, 1999, 59 p. (In Russian).

4 Selimov MA: Modern achievements in rabiology. Review information. Moscow: VNIIMI 1987; 4: 35-44. (In Russian).

5 Selimov MA, Fodor II, Grabko VI: On the problem of a gene-engineering antirabic vaccine. Gene-engineering and synthetic vaccines. Pushen? 1990, pp 64-70. (In Russian).

6 Sedov VA, Koromyslov GF, Kulikovskiy AV: Seminar of the WHO in rabies control in the wild. Bulletin s.-hk. Sciences 1991; 4: 172-173. (In Russian).

7 Rupprecht CE, Hanlon CA, Niezgoda M, Buchanan JR, Diehl D, Koprovski H: Recombinant rabies Vaccines-Efficacy Assessment in Free-Ranging Animals//Onderstepoort J Vety Res 1993; 60 (4): 463-468.

8 Tsiang H: Current concept in rabies//Adv Virus Res 1995; 2: 2-4.

9 Khisamutdinov FF, Khismatullina NA, Jusupov RH, Burganov EG: New method of natural rabies control. ??z Report Repub. Scientific – product. Conf. Kazan, 1996, 52 p. (In Russian).

10 Khismatullina NA, Chernov AN, Tjatigachev SA et al: The organization of an oral immunization of foxes. ??z report Repub scientific – product Conf. Kazan, 1997, 56 p. (In Russian).

11 Khismatullina NA: Development of agents and methods of immunological monitoring and control in rabies and Q fever: Autoref. dis.... dr. biol science Kazan 2000: 45. (In Russian).

12 Cherkasskiy BL: Epidemiology and prophylaxis of rabies. Moscow, Medicine, 1985, 288 p. (In Russian).

Dr. N. Khismatullina, Federal State Scientific Institute "All-Russian Research Veterinary Institute", Nauchniyi gor. 2, RU-420075 Kazan, Russia.
E-mail: naanhis@mail.ru

Appendix: Plan of preventive measures to reduce rabies in foxes

1. Study of geographical features of district

1.1 To study landscape features of the locality.

1.2 To determine fox population density.

2. Investigation of epizootological factors

No later than 12 months prior to immunisation, a district should be put under epizootologic surveillance. Residents should be informed of the forthcoming programme.

2.1 To carry out the registration and mapping of rabies foci (the determination of specific structures and the number of infected animals and their distribution over the territory).

2.2 To carry out the localisation and mapping of foxholes in rabies foci.

2.3 To examine all dead wild animals as well as suspected infected animals for rabies by virological and serological methods.

2.4 To cull foxes with the aim of eliminating rabies by population control.

2.5 To carry out prophylactic immunisation of cattle, dogs and cats in affected districts.

3. Immunisation

3.1 Oral immunization should take place in autumn and/or winter (November-December) and in spring (March-April).

3.2 Oral vaccine should be laid in baits in known fox habitats, on average 15-20 baits per square kilometre, or at 10-15 metres from mapped, inhabited foxholes.

3.3 The record of baits eaten by wild animals should be kept daily during 5-8 days.

3.4 The control of vaccine-induced immunity should be estimated according to the titres of specific virus neutralizing antibodies in the blood of culled animals and according to epizootological indices.

3.5 Rodents should be trapped to study their virus carrier state along with a study of dead rodents in order to examine a possible negative impact of the vaccine virus on small rodents.

3.6 Conduct immunisation and epizootological inspection every 3-5 years to evaluate oral immunisation programmes.

Dodet B, Schudel A, Pastoret PP, Lombard M (eds): Rabies in Europe.
Dev Biol (Basel). Basel, Karger, 2006, vol 125, pp 51-58.

Epizootiological Characteristics of Rabies in Serbia and Montenegro, 1993-2004

B. Djuricic[1], *O. Vukelic*[2], *N. Knezevic*[3], *S. Radojicic*[1], *U. Ungurovic*[5], *Z. Debeljak*[4], *R. Ignjatovic*[4], *L. Simonovic*[4], *M. Zivojinovic*[4], *A. Zivulj*[4], *D. Lausevic*[4]

1 Veterinary Faculty, Belgrade, Serbia
2 Ministry of Agriculture, Veterinary Sector, Belgrade, Serbia
3 Veterinarski zavod, Zemun, Serbia
4 Veterinary Institut Kraljevo, Serbia
5 Pasterov zavod, Novi Sad, Serbia

Introduction

Rabies is an acute infectious disease of animals and humans characterised by the appearance of encephalitis which is invariably fatal. The cause is a virus of the family *Rhabdoviridae*, genus *Lyssavirus*. The illness occurs, to a greater or lesser extent, on all continents. In Europe, rabies is still present in the east, while it has been eradicated in western countries. In some countries (Holland, Germany, France etc.) rabies is present only in bats. In the majority of other countries, the sylvatic form predominates over urban rabies which occurs only in Turkey and Russia. Forty to fifty thousand cases of human rabies are reported every year (WHO estimates). Western European countries have gone to great lengths to eradicate rabies, applying oral vaccination to the natural animal reservoir (red fox – *Vulpes vulpes*). The course to the planned final eradication of the illness in Europe by 2010 will be uncertain, because of the lack of financial and organizational resources in the countries of Eastern Europe [1].

Rabies in Yugoslavia (Serbia and Montenegro – SCG)

Until 1991, epizootics of rabies in the central Balkans (Yugoslavia, Serbia and Montenegro — SCG), which began in the early seventies from northern Europe, were present only in the northern part of country (up to the Sava and Danube rivers). From 1991 to 1992, the infection crossed this border and was registered in the Southeast of SCG. Since then rabies has spread in SCG due to the migration of the natural reservoir species [2]. Similar epizootiological data can be found in the surrounding countries (cat rabies in Skopje, FYR Macedonia in 2000, the appearance of rabies in the south of Montenegro in 2001, two cases of rabies in foxes in Albania on the border of SCG (Kosovo and Metohija) in 2003 etc.). Epizootiological data show that the sylvatic form of rabies is dominant in the area and foxes are the main reservoir. The number of infected foxes has been relatively constant and accounts for over 78 % of rabies cases per year [2,3] (Table 1).

Table 1: Rabies cases (n = 202) in SCG in 2004.

	Wild animals			**Domestic animals**						
(%)	163 (80.7%)			39 (19.3%)						
Animals	W. cat	**Fox**	Wolf	Sheep	Dog	Cow	Horse	Goat	Pig	Cat
Total	1	161	1	3	15	3	1	1	1	15
%	0.5	**79.7**	0.5	1.5	7.4	1.5	0.5	0.5	0.5	7.4

On this basis, in the territory of Serbia and Montenegro as well as in other parts of Europe, the fox population is an indicator of the expected appearance of the disease in a given locality. It is known that in certain territories where sylvatic rabies is endemic, a considerable reduction in the number of foxes can end the epizootic. Then, several years later, when the fox population is restored, the epizootic can flame up again, with the arrival of infected foxes from surrounding territories.

The epizootiological picture of rabies in SCG has been unfavourable for many years. The territorial spread of rabies in the country from 1993 to 2003 (Fig. 1: maps 1-12) show that the infection has spread among wild animals due to the migration of reservoir species (fox and other wild animals).

The number of infected regions has increased from 30 in 1994 to 81 in 2004. The overall number of registered cases of rabies was 1,517 with fluctuations from year to year: from 46 cases in 1994 to 245 cases in 2001. The real epizootiological situation in the field is certainly different since the number of registered cases depends on the number of samples gathered and the impact of disease control programmes in a given area.

With respect to the temporal distribution of diagnosed cases, the majority were registered in the winter period, November – December and February – March, and accounted for approximately 45 % of the annual total of diagnosed cases. Epizootiological data on rabies in the region of Kosovo and Metohija 1999 – 2004 are missing, due to organisational and technical inspection problems, but it is certain that even that territory is infected with sylvatic rabies.

Regarding animal species distribution, a worrying increase in the number of infected dogs and cats in direct contact with people was registered.

This fact is a warning that the situation must be taken seriously and that vigorous steps must be taken to implement the measures, established by law, concerning compulsory, prophylactic vaccination of animals. The programme of compulsory vaccination of dogs and cats in Serbia and Montenegro is achieved through the use

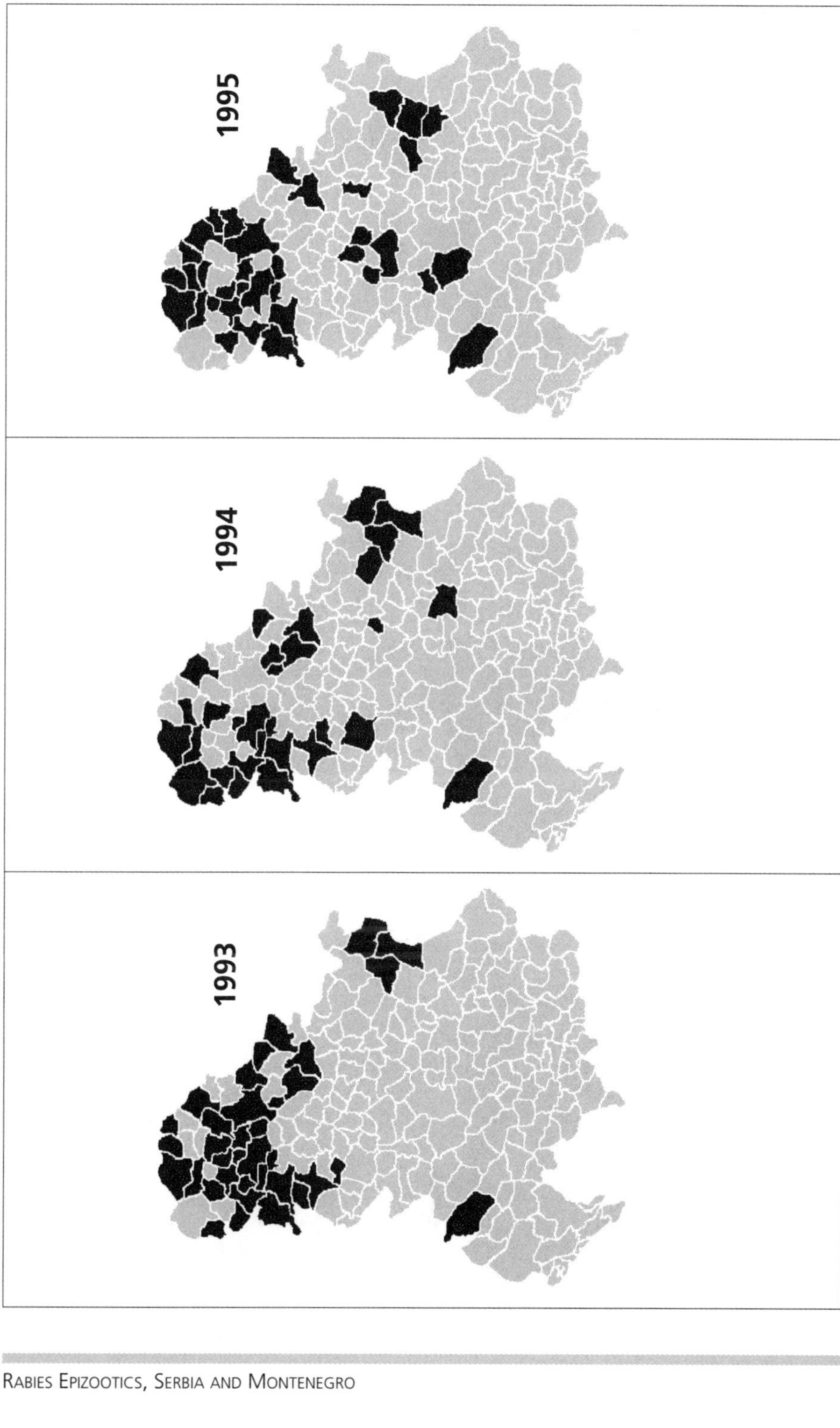

Fig. 1: Maps 1-12: The spread of rabies in Serbia and Montenegro 1993-2004.

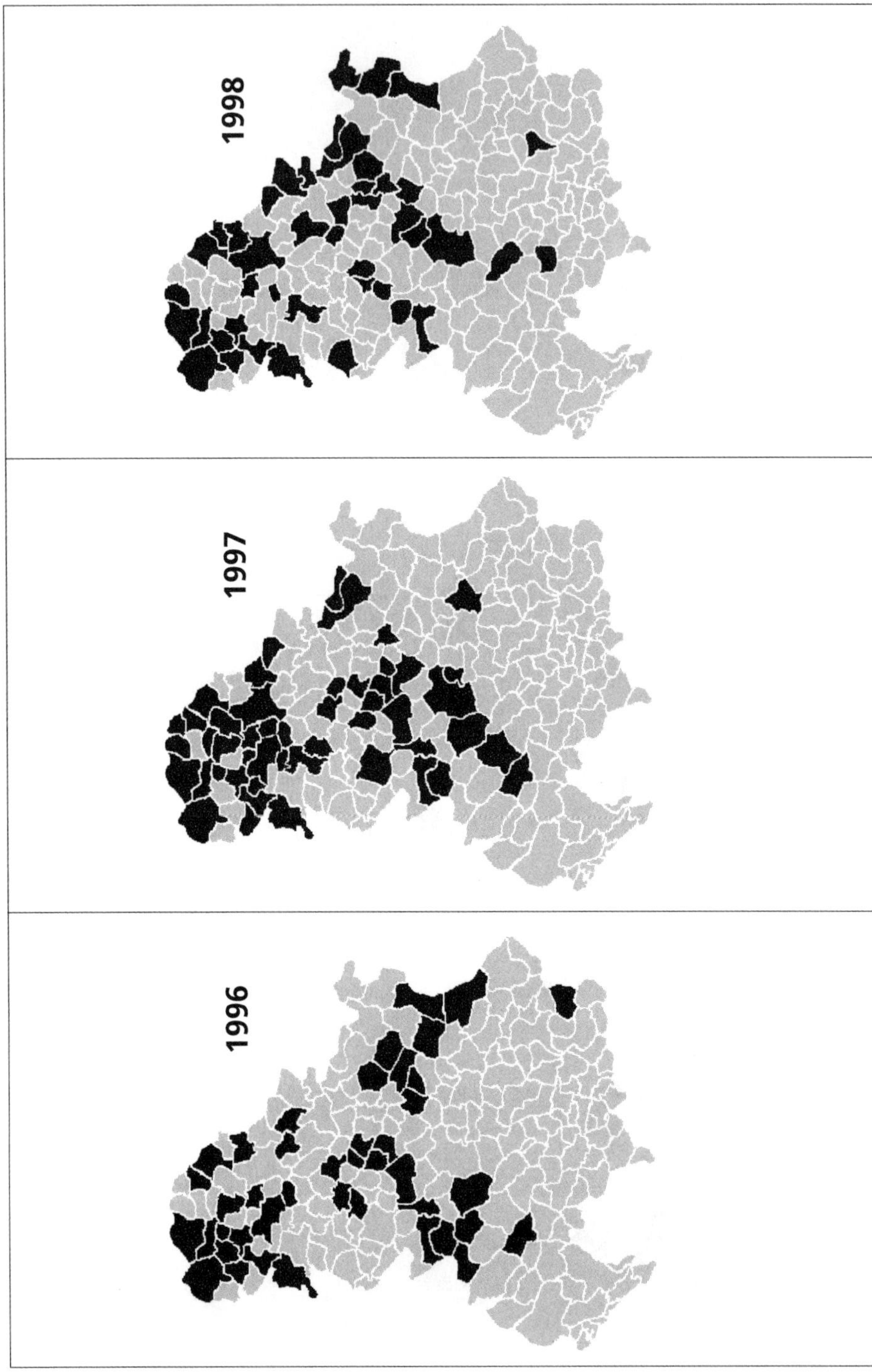

Fig. 1 : Maps 1-12 : The spread of rabies in Serbia and Montenegro 1993-2004.

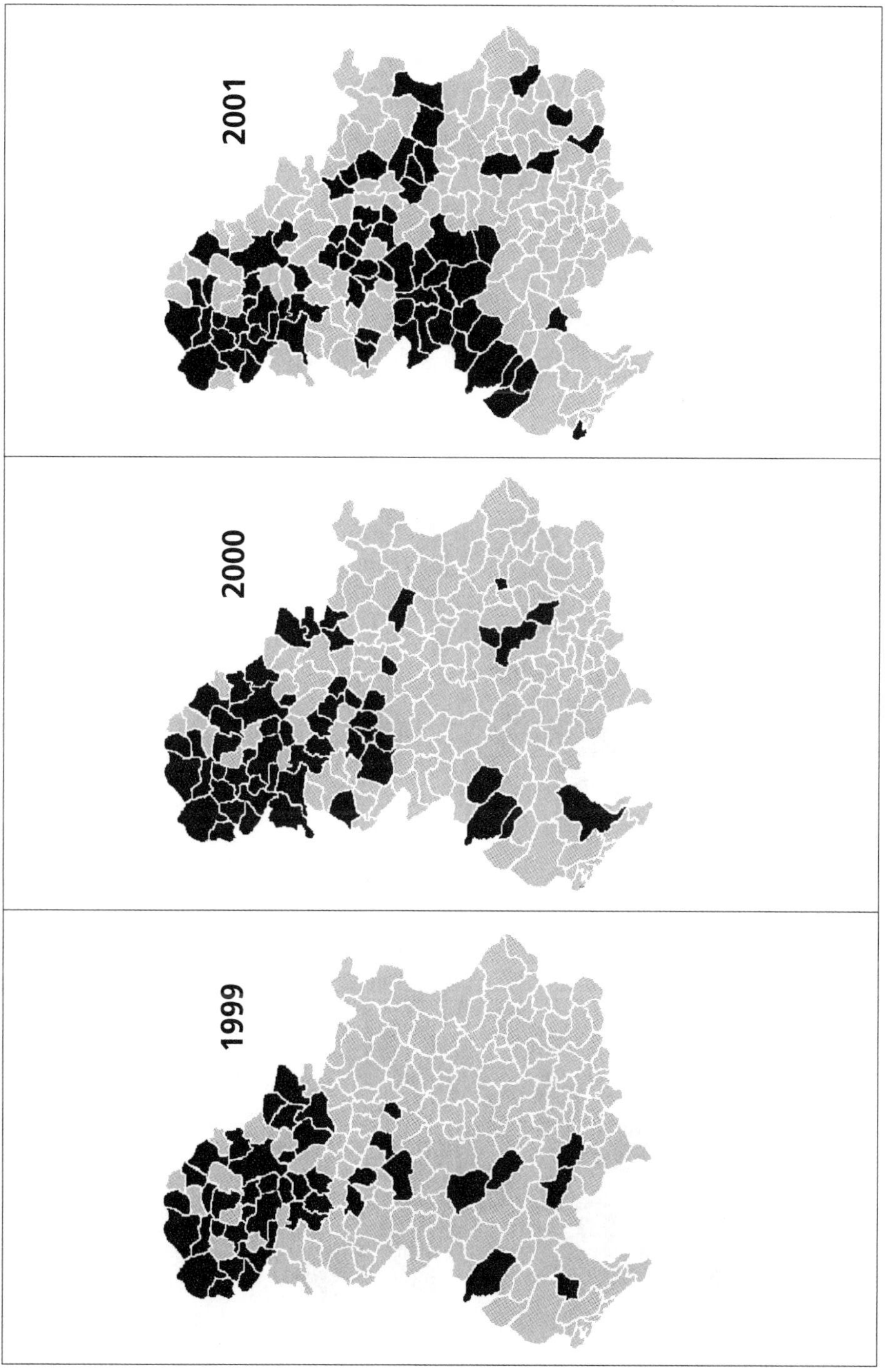

Fig. 1 : Maps 1-12 : The spread of rabies in Serbia and Montenegro 1993-2004.

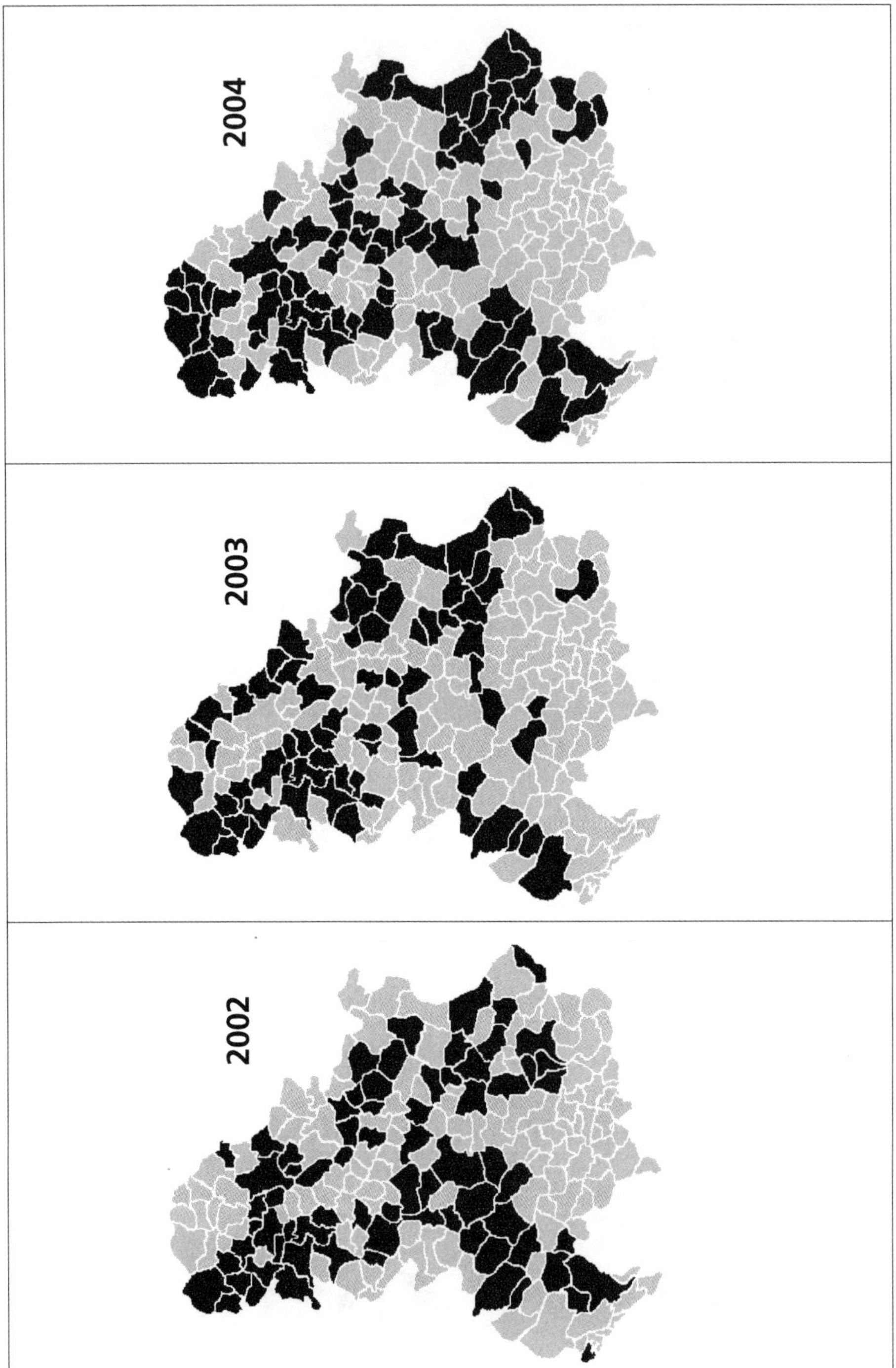

Fig. 1 : Maps 1-12 : The spread of rabies in Serbia and Montenegro 1993-2004.

Table 2: Total number of diagnosed rabies cases in Serbia and Montenegro.

No. areas	Year	N° of animals	Domestic animals	Wild animals	Vaccination*	Inactivated vaccines
37	1993	82	29	53	525 300	
30	1994	46	21	25	507 755	
37	1995	118	18	100	613 935	
45	1996	110	29	81	407 041	
51	1997	98	31	67	456 464	
47	1998	103	31	72	566 190	
51	1999	113	29	84	407 810	
58	2000	152	40	112	426 435	
74	2001	245	60	185	483 093	
72	2002	218	36	182	319 125	150 000
72	2003	232	48	184	362 307	75 000
81	2004	202	39	163	356 243	235 000

* Locally produced attenuated vaccine.

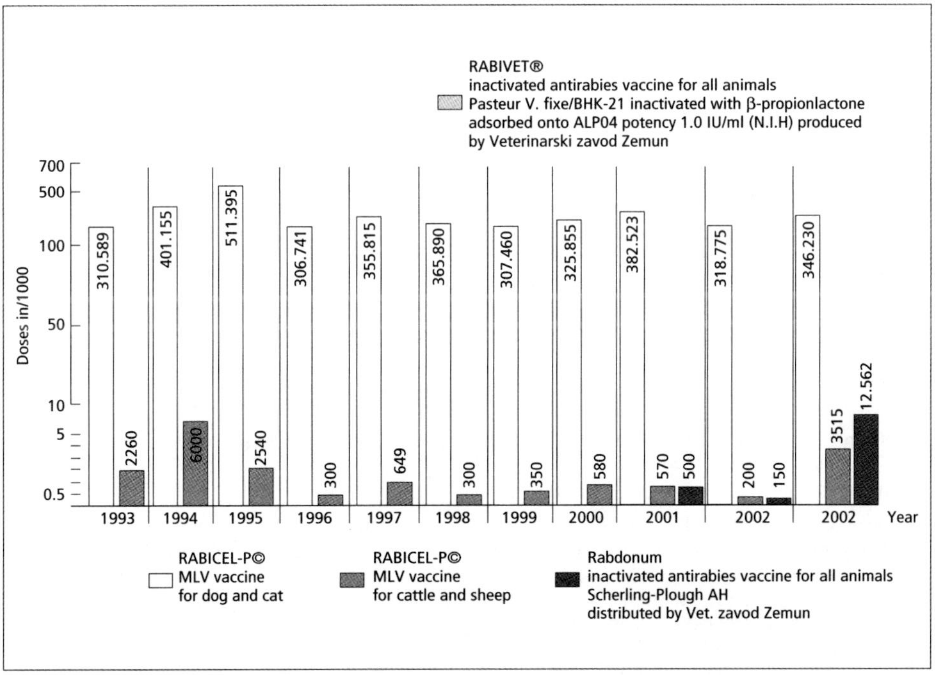

Fig. 2: Ten years of production and distribution of antirabies vaccines by Veterinarski zavod Zemun (VZZ).

of a locally produced attenuated vaccine (HEP FLURY strain) and about 52 % of dogs have been vaccinated (Fig. 2).

The increased number of infected dogs and cats is directly correlated with the increased number of foxes in spring and autumn-winter months, which is related to the life cycle of foxes ("spill-over" effect). This spill-over of rabies from foxes to domestic animals, bearing in mind the increased risk to man in such circumstances, is a further indication of the need to apply adequate measures to wipe out rabies in foxes. In the first place the number of foxes should be reduced, and then the proven method of eradicating rabies by oral vaccination of foxes should be applied.

Vaccination of wild animals in Serbia and Montenegro has been carried out in two trial programmes in two small areas, but the results of the programmes have not yet been studied.

As Western European countries have shown, oral vaccination is an efficient way of fighting rabies. However, it requires considerable financial resources as well as the coordinated action of all interested parties; veterinary services, rabies diagnostic laboratories and the appropriate ministries must all act together. A very important aspect which must be considered is the implementation of joint programmes with surrounding countries which will help decrease the number of cases and finally eradicate rabies.

Conclusion

Rabies remains endemic in SCG. Areas with the lowest numbers of registered cases are probably not spared from rabies, but have collected fewer samples for laboratory examination. The lack of data on the epizootiological situation in Kosovo and Metohija also does not mean that this territory is free from rabies. Considering the epizootiological situation in SCG, surveillance of this deadly zooanthroponosis remains an imperative, along with the introduction of preventive measures aimed at the eradication of rabies.

References

1 Pastoret PP, Kappeler A, Aubert A: European rabies control and its history, in King AA, Fooks AR, Aubert M, Wandeler AI (eds): Historical Perspective of Rabies in Europe and the Mediterranean Basin. Paris, OIE (World Organization for Animal Health), 2004, pp 337-350.

2 Bosiljka D, Stankov S, Radenković B, Janković L: Significance of bats for the human aerogenic rabies infection, Veterinarian Symposium Republic of Serbska, Bosnia and Herzegovina, Banja Vrucica, Teslic, June 1999:12-22,

3 Bosiljka D, Stankov S: Rabies – new aspects on the pathogenesis and antigenic structure of rabies virus, First Symposium of veterinary praxis and science, Zlatibor, November 1999:93-97.

Koprowski H: The mouse inoculation test, in Meslin FX, Kaplan MM, Koprowski H (eds): Laboratory Technique in Rabies. 4th ed Geneva, WHO (World Health Organization), 1996, pp 88-95.

WHO: Rabies Bull Europe 2003; 27 (4).

Dean DJ, Abelseth MK, Atanasiu P: The fluorescent antibody test, in Meslin FX, Kaplan MM, Koprowski H (eds): Laboratory Technique in Rabies. 4th ed Geneva, WHO (World Health Organization), 1996, pp 88-95.

Crawford-Miksza LK, Wadford DA, Schnurr DP: Molecular epidemiology of enzootic rabies in California. J Clin Virol 1999; 14 (3): 207-219.

Dr. B. Djuricic, Veterinary Faculty, Belgrade, Bul. JNA 18, Serbia.
E-mail: bosa@beotel.yu

Dodet B, Schudel A, Pastoret PP, Lombard M (eds): Rabies in Europe.
Dev Biol (Basel). Basel, Karger, 2006, vol 125, pp 59-68.

Rabies in Europe – Trends and Developments

C.J. Pötzsch[1], A. Kliemt[1], D. Klöss[1], R. Schröder[1], W. Müller[2]

[1] Institut of Epidemiology, Friedrich-Loeffler-Institute, WHO Collaborating Centre for Rabies Surveillance and Research, Wusterhausen, Germany

[2] Veterinary Consultant, Tübingen, Germany

Abstract: Rabies continues to be a major public health concern both in Europe and worldwide. In the greater part of the European continent the disease has been eradicated, or its incidence drastically reduced, by oral vaccination of wildlife reservoirs. Yet, 'hot spots' still remain in north-eastern and south-eastern Europe with a high temporal variation of disease distribution in the previous decade.

Rabies is predominantly transmitted by the red fox; but in recent years, especially in Eastern European countries, an independent infection cycle in raccoon dogs seems to have developed. Although countries such as the Czech Republic, Slovenia and Poland achieved very impressive rabies control results and trend analyses of rabies occurrence showed a long- and short-term decrease, there is still need for improved rabies surveillance and control in Europe. The Rabies Bulletin Europe (RBE), a quarterly, printed and on-line publication, aims to improve this situation. Besides the need to improve the quality of data in some countries, it will provide a public domain rabies database in the near future. Further strategic cooperation is necessary to control the disease in areas of European public health concern.

INTRODUCTION

Classical rabies, caused by *Lyssavirus* genotype 1, is a zoonosis that claims more then 55,000 human victims worldwide, over 99.8 % in Asia and Africa [1]. In Europe, rabies also continues to be major public health concern; mainly in the eastern countries, where rabies is still endemic in vast territories.

In Europe, rabies is predominantly propagated and maintained by the red fox (*Vulpes vulpes*), while in the eastern parts the raccoon dog (*Nyctereutes procyonoides*) may also sustain the chain of infection. The disease is also frequently detected in a wide range of other wildlife and domestic species, usually in spatial and temporal association with fox rabies.

Before the 1980s the disease was endemic in large parts of Europe, with annual case figures between 16,000 and 25,000 [2,3]. The situation has improved since the application of oral vaccination of foxes in the late 1980s in affected countries. As a result, the annual number of cases reported has decreased to below ten thousand for the first time in 1993. Countries such as Finland, the Netherlands, Italy, Switzerland, France, Belgium, Luxemburg and the Czech Republic have been rabies-free since then. However, rabies is still endemic in large parts of Europe, as oral vaccination is an expensive and logistically difficult task. Apart from the high cost of rabies control in wildlife, another major factor for the low level of commitment to rabies control in many countries is the lack of accurate data on the distribution and true impact of the disease [1]. The Rabies Bulletin Europe (RBE), a quarterly, printed and on-line publication, aims to improve this situation and has provided rabies data and disease information since 1977 [2]. The data are obtained from reports of the European veterinary authorities, which are then summarized and published in the public domain. The RBE is probably the most comprehensive international rabies data source. It is edited and published by the World Health Organization "Collaborating Centre for Rabies Surveillance and Research" in Wusterhausen, Germany.

This paper describes the situation of classical rabies in Europe from 1994 to 2004 and analyses recent trends.

Materials and Methods

Data were derived from the national rabies reports to the RBE. National veterinary authorities report the number of rabies cases and animals tested per species at the end of each quarter to the RBE. The geographical units on which these reports are based are districts or comparable areas. Data were analysed for the years of 1994 to 2004. To demonstrate temporal trends in wildlife rabies, the percentage of the number of wildlife cases was calculated from 2002 to 2004 and compared with the average during the corresponding previous 10 years. In the trend analyses, the averages over 10 years were based on the period from 1992 to 2004. When describing rabies in raccoon dogs and domestic dogs, ratios were calculated comparing rabies in these two species with fox rabies, as foxes are the main reservoir species in Europe. Data were analysed using descriptive statistical methods with a significance level of $p \leq 0.05$ [4].

In evaluating the data presented, the existence of different national surveillance and reporting systems with their particular characteristics must be taken into account. The data from the Russian Federation covered only the European part of the country.

Results

The distribution of rabies in Europe in wildlife and domestic animals is shown in Figure 1. After a low level of 5,039 cases in wildlife and domestic animals in 1997, the number increased to 11,046 in 2003, the highest number since 1992. In the following year, the figure dropped sharply to 5,393 cases. The majority of cases (76 %) were reported in 2004 from the Eastern European countries: Russia, Ukraine, Lithuania, Latvia, Estonia, Belarus and Poland (Fig. 2). In south-eastern Europe, Croatia, Serbia/Montenegro, Hungary, Turkey, Romania and Bosnia/Herzegovina accounted for another 22 % of rabies cases. The remaining countries contributed less than 2 % in 2004. Thirteen human rabies cases were reported in 2004. Since 1994, fewer than 15 cases were reported annually in Europe.

Rabies in wildlife

Wildlife accounted for 60 % of all rabies cases. The red fox remained the main rabies reservoir accounting for 78 % of all wildlife cases in 2004. This represents a significant drop of 12 % since 1994. During this period, rabies in raccoon dogs has increased more than six-fold from 183 cases in 1994 to 1,163 cases in 2003, and 500 in 2004. Among the countries with raccoon dog rabies in 2004, the raccoon dog rabies/fox rabies ratio was highest in Estonia (1.67), Latvia (0.77) and Lithuania (0.83), while it was considerably lower in Poland (0.14), Belarus (0.13) and Russia (0.05). In the three Baltic States, Estonia, Latvia and Lithuania, raccoon dog rabies has increased from 19 % of all wildlife cases in 1994 to 45 % in 2004. The annual increase was significant for the averages over two-years, except 1996/97 and 2001. Fox and raccoon dog rabies together accounted for 90 to 94 % of wildlife rabies in these countries between 1994 and 2004; with no significant differences between consecutive years. Other species were less important in the whole of Europe and contributed between only five to seven percent to wildlife rabies.

Long-term and short-term trends in wildlife rabies are presented in Table 1. A value above 100 % represents a long-term increase, while values below 100 % show a reduction and therefore a positive trend. Positive, short-term trends were characterised by consecutively decreasing percentages between 2002 and 2004. In Austria, Germany and Hungary a positive long-term trend in wildlife rabies could be demonstrated for 2002 to 2004 as the number of cases had decreased, while in the Slovak Republic and Croatia such a drop was noticeable in two of the three years. This positive development can be explained by the fact that the first four named countries engage in regular oral vaccination of foxes. Both, positive long- and short-term trends were observed in Bulgaria, the Czech Republic, Poland and Slovenia. Here also, the last three of the four countries listed regularly carried out oral vaccination of foxes. In Bulgaria however, rabies has always occurred at a low level, with the number of annual cases never exceeding 32 since 1991. In Belarus, Lithuania, Moldova and Turkey, positive short-term trends were recognizable, as the percentage investigated decreased between 2002 and 2004. Associations with rabies control measures in these countries have yet to be established.

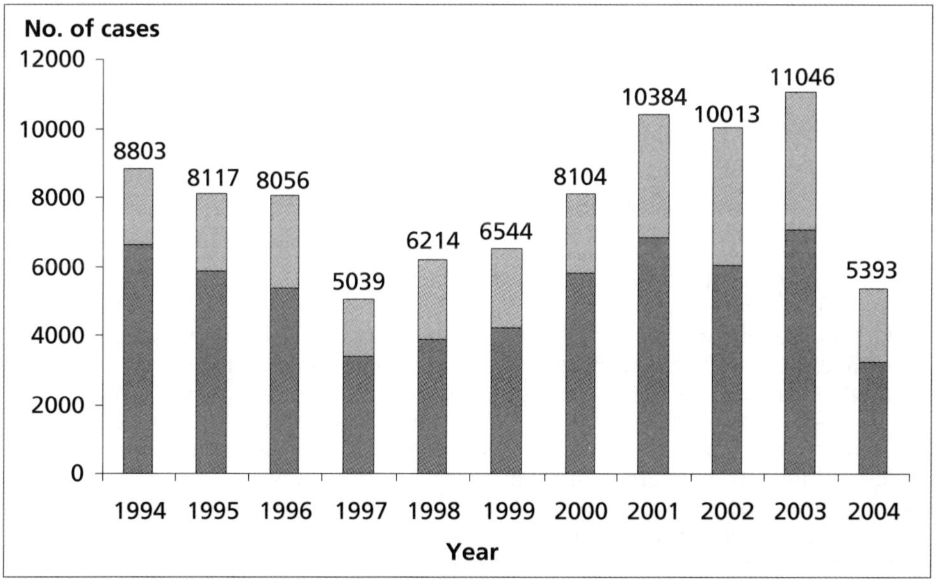

Fig. 1: Number of reported rabies cases in wildlife (dark), domestic animals (light) and totals (column top) in Europe 1994-2004.

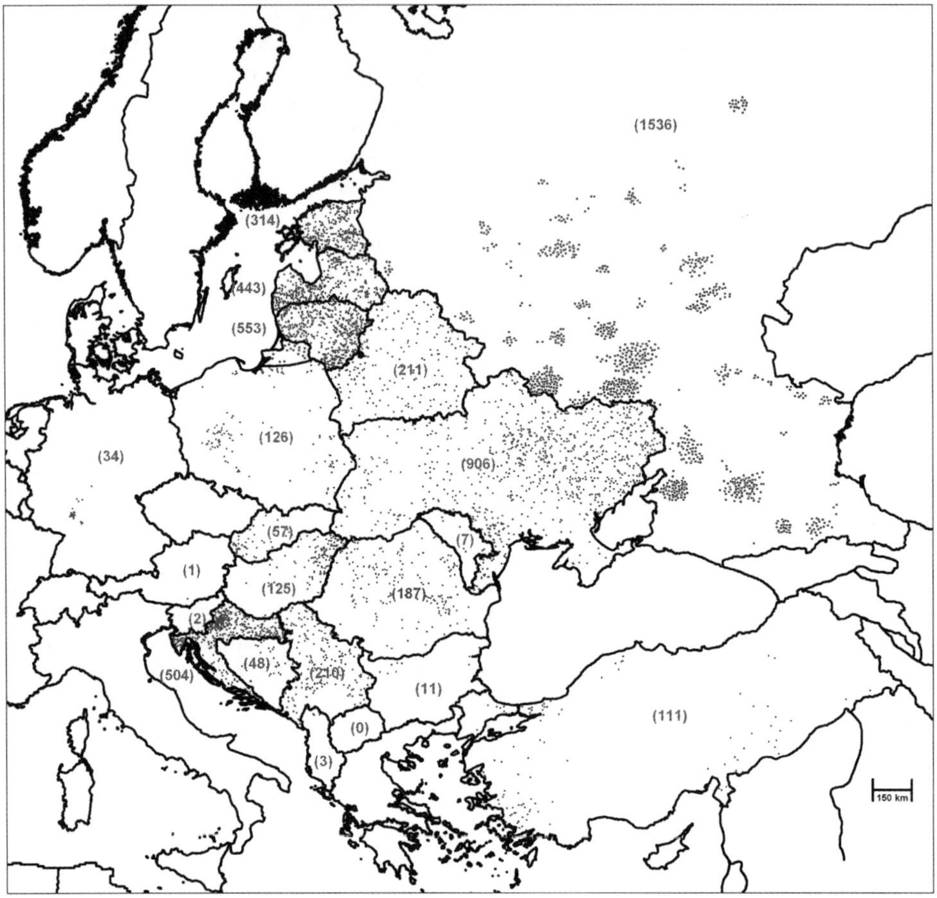

Fig. 2 : Distribution of rabies in Europe, fourth quarter of 2004.

Rabies in domestic animals

Dogs, cats and cattle together accounted for 96 % of all rabies cases in domestic animals in 2004 and for 89 to 95 % during the last decade. The proportional contribution of these three species was 36 %, 33 % and 28 %, respectively, in 2004. Since 1994, this proportion was 32 % for dogs and 34 % for cattle, with a range from 27 to 37 % and 28 to 39 %, respectively. No clear temporal changes were observed. This was different for cats. Their proportion increased significantly from 24 % (range 22- 27 %) in 1994 to 1999, to 29 % (range 26-33 %) in 2000 to 2004.

Apart from foxes and raccoon dogs, domestic dogs are potential reservoir hosts for rabies and able to maintain their own infection cycles. The average dog rabies/fox rabies ratio in Europe was 0.25 in 2004 and between 0.10 and 0.21 in the previous decade. Some countries had ratios higher than the average; it was highest in Turkey with 23.0; 0.72 in Russia, 0.50 in Moldova and 0.35 in Ukraine. Yearly fluctuations of dog rabies cases were high between 1994 and 2004 and could reach about 500 to 600 %, e.g. in Turkey and Russia. No clear temporal trends were recognisable.

Table 1: Long- and short-term trends of wildlife rabies distribution in countries with rabies reports in 2002-2004. (Columns 2-4 show the percentage of cases compared to the preceding 10-years average, a figure > 100 = an increase in case numbers, while < 100 = a reduction and therefore a positive long-term trend; positive short-term trends are characterised by consecutively decreasing percentages in columns 2-4).

Country	Percent cases in 2002-2004, compared with preceding 10-years average			Positive long-term trends*	Positive short-term trends*	Reporting since
	2002	2003	2004			
Albania**						1997
Austria	3.2	no cases	2.7	+		
Belarus	580.0	515.9	62.0		+	1993
Bosnia/Herzegovina	161.5	185.3	77.9			2001
Bulgaria	85.1	76.1	19.0	+	+	
Croatia	98.0	114.5	87.0	(+)		
Czech Republic	1.6	No cases	No cases	+	+	1993
Estonia	380.1	575.1	141.3			
Germany	2.8	7.7	13.6	+		
Hungary	16.6	23.1	22.9	+		
Latvia	218.6	374.7	120.1			
Lithuania	405.8	340.3	131.2		+	
Moldova	156.6	111.8	17.0		+	1995
Poland	48.3	19.1	7.1	+	+	
Romania	131.8	122.5	207.0			
Russian Federation	203.1	262.2	87.8			
Serbia/Montenegro	212.4	225.5	155.8			
Slovak Republic	31.8	103.0	19.8	(+)		1993
Slovenia	4.9	2.8	0.8	+	+	
Turkey	507.9	239.4	96.4		+	
Ukraine	103.5	142.8	57.5			2001

* + = reduction of case numbers in three years 2002-2004; (+) = reduction of case numbers in two years 2002-2004.

** Since 1997, Albania has reported only one case in 2002, two in 2003 and one in 2004.

European rabies surveillance – the Rabies Bulletin Europe

The national rabies data coverage of the RBE for the 32 European countries which regularly report is nearly complete. Since 2002, quarterly rabies reports were missing on average from only one country or two at most. Three to four countries did not supply data on animals tested for rabies.

An important indicator for disease surveillance, in addition to case figures, is the number of animals tested. To improve the assessment and analysis of the epidemiological rabies situation in Europe, the number of animals tested for rabies was provided in the RBE for the first time in 2003. The possibility to compare case numbers with the numbers of animals tested greatly improves the quality of information. As shown in Figure 3, the numbers of wildlife tested for rabies varied greatly across Europe. According to previous WHO recommendations, countries applying oral vaccination should test eight foxes/other main rabies vectors per 100 km^2 [5]. This recommended surveillance density has only been achieved by Austria and the Czech Republic in 2004. As of mid-2005 a minimum of four target animals per 100 km^2 are now recommended for monitoring the efficacy of oral vaccination programmes (biomarker detection, serological testing and rabies incidence) [1]. This lower testing level was met by Croatia, Germany, Poland and Slovenia; in addition to the countries mentioned above, in 2004.

To enhance European rabies surveillance, the RBE has constantly been modified and improved. In the near future a new concept will be implemented and the RBE will then consist of an Internet based rabies database as well as the journal. The journal will continue to be published in print and on-line. The database is currently being developed at the WHO Collaborating Centre in Wusterhausen and aims to provide better quality data and improve data analysis. It will therefore greatly assist the evaluation of the epidemiological rabies situation as well as the planning and coordination of European rabies control. In the database, summary

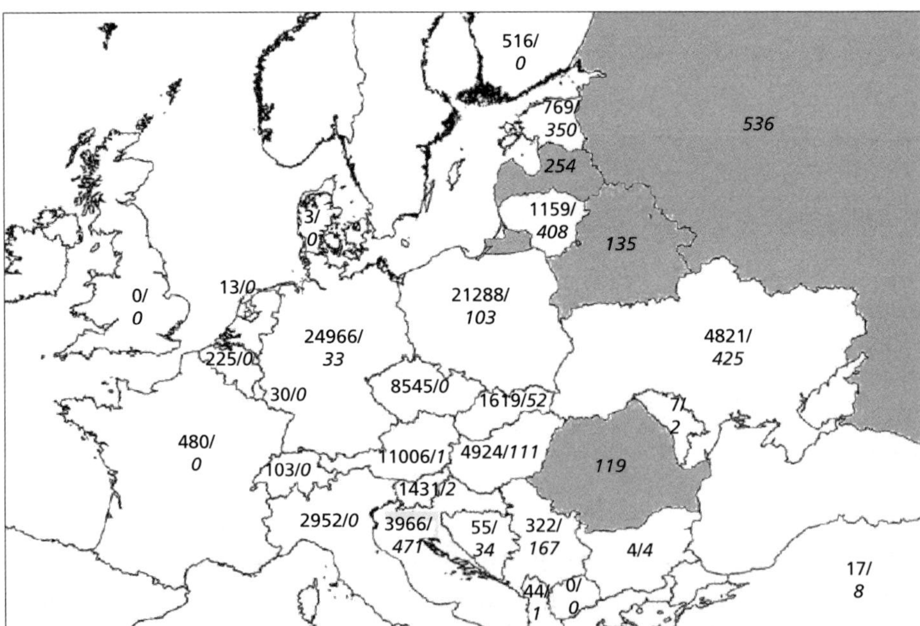

Fig. 3: Number of wildlife rabies cases and wildlife tested (italic) in Europe in 2004. Grey countries: no wildlife testing reported.

tables and graphs can be generated. Output data will be stratified by location (country, groups of countries or national administrative units), time (quarter, year or other reporting periods) and animal species. Also trends, both long- and short-term, can be displayed. A geographical information system component will be included which enables the generation of rabies distribution maps according to selected parameters. Data analysis and visualisation is HTML-based and uses the Internet browser. Concerning the journal, data are entered at the WHO Collaborating Centre in Wusterhausen and reading access to the database will not be restricted. The database is anticipated to be available on-line in late 2005.

Discussion

Never since the devastating spread of sylvatic rabies in Europe during the second half of the 20th century, have so many countries been rabies-free. Yet, rabies hot spots still exist in north-eastern and south-eastern Europe. Here, disease occurrence is almost hyper-endemic, surveillance systems are mainly passive and large-scale, long-term oral rabies vaccination has not yet been practised.

In 2004, the number of rabies cases throughout Europe dropped to about half the 2003 peak level. This was largely due to a decreased incidence in the north-eastern countries. Rabies occurrence in a region can increase and decrease in a cyclic manner. The reduction of rabies described was probably caused by the reduction of reservoir animal populations due to previous high rabies incidence in these animals. Fluctuations in the occurrence of rabies or the reservoir species populations could also have contributed to or caused the 2004 reduction. Rabies control by means of oral vaccination may additionally have reduced case numbers in some of these countries, e.g. in Poland. Low surveillance and reporting levels can also artificially reduce the incidence of rabies in a country. This did not seem to be the case as the drop in rabies cases occurred in the region at about the same time, and case figures began to increase in the north-eastern region again in early 2005 [2]. It must be taken into account that during the 1990s surveillance and rabies reporting in Eastern Europe could have been negatively influenced by political and economic changes [6].

In the whole of Europe the red fox remains the main rabies reservoir, but its share has decreased since 1994. At the same time, raccoon dog rabies has increased in north-eastern Europe and more than doubled in the Baltic States. Red fox and raccoon dog rabies together accounted for a constant level of 90 to 94 % of wildlife rabies in the last decade. This could imply an independent raccoon dog infection cycle competing with the fox rabies cycle. Epidemiological, diagnostic and molecular investigations could help to provide an answer.

Besides fox rabies, the dynamics of rabies in other species should be carefully monitored and more intensively researched. This also includes domestic dogs. The dog rabies situation in Europe is very inconsistent. Turkey is the only country in Europe where urban dog rabies infection cycle predominantly occurs [7,8]. Whether this type of rabies, or spill-over infections from foxes, are mainly responsible for the dog rabies problems in other eastern countries, should be investigated in more detail. The increase of cat rabies in the last decade could indicate that, although most countries do advocate dog vaccination, rabies prevention in cats should receive more attention.

In parts of the continent the disease has been eradicated or its occurrences drastically reduced by oral vaccination of the wildlife reservoirs. Countries such as the Czech Republic, Slovenia and Poland achieved very impressive rabies control results in previous years.

Successful oral vaccination of wildlife reservoirs also controls rabies in domestic animals and spill-over to other wildlife species. Rabies in raccoon dogs can successfully be controlled by oral vaccination. This has been demonstrated in experimental and field studies, as well as during the oral vaccination campaigns in Poland [2,9,10]. However, further studies are needed to examine whether vaccination strategies for foxes could be optimised to control the disease in raccoon dogs more effectively. Successful strategies to control dog rabies in affected countries have yet to be applied.

To monitor the national rabies situation and developments effectively, surveillance needs to be improved, especially in countries with endemic occurrence. The data and analyses provided in the RBE and in this paper are based on national rabies reports. As the reporting and surveillance systems in Europe differ greatly, comparing countries is nearly always prone to bias. Therefore, national surveillance characteristics should be taken into account. For instance, a large proportion of Europe is free of classical rabies [11] and potential reservoir species in these countries are often not routinely tested. On the other hand, in many countries financial and logistical constraints hamper widespread and routine surveillance, testing and reporting, and therefore the generation of good quality data.

With our new concept, including a user-friendly Internet based rabies database, the RBE will in future be able to provide even better support for European rabies surveillance and control. It will constitute a much more powerful data source for decision makers, rabies scientists and the public. Also, communication with other rabies data sources, such as the World Health Organization (WHO) website Rabnet [12], will be improved.

Rabies control is a costly and long-term commitment. The financial support of the European Union has largely contributed to the achievements of rabies control in Europe.

Although the situation has improved in recent years, it is by no means under control. Many countries in Eastern Europe still do not apply oral vaccination to wildlife reservoir animals. Positive developments have been seen in central Europe, where large-scale oral vaccination is carried out. Western Europe, apart from one pocket in Germany, is free of classical rabies. The western countries are for this reason very susceptible to the re-introduction of the disease. The current positive trend of low rabies incidence could well be a passing phenomenon and will perhaps be replaced by future negative developments. As the improvement of the overall situation would benefit all European countries, the European Union and the member states should mobilise all possibilities of financial, logistical and other support for affected countries. A range of activities, including expert meetings and conferences, and the dissemination of guidelines are organised by the WHO, the World Organisation for Animal Health (OIE) and the European Union (EU) [1,11,13,14]. However, larger scale practical bilateral cooperation in rabies surveillance and control, especially oral vaccination of wildlife, hardly exists. This, however, would be urgently necessary for controlling rabies, especially in highly endemic regions with no effective natural barriers, such as in north-eastern Europe. More research should also focus on strategic and cost-effective methods of oral vaccination and additional control methods to reduce the public health risk of rabies, especially in eastern and southern Europe.

The years to come will show whether currently practised rabies control can keep the rabies figures down, despite continuing rabies pressure.

Conclusions

- The low reservoir population in parts of Europe could provide a period for intensified, more cost-effective rabies control.
- The dynamics of rabies distribution in reservoir species needs constant monitoring and additional research.
- The quality of surveillance and reporting in Europe needs improvement.
- The new Rabies Bulletin Europe will provide improved support for European rabies surveillance and control.

Acknowledgements

We are grateful to the national veterinary authorities for their high level of cooperation and their quarterly reports to the Rabies Bulletin Europe.

Our surveillance work is supported by the World Health Organization and the World Organisation for Animal Health.

References

1 WHO: WHO Expert Consultation on Rabies. WHO Technical Report Series 931, 2005; http://www.who.int/rabies/trs931_%2006_05.pdf].

2 Rabies Bulletin Europe, www.who-rabies-bulletin.org.

3 King AA, Fooks AR, Aubert M, Wandeler AI (eds): Historical perspectives of rabies in Europe and the Mediterranean Basin. Paris, World Organisation for Animal Health, 2004.

4 Kirkwood BR: Essentials of Medical Statistics. Blackwell Scientific Publications, 1988.

5 WHO: Expert Committee on Rabies 8th Report. WHO Technical Report Series 1992:824.

6 Pötzsch CJ, Müller T, Kramer M: Summarizing the Rabies Situation in Europe 1990-2002 from the Rabies Bulletin Europe. Rabies Bull Europe 2002; 26 (4): 11-17.

7 Aylan O, Yörük I, Ün H: Rabies in Turkey, 1987-1996. J Etlik Vet Microbiol Ankara 1998; 9: 35-59.

8 Müller WW: Rabies in Europe – epidemiological cycles and the impact of oral vaccination of foxes. Rabies Bull Europe 2000; 24 (1): 8-12.

9 Schuster P, Müller T, Vos A, Selhorst T, Pommerening E: Comparative immunogenicity and efficacy studies with oral rabies virus vaccine SAD P5/88 in raccoon dogs and red foxes. Acta Vet Hung 2001; 49 (3): 285-290.

10 Nyberg M, Kulonen K, Neuvonen E, Ek-Kommonen C, Nuorgam M, Westerling B: An epidemic of sylvatic rabies in Finland – descriptive epidemiology and results of oral vaccination. Acta Vet Scand 1992; 33 (1): 43-57.

11 OIE: Terrestrial Animal Health Code 2004. Chapter 2.2.5. Rabies. 2004; http://www.oie.int/eng/normes/mcode/en_chapitre_2.2.5.htm#rubrique_rage.

12 WHO: http://www.who.int/rabies/rabnet.

13 OIE: First international conference "Rabies in Europe". Kiev, Ukraine, 15 – 18 June 2005. Conclusions and recommendations. 2005; http://www.oie.int/downld/Rabies_Conclusions%20and%20Reccomendations_05.pdf.

14 European Commission, The oral vaccination of foxes against rabies. Report of the Scientific Committee on Animal Health and Animal Welfare. Adopted on 23 October 2002; http://europa.eu.int/comm/food/fs/sc/scah/out80_en. pdf.

Dr. C.J. Pötzsch, Institut of Epidemiology, Friedrich-Loeffler-Institute, Seestr. 55, DE-16868 Wusterhausen, Germany.
E-mail: carsten.poetzsch@fli.bund.de

Dodet B, Schudel A, Pastoret PP, Lombard M (eds): Rabies in Europe.
Dev Biol (Basel). Basel, Karger, 2006, vol 125, p 69.

SESSION II

Rabies Diagnosis

Chairperson: *S. Edwards* (VLA, United Kingdom)
Rapporteur: *P. Hostnik* (University of Ljubljana, Slovenia)

Dodet B, Schudel A, Pastoret PP, Lombard M (eds): Rabies in Europe.
Dev Biol (Basel). Basel, Karger, 2006, vol 125, pp 71-77.

Rabies Diagnosis

J. Barrat, E. Picard-Meyer, F. Cliquet

AFSSA-LERRPAS, Domaine de Pixérécourt, Malzéville, France

Abstract: A reliable diagnosis of rabies can only be made based on laboratory examination of specimens collected from suspected animals. Without data from diagnostic tests, it is not possible to establish rabies control policies. These data are also necessary for evaluating the impact of control measures on the disease and to adapt veterinary and human health policies to the rabies situation.

This paper presents the routine laboratory techniques for rabies diagnosis that are published and recommended by both the OIE and WHO and which form the basis of rabies surveillance. They are presented along with more recent techniques which have proved useful in epidemiological and phylogenetic studies.

The first step in controlling a disease is to be able to identify it consistently. A reliable and sensitive diagnostic test is therefore essential for use in epidemiological studies and disease control. Reliable diagnosis is also needed by official medical and veterinary services to decide how to deal with infected humans or animals. Without knowing where rabies is present in a country, it is difficult to establish a solid, long-term control policy.

A viral disease may be diagnosed on the basis of clinical signs or after laboratory examination. Clinical diagnosis is based on the observation of symptoms and on observation of specific or at least highly evocative signs. Laboratory tests reveal the presence of infection using either indirect or direct methods. The most frequently used indirect methods are based on serological testing. Direct methods aim to detect the virus itself, its proteins, genetic material or traces of its replication in tissues.

Clinical Diagnosis

Rabies is due to the infection of a susceptible animal by the neurotropic rabies virus. The signs observed during the clinical phase mainly reflect central nervous system disorders induced by the replication of the virus. Major clinical signs include:

- changes in behaviour (e.g. wildlife not showing fear of humans, an increase or decrease of aggressiveness);
- lack of muscular coordination or paralysis;
- hydrophobia in infected humans;
- swallowing difficulties in animals due to pharynx paralysis; and
- bi-tonal barking in infected dogs.

Field and experimental observations have shown that these signs are generally not expressed simultaneously in the infected individual. Even if some signs are strongly evocative of rabies, there is no definitive sign to allow reliable clinical diagnosis of rabies and it cannot be recommended for definitive diagnosis.

Laboratory Diagnosis

Indirect methods: serological testing

Seroconversion of infected individuals is not constant and when it does occur it is generally at the end of the course of disease. Serological testing of cerebrospinal fluid may be carried out for ante-mortem diagnosis in humans but, as is often the case in ante-mortem diagnosis, only a positive result can be judged reliable. Due to their unreliable responsiveness and lack of sensitivity when used for disease diagnosis, serological tests cannot be considered for routine testing.

Direct diagnosis: histology

In 1903, Negri described eosinophilic inclusions in the cytoplasm of infected cells. Negri bodies are aggregates of viral proteins and their structure is therefore specific to rabies virus, but the method of detection, based on dye affinity, is not. Two methods are still sometimes used in diagnosis:

- Seller's test is performed on unfixed smears. It gives a response within one hour but it is very difficult to read and interpret if the specimen is not very fresh.
- More traditionally, fixed specimens are embedded in paraffin and slices are stained according to different procedures, such as Mann's. It takes up to four days to get a result. When the test is done on fresh specimens, its sensitivity reaches 95 %, but as soon as autolysis begins the sensitivity drops to 50-60 %. Once again, for best results specimens must be very fresh.

Regular training of technicians is necessary both for technical reasons and to maintain their interpretation skills; slides derived from cattle, for instance, may show intracytoplasmic corpuscles that are difficult to differentiate from Negri bodies. Because of these technical reasons, and the fact that Mann's test is more expensive than the fluorescent antibody test (FAT), classical histological methods can no longer be recommended for routine diagnosis.

Direct diagnosis: antigen detection

Of the different antigens produced in infected cells, the most abundant is the N protein which makes it the preferred target for diagnostic purposes. Antigen detection methods use a specific antibody (or a mix of antibodies) labelled with FITC, an enzyme or biotine, or an anti-species antibody in indirect tests. Tests may be conducted on tissue samples with specimens fixed in acetone in the fluorescent antibody test (FAT) or embedded in wax (immunohistochemical tests) or on homogenised tissues in enzyme-linked immunosorbent assay (ELISA).

Fluorescent antibody test (FAT)

FAT uses a fluorescent conjugate to detect rabies antigen in the sample. It may be used on prints, on smears or on cell layers. It is the gold standard for laboratory diagnosis of rabies and the reference method for the OIE and WHO. The FITC-labelled conjugate is preferably based on a polyclonal antibody against the N protein of the rabies virus. Some other commercially available conjugates are a mix of several monoclonal antibodies. It is the core test of routine laboratory diagnosis:

- it alone gives an answer from a tissue sample;
- it confirms replication of rabies virus in cells, and
- it can be used in mouse inoculation tests to confirm that the cause of death was rabies.

Each technical step in the procedure is important for the quality and reliability of the final result.

- Fixation is done in cold, pure, high-grade acetone (30 min at -20° C).
- Staining uses the fluorescent conjugate at its correct working dilution in a humid, incubation chamber.
- Mounting medium should be alkaline because the energy efficiency of FITC is better at pH # 8.5.
- A double reading of the slides is important to increase the reliability of the test.

The major advantages of the technique are: high sensitivity (97 to 99 %), rapidity (response in a few hours) and low cost. However, FAT carried out on putrefied specimens may be difficult to read and give inconclusive results, which underlines the need for regular practice to maintain high standards.

Enzyme-linked immunosorbent assay (ELISA)

ELISA techniques may be useful in large epidemiological studies because they are more rapid than FAT. A commercial test the Rapid Rabies Enzyme ImmunoDiagnosis (RREID), used to be available. The advantages of the test were its fast answer (40 samples, in duplicate, within four hours), easiness to read and its tolerance to putrefaction of the sample. The main disadvantage was that its detection range was limited to genotype 1 virus, and it is no longer available.

Results of an inter-laboratory test on rabies diagnosis conducted in 2001

For the reliable exchange of epidemiological data, it is important to standardise the way information is collected. To investigate the current situation, a voluntary, inter-laboratory test was carried out in 2001. Three years earlier, a technical questionnaire on rabies diagnosis had been sent to European laboratories which revealed that important technical variations in fixation methods (heat/acetone, time, temperature), conjugate (commercial, homemade, working dilution), mounting medium, microscope magnification and equipment existed between laboratories. Some less important variations existed at the organisational level (e.g. daily number of specimens tested, routine practice of technical staff).

Overall, results were obtained for 17 procedures from 14 participating countries. Each laboratory received a panel with three controls (one negative, one strong positive, one weak positive) and eight coded slides (three negative, one strong positive fox strain, one weak positive fox, one EBL1, one polar fox, one atypical fox strain) that had to be tested in two independent staining sessions. Three laboratories performed a single test, 14 tested the samples twice, and in two cases there were discrepancies between the tests.

Five out of the 14 laboratories (or out of the 17 procedures tested) made errors:

- laboratory A: one single test, one false positive;
- laboratory C1: two false negatives (weak fox, atypical fox);
- laboratory C2: three false negatives (weak fox, EBL1, weak positive control), discrepancies between tests;
- laboratory G: one false positive, discrepancies between tests;
- laboratory H: one single test, one false negative (weak fox), two false positives.

The errors in positive samples corresponded to samples that may have been more difficult to stain with over-diluted conjugates or did not fall within the range of detection of the conjugate used in the laboratory.

Direct diagnosis: virus detection

Inactivated virus detection can be undertaken on cells or in animals. A rabies tissue culture inoculation test (RTCIT) uses Neuro2a cells (ATCC no = CCL131). As replication of rabies virus generally does not induce any cytopathic effect, FAT is needed to detect rabies virus replication in cells. This in vitro inoculation test is very sensitive (96-97 %), gives a rapid answer (one to five days according to the incubation period used in the laboratory) and is much cheaper than the mouse inoculation test. However, the cells are quite sensitive to putrefied specimens (the action of bacteria that are not destroyed by the antibiotics added to the medium and action of cytolytic toxins).

The mouse inoculation test (MIT) uses intracranial injection of the supernatant of a 10 % brain suspension to anaesthetised mice. OF1 mice are used, either five mice two to three weeks old, or a litter of 48 hr-old suckling mice to obtain a more rapid response. This inoculation test is sensitive (92-99 %), robust and allows for easy isolation of the strain for further studies.

Among the disadvantages, the delay in response is lengthy (positive fox specimens generally respond between nine and 14 days, bats around 20 days, and the negative response is obtained 28 days post-injection). It is also a costly method that requires animal experimentation facilities.

RTCIT is an alternative to this test, is as sensitive as MIT and fulfils the "Replacement" requirement of the "3Rs" rule. A change-over from MIT to RTCIT should be done whenever possible.

Direct diagnosis: RNA detection

Reverse transcriptase-polymerase chain reaction (RT-PCR) was first used for the diagnosis of rabies in the 1990s. Under some conditions, the techniques described above may have limits. For instance, FAT has reduced sensitivity when applied to putrefied samples and its sensitivity may also be reduced with viruses other than genotype 1. Inoculation tests are also difficult with putrefied specimens. However, molecular tools may be a useful research complement to the routine diagnosis reference methods.

Hemi-nested RT-PCR [1] is a rapid, specific and sensitive technique that allows for the identification of viral strains by sequencing the PCR products. Phylogenetic analyses may then be performed to investigate rabies epidemiology, establish species, geographical links and differentiate between the seven genotypes and their potential sub-types. The technique is highly sensitive, up to 300,000 (5.5 log) times more than MIT or RTCIT. It is also not very sensitive to putrefaction; a mixture of rabies positive brain tissue aliquoted and conserved at - 80° C (control) and in a 37° C incubator (test) gave the following results:

- FAT became negative after three to four days;
- inoculation tests both on cells or in mice became negative after one week; and
- RT-PCR was still positive on day 66.

While these results are interesting, the high sensitivity of the test also means that there is a high risk of laboratory contamination and the tests have to be checked by adequate controls at every step. One way to reduce this risk is to have a room equipped for molecular work and to use experienced, trained staff. The primers also have to be regularly checked against new sequences.

On the downside, this technique is too expensive for routine use and it is not recommended for routine laboratory diagnosis either by the OIE or by WHO.

Samples to be Tested

Post-mortem diagnosis of rabies is conducted on brain tissue. Different techniques are available but the sensitivity of the results depends upon the amount of virus present in the piece of brain tested. J. Bingham [2] studied the sensitivity of laboratory diagnosis of rabies carried out on different portions of the central nervous system. The "best" portions are the hippocampus (Ammon's horn), thalamus and medulla oblongata; the cortex is less sensitive and the cerebellum less again (Fig. 1).

Choice of Tests

The choice of which test to use depends on the purpose of diagnosis. A summary of considerations is shown in Table 1.

Exchange of Information

At a national level, data collected on rabies diagnosis should be rapidly and regularly exchanged between the different administrative structures involved in rabies. The information should be centralised in a single laboratory that edits a regular epidemiological bulletin reporting both positive and negative results. At an international

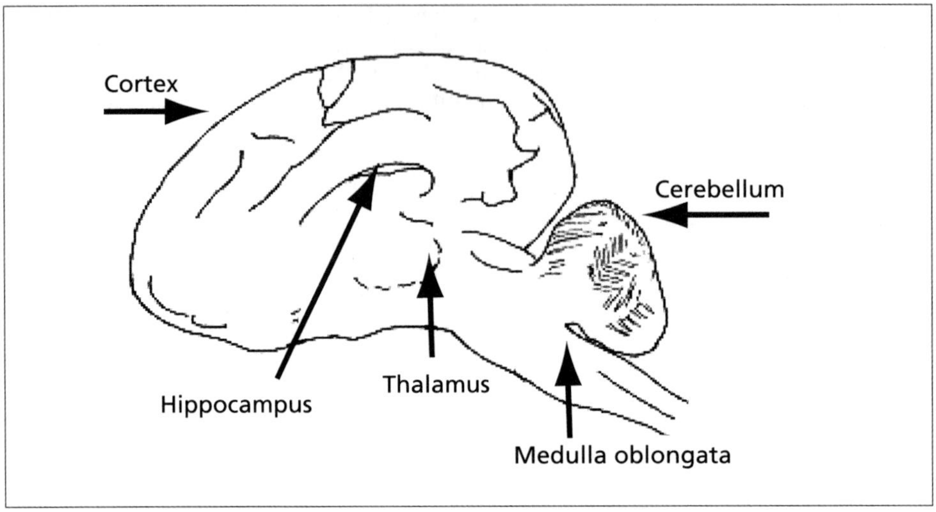

Fig. 1: Longitudinal section of the dog brain showing the different parts of brain preferentially collected for rabies diagnosis.

Table 1 : Choosing a rabies diagnostic test.

Purpose of diagnosis	FAT	RTCIT	MIT
Human infection	YES	At least if FAT negative	Possible alternative
Animal infection	YES	Possible if FAT negative	Possible alternative but not recommended
Epidemiological diagnosis	YES	Possible if FAT negative	Not for routine

level, epidemiological data should be regularly exchanged between neighbouring countries to facilitate regional control of the disease. Rabies Bulletin Europe should be regularly updated with positive and negative data.

Conclusions

The clinical diagnosis of rabies is not reliable. Definitive diagnosis can only be made based on laboratory investigations. Routine rabies diagnosis should be undertaken using only the techniques recommended by WHO and the OIE, closely following the procedures described in official publications.

The principal "gold-standard" diagnostic test for rabies is the FAT.

Confirmatory diagnosis should be undertaken using RTCIT. MIT remains a possible alternative for virus isolation.

Methods for rabies diagnosis should be harmonised across Europe. The techniques should be standardised via inter-laboratory tests.

The use of molecular techniques is not currently recommended for routine diagnosis. These techniques are useful in epidemiological surveys. They should be used under strict quality controls in national reference laboratories that routinely use these techniques.

Attempts should be made to isolate viruses for characterisation of prevalent strains. The strains should be typed and compared with isolates from neighbouring countries. The data should be rapidly exchanged and the original isolates submitted to an independent laboratory for further characterisation.

Serological methods should not be used for routine rabies diagnosis.

Acknowledgements

The authors wish to acknowledge those who made this work possible, mainly the previous and the more recent diagnostic teams in Malzéville: J. Ambert, M.J. Barrat, C. Bujack, J.M. Bousset, C. Patron, M. Ritleng, J.L. Schereffer, N. Stroucken, E. Tissot and A. Verdot, the participating laboratories and those willing to participate in the ring test, M.J. Duchêne for her documentation work and G. Farré for his photographic work.

References

The reference techniques are described in the following two books that should be made available in diagnostic laboratories:

- Manual of diagnostic tests and vaccines for terrestrial animals (mammals, birds and bees), 5th ed OIE, Paris, 2004.
- Meslin FX, Kaplan MM, Koprowski H (eds): Laboratory techniques in rabies, 4th ed, World Health Organization, Geneva, 1996, 476 p.

1 Picard-Meyer E, Bruyère V, Barrat J, Tissot E, Barrat MJ, Cliquet F: Development of a hemi-nested RT-PCR method for the specific determination of European bat lyssavirus 1. Comparison with other rabies diagnostic methods. Vaccine 2004; 22: 1921-1929.

2 Bingham J, Van der Merwe M: Distribution of rabies antigen in infected brain material: determining the reliability of different regions of the brain for the rabies fluorescent antibody test. J Virol Methods 2002; 101: 85-94.

Dr. J. Barrat, AFSSA-LERRPAS, Domaine de Pixérécourt, BP 9, FR-54220 Malzéville, France.
E-mail: j.barrat@afssa.fr

Dodet B, Schudel A, Pastoret PP, Lombard M (eds): Rabies in Europe.
Dev Biol (Basel). Basel, Karger, 2006, vol 125, pp 79-90.

The Diversity of Rabies Virus in Russia Demonstrated by Anti-Nucleocapsid Monoclonal Antibody Application and Limited Gene Sequencing

A.D. Botvinkin[1], *I.V. Kuzmin*[2], *L.M. McElhinney*[3], *N. Johnson*[3], *A.R. Fooks*[3]

[1] Irkutsk State Medical University, Irkutsk, Russia

[2] Research Institute for Natural Foci Infections, Omsk, Russia

[3] Rabies and Wildlife Zoonoses Group, Veterinary Laboratories Agency, Weybridge, WHO Collaborating Centre for the Characterisation of Rabies and Rabies-Related Viruses, Addlestone, Surrey, UK

Abstract: A comparative analysis of anti-nucleocapsid monoclonal antibody (N-mAb) reaction profiles and DNA sequences was performed on 97 selected rabies virus (RABV) isolates from Russia and neighbouring states. A panel of 73 N-mAb from the Wistar Institute (Philadelphia, PA, USA), Veterinary Laboratories Agency (Weybridge, UK) and P-41 (Tübingen, Germany) was used. The sequence of a 400 bp fragment of the N gene was generated for all available isolates and a phylogenetic analysis of the fragment was carried out. The results of genetic and antigenic typing were in concordance, except for a few deviations. Three RABV variants with distinct antigenic patterns corresponded to well characterised genetic groups. The phylogenetic analysis also allowed the discrimination of RABVs with similar antigenic profiles originating from distant geographical locations in Russia and other states of the former Soviet Union. In some instances, more than one specific antigenic variant was detected within a phylogenetic group. A number of antigenic and genetic variants were associated with a specific host species (such as red fox, raccoon dog, wolf or polar fox) in different parts of Russia. A single, antigenically divergent, P-41-positive, rodent isolate from Siberia was described.

INTRODUCTION

During the past 25 years, the diversity of the rabies virus (RABV) has been successfully studied using two approaches: antigenic methods using monoclonal antibodies (mAbs) and genetic methods based on DNA sequencing and phylogenetic

The article is devoted to the memory of Professor M.A. Selimov (Institute of Polio and Viral Encephalitides, Moscow, Russia) and Dr A.A. King (CVL, Weybridge, UK) who created the foundations for the development of molecular epidemiology of rabies in Russia and the former Soviet Union.

analysis. As a result, substantial progress in the molecular epidemiology of rabies has been achieved. A number of studies have identified the N gene and nucleoprotein as the most suitable targets for epidemiological studies of RABV variation [1-7].

In the former Soviet Union, antigenic typing using mAbs has been performed since 1982 at the WHO Collaborating Centre for Rabies Surveillance and Research by teams led by Professor Midat Selimov of the Institute of Polio and Viral Encephalitis, Moscow [8]. In 1988, Dr Arthur King of Central Veterinary Laboratories (currently VLA Weybridge), UK first visited Moscow bringing with him a panel of mAbs, and collaboration between the two laboratories began. More than 350 field isolates of RABV have been studied, and a number of antigenic variants within serotype 1 have been identified [8-11]. The results of the mAb typing indicated that certain antigenic variants of RABV predominated and that they were widely distributed among different host species in Russia. These data did not correlate with the epidemiological knowledge of the time, which anticipated finding only a few antigenic variants that shared a local distribution and a more or less definitive, single host species.

The data collected using mAbs have now been complemented by genetic studies of RABV isolates from the former Soviet Union [5,12-14]. Genetic data have sometimes confirmed, but occasionally contradicted, early theories of the molecular epidemiology of RABV in Russia and the former Soviet Union that were based on mAb typing. Comparative analyses of mAb patterns and phylogenetic typing are useful to support previous conclusions and may help future research.

Material and Methods

Viruses

In total, 97 terrestrial RABV isolates for which antigenic or genetic patterns were available were selected for comparison (Tables 1 and 2). The isolates were obtained from brain samples received by local veterinary and medical laboratories in various Russian provinces ($n = 79$) and neighbouring states ($n = 18$). The majority of the isolates had been collected during 1977-1991, before the implementation of the campaigns for oral vaccination against rabies in Eastern Europe and Siberia. RABV isolates were recovered from humans, domestic animals (six species) and wild, terrestrial mammals (eight species). The most common host species among wild mammals were the red fox (*Vulpes vulpes*), polar fox (*Alopex lagopus*), steppe fox (*Vulpes corsac*), wolf (*Canis lupus*), raccoon dog (*Nyctereutes procyonoides*) and badger (*Meles meles*). Rare cases of rabies in wild cat (*Prionalurus bengalensis*) and suslik (*Spermophillus undulatus*) were also described.

Virus isolation was performed by the mouse inoculation test [15], and primary rabies diagnosis was undertaken by direct fluorescent antibody test (FAT) [16].

Antigenic typing using mAbs

The isolates on which antigenic typing was performed are listed in Table 1. A panel of 73 mAbs against lyssavirus nucleoprotein was used: 36 mAbs from the Wistar Institute of Anatomy and Biology, Philadelphia, PA, U.S.A (Wistar panel) [1]; 36 mAbs from the Central Veterinary Laboratory, Weybridge, UK (CVL panel) [10]; and mAb P-41 from the Federal Research Centre for Animal Virus Diseases, Tübingen, Germany [17]. Sections of brain from infected mice were mounted on glass slides and tested by indirect FAT. About 30 % of the isolates were also tested in infected BHK-21 cells [10]. Working dilutions of the mAbs were prepared in minimum essential medium (MEM), supplemented with 10 % calf serum. Fluorescein-5-isothiocyanate (FITC)-labelled anti-mouse IgG from goats or rabbits was used as the second antibody. Fluorescence was measured using ultraviolet (UV) microscopes (LOMO, USSR, or Leitz, Germany) with objectives of magnification × 90, × 40, or × 25 and eyepieces of × 5 or × 6.3. Samples showing bright, specific fluorescence were considered to be positive; a sample showing weak fluorescence or no fluorescence in any sample of a series was considered to be variable, and in the absence of any reaction the sample was considered to be negative for viral antigen. All isolates were tested at least twice.

Table 1 : Rabies virus isolates from Russia and neighbouring states, tested by anti-nucleocapsid mAbs.

Country, area (town)	**Year(s) in which samples were isolated**	**Host species**	**No. of isolates tested**	**mAb groups**
Russia, South-East (Spassk, Birobidzhan)	1980-1988	Raccoon dog	5	
		Wild cat	1	2
		Human (dog)	1	
Russia, North-East (Ykutsk, Nizhne-Kolimsk)	1986-1990	Polar fox	12	
		Raindeer	3	7
		Unknown	1	
Russia, South of East Siberia (Chita)	1977-1980	Red fox	1	
		Steppe fox	2	5
Russia, Tuva (Kizil)	1980-1989	Wolf	2	2
		Rodent	1	9
Russia, South of West Siberia and Ural (Omsk, Novosibirsk, Orenburg)	1981-1888	Red fox	7	2 + 8 + 6
		Badger	1	6
		Cat	1	2
		Human (unknown)	1	8
Russia, South of European Russia (Krasnodar, Belgorod, Voronezh)	1990-1991	Red fox	5	8 + 2
		Cat	2	8 + 2
		Cow	1	8
Russia, West (Tula, Bryansk, Kaluga)	1988-1991	Red fox	10	1 + 2
		Raccoon dog	1	1
		Wolf	1	1
		Dog	4	1
		Cow	2	1 + 2
		Human (dog, raccoon dog)	3	1 + 2
Russia, North-West (Pskov, Leningrad, Kaliningrad)	1990-1991	Raccoon dog, dog, human (dog)	3	4
Russia, Kolsk peninsula (Murmansk)	1988	Polar fox, dog	2	3
Estonia	1990-1991	Red fox	2	3 + 4
		Wolf	2	3 + 4
		Raccoon dog	1	4
Georgia	1988-1990	Dog, cow	2	2
Kazakhstan	1988	Red fox, goat	2	2
Uzbekistan	1990	Human (dog)	3	2
Total			**85**	

[a] The source of human infection is given in parentheses.

Table 2: Rabies virus isolates from Russia and neighbouring states, used for phylogenetic analysis.

Isolate No.	Country	Area (town)	Year of isolation	Host species	mAb group	Genbank accession No.
RV234	Russia	Tula	1988	Dog	1	AY352476
RV236	Russia	Tula	1988	Red fox	1	AY352506
RV237	Russia	Tula	1988	Dog	1	AY352507
RV238	Russia	Tula	1988	Dog	1	AY352508
RV240	Russia	Tula	1988	Human (raccoon-dog)	1	DQ317516
RV247	Russia	Tula	1988	Red fox	1	AY352511
RV299	Russia	Tula	1990	Red fox	1	AY352479
RV239	Russia	Tula	1989	Human (dog)	2	AY352509
RV246	Russia	Tula	1988	Red fox	2	AY352510
RV241	Russia	Tula	1988	Red fox	2	AY352477
RV253	Russia	Tuva	1989	Wolf	2	AY352483
RV260	Russia	Omsk	1987	Red fox	2	AY352465
RV298	Russia	Tula	1990	Cow	2	AY352478
RV300	Russia	Orenburg	1990	Cat	2	AY352473
RV303	Russia	Spassk	1980	Raccoon-dog	2	AY352505
RV304	Russia	Birobidzhan	1988	Human (dog)	2	AY352502
RV434	Russia	Belgorod	1991	Cat	2	AY352456
RV259	Kazakhstan	Celinograd	1988	Fox	2	AY352491
RV305	Georgia	–	1989	Dog	2	AY352515
RV307	Georgia	–	1989	Cow	2	AY352516
RV245	Russia	Pscov	1990	Human (dog)	4	AY352475
RV309	Russia	Leningrad	1990	Raccoon-dog	4	AY352504
RV248	Russia	Chita	1977	Red fox	5	AY352460
RV251	Russia	Yakutia	1988	Polar fox	7	AY352512
RV293	Russia	Yakutia	1990	Reindeer	7	AY352513
RV255	Russia	Yakutia	1988	Polar fox	7	DQ010125
RV294	Russia	Yakutia	1990	Polar fox	7	AY352514
RV257	Russia	Omsk	1987	Red fox	8	AY352464
RV290	Russia	Krasnodar	1990	Cat	8	AY352503
RV291	Russia	Krasnodar	1990	Red fox	8	AY352461

Table 2: continued.

RV442	Russia	Orenburg	1990	Human (unknown)	8	AY352472
RV250	Russia	Tuva	1983	Rodent (Suslik)	9	AY352480
RV439	Russia	Pscov	1990	Red fox	ND	AY352474
RV440	Russia	Pscov	1990	Dog	ND	AY751535
RV443	Russia	Yakutia	1990	Horse	ND	DQ010127
RV448	Russia	Pskov	1990	Red fox	ND	DQ317520
RV449	Russia	Pskov	1990	Dog	ND	DQ317521
RV1334	Russia	Krasnoyarsk	2002	Wolf	ND	DQ010128
RV1336	Russia	Yakutia	1996	Polar fox	ND	DQ010129
RV295	Estonia	–	1989	Raccoon-dog	ND	DQ317517
RV296	Estonia	–	1989	Raccoon-dog	ND	DQ317518
RV437	Estonia	–	1990	Raccoon-dog	ND	AY091627
RV118	Finland	–	1988	Dog	ND	AY751534
RV306	Georgia	–	1989	Cow	ND	DQ317519
RV308	Georgia	–	1989	Human (dog)	ND	AY352497
U42714[1]	Estonia	–	1991	Raccoon-dog	ND	U42714
U43432[1]	Estonia	–	1991	Raccoon-dog	ND	U43432
02LAT[3]	Latvia	–	–	–	ND	AY277571
04LAT[3]	Latvia	–	–	–	ND	AY277572
12LAT[3]	Latvia	–	–	–	ND	AY277574
18LAT[3]	Latvia	–	–	–	ND	AY277576
Nishigahara[2]	Japan	–	–	Dog	ND	AB128149

ND, not done.

1 Bourhy et al, 1999 [6].

2 Ito et al, 2001 [23].

3 Vanaga et al, 2003 [13].

Polymerase chain reaction (PCR), sequencing and phylogenetic analysis

The isolates on which phylogenetic analysis was performed are listed in Table 2. Total RNA was extracted from clinical samples using the TRIzol method (Invitrogen, Life Technologies, MD, USA) following the manufacturer's instructions. The reverse transcription reaction and PCR were performed as previously described [18] using the sense primer JW12 and anti-sense primer JW6. The PCR products were sequenced with primers JW12 and JW10 using the BigDye Sequencing Kit (Applied Biosystems, Warrington, UK).

The 400 nucleotide sequence of the N gene (positions 71 to 470 according to the Pasteur virus genome) obtained from each sample was edited using the EditSeq software (DNAstar Inc., Madison, USA) and aligned using the ClustalW programme (Version 1.5). Phylogenetic analysis was performed using the neighbour-joining module of the PHYLIP package (Version 3.5) for 100 bootstrap replicates, as described previously [7]. A phylogenetic tree was visualized using the TREEVIEW program. Bootstrap values greater or equal to 70 % were considered to be significant.

RESULTS

Typing using mAbs discriminated the isolates into nine antigenic variants within serotype 1 (Table 3). Almost two-thirds of the isolates were positive for all mAbs of the Wistar panel, except mAb 422-5 for which all were negative. Approximately 30 % of isolates were negative for mAb 102-27. Most of the isolates in this group originated from the Northern Territories of Russia. The majority of the isolates differed in reactivity to only one or two "key" mAbs from the Wistar panel. For example, an absence of reaction to mAb 701-9 was selective for Arctic strains from North East Russia, while an absence of reaction to mAb 590-2 and 103-7 was characteristic of some isolates from red fox from steppe and forest-steppe zones. The reactions with mAb 714-3 were highly variable. The single, rodent isolate (RV250) was the most divergent and demonstrated a negative reaction with seven mAbs in addition to 422-5. In total, the Wistar panel identified only five RABV variants in this study.

The isolates that gave a positive reaction with P-41 were obtained from polar foxes and other mammals from the tundra zone, close to the polar circle, in the former Soviet Union. Isolates obtained from raccoon dogs, wolves and foxes in mod-

Table 3: Antigenic variants of rabies virus in Russia, detectable by anti-nucleocapsid monoclonal antibodies.

mAbs		**Antigenic variants (mAb groups) of rabies virus**								
		1	2	3	4	5	6	7	8	9
Wistar	102-27	+	+	+	-	-	-	-	+	-
	701-9	+	+	+	+	+	+	-	+	-
	590-2	+	+	+	+	+	+	+	-	+
	364-11	+	+	+	+	+	+	+	v	+
	103-7	+	+	+	+	+	+	+	-	+
	389-1	+	+	+	+	+	+	+	+	-
	805-3	+	+	+	+	+	+	+	+	-
	816-1	+	+	+	+	+	+	+	+	-
	111-2	+	+	+	+	+	+	+	+	-
	111-14	+	+	+	+	+	+	+	+	-
CVL	L-4	+	-	-	-	-	-	-	-	-
	L-18	+	-	-	v	-	-	-	-	-
	L-25	+	-	-	v	-	-	v	-	+
	L-28	+	-	-	v	-	-	v	-	-
Tübingen	P-41	-	-	+	+	+	-	+	-	+
Isolates tested (%)	85	16	30	4	6	3	2	16	8	1
	100	18.8	35.8	4.7	7.0	3.5	2.3	18.8	9.4	1.2

+, positive **reaction**; -, negative **reaction**; v, variable **reaction.**

erate latitudes of the North West region of Russia, the Baltic states and Eastern Siberia were also P-41-positive. The rodent isolate also demonstrated a positive reaction to the P-41 mAb. Some isolates that were not discriminated by the Wistar panel could be typed by the P-41 mAb.

Whilst the CVL panel was originally developed for the identification and discrimination of non-RABV bat lyssaviruses, it was shown to also differentiate between terrestrial RABV isolates. In this study, mAbs produced against Lagos bat virus (serotype 2) were effective for the discrimination of terrestrial isolates. For example, variants 1 and 2, and 4 and 5 could only be separated by the CVL panel. A number of CVL mAbs (M5-M7, M11, D1, D3, DB2, DB9, DB10, L1, L2, L7-L9, L11, L16, L20, L22, L27) gave no reaction, while others (M2, DB1, DB3, DB4, DB11, L3, L26) gave strongly positive results with all the isolates tested. The mAbs D2, D3, D9, DB6, DB14 and L23 gave very varied results.

Fifteen of the 73 mAbs used (Table 3) discriminated the isolates from Eastern Europe and Northern Asia. The mAbs that gave positive or negative reactions with all isolates, and mAbs that demonstrated highly variable reactions without any correlation to the geographical origin of the isolate or the host species, were excluded from the comparisons. The most important differences were obtained for mAbs P-41, 701-9 (frequently correlated with 102-27), 590-2 (correlated with 103-7 and 364-11), L-25 and L-28 (correlated with L-4 and L-18). Hence, only a small part of the panel could be used to discriminate the isolates in this study.

Partial N-gene sequences were obtained for all antigenic variants, except rare variants 3 and 6. As expected, all isolates belonged to genotype 1. Two highly divergent clusters were identified (Fig. 1). The first cluster grouped Arctic and Arctic-like viruses from the Arctic zone, East Siberia and the Far East. The second cluster grouped isolates originating from moderate latitudes of the European region of the former Soviet Union, the Ural Mountains and West Siberia. These have been subdivided into well-differentiated genetic groups, as described previously [14].

In general, the results of phylogenetic analysis were in concordance with the mAb typing. Separated branches on the phylogenetic tree corresponded to specific antigenic variants, with only a few deviations. The phylogenetic origin of antigenic variants 1, 4 and 7 was confirmed. The widely distributed antigenic variant 2 was additionally subdivided into a number of phylogenetic lineages resolved at a geographic level, some of which belonged to different phylogenetic clades. Isolates from the Baltic region (variant 4) that were P-41-positive could only occasionally be differentiated from Eastern Siberian isolates (variant 5), owing to weak binding with three CVL mAbs. However, phylogenetic analysis separated these variants into quite different lineages at the genetic level.

Discussion

The geographical distribution and host specificity of certain antigenic variants of RABV have been described in several studies [9-11,19]. The variants 1, 2 and 7 predominated among the samples examined in this study; however, variant 2 had a very wide geographical distribution, while variants 1 and 7 were found only in limited areas. Variant 7 predominated in Asian Arctic regions and had a different antigenic pattern from that of isolates from polar fox from the Kolsk peninsula. Two or more antigenic variants of RABV were sometimes found within the same geographical

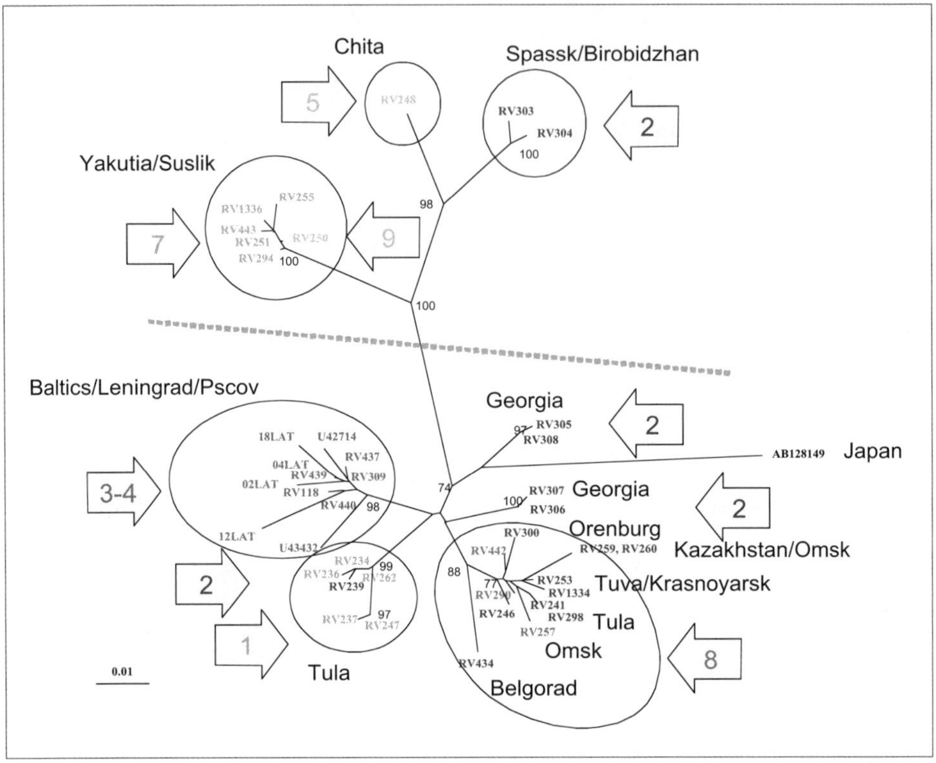

Fig. 1: Neighbour joining phylogenetic tree of 74 rabies virus isolates according to 400bp of nucleoprotein (N) gene. Genbank accession numbers are given when strain names are unavailable. Bootstrap values considered significant (> 70%) are presented and branch lengths are drawn to scale (substitutions/site). The antigenic (Mab) variants 1, 2, 4, 5, 7, 8 and 9 are represented on the tree. Individual isolate labels are shown to represent the respective Mab variant (if known) and the distribution of the Mab variants is indicated by the arrows.

area. Antigenic variants specific to a particular geographical area were commonly recovered from a range of wild and domestic animals.

The wide geographical distribution of some antigenic variants may indicate insufficient resolution by mAb typing. In some cases, genetic data resolved some of the more debatable assumptions made on the basis of mAb typing. For example, phylogenetic analysis distinguished the widely distributed antigenic variant 2. In a previous study [17], we described this variant as a dog RABV of Asian origin. Similar conclusions about isolates that gave a positive reaction with all mAbs of the Wistar panel, excluding mAb 422-5, were reached in other studies [5,20]. However, it is now apparent that this phenotype is present in divergent genetic groups and the antigenic variant 2 is not limited to RABV in dogs as previously thought. For example, the isolates from raccoon dogs originating from true Asian habitats also belonged to this antigenic variant, and represented an "Arctic-like" group (RV303 and RV304), which was genetically distant from the isolates from the European raccoon dog.

As previously shown, mAb P-41 is a very specific marker for Arctic RABV: a positive reaction with this mAb was observed for nearly all isolates from the Northern Territories [17]. Genetic methods provided an insight into the diverse distribution of P-41-positive RABV isolates from Russia and neighbouring countries. It was difficult to explain the discovery of P-41-positive viruses in moderate latitudes of the former Soviet Union. Long-distance migrations by the polar fox and historic conditions related to the ice age have been proposed [9]. Genetically, such isolates from the North West of Russia are closely related to those from Estonia, Latvia, Finland and Poland [6,21] and are represented in the North Eastern European phylogenetic group (NEE), which is most closely related to non-Arctic European RABV lineages. The P-41-positive isolates from the Asian part of Russia (sometimes indistinguishable from the European isolates on the basis of mAb patterns) belonged to the phylogenetic cluster of Arctic and Arctic-like viruses.

As shown in Table 4 and Figure 1, some phenotypes that are detectable by mAbs may be found in divergent phylogenetic groups and vice versa. For example, isolates with a very characteristic antigenic profile (variant 8) were found within a genetic group that is broadly distributed in Russia (Siberia, the Ural Mountains and the Northern Caucasus). This antigenic variant predominated in the Northern Caucasus in around 1990. Moreover, the same antigenic variants had been described in France and in parts of Africa [20, 22]. Following other studies [20] we proposed that this antigenic group represented a fox variant of RABV [19]. However, King et al [22] described the same phenotypic signs in RABV isolates of African viverrid origin. But it is still unclear whether this antigenic pattern is evidence of ancestral homology, convergent evolution, or just an arbitrary effect resulting from a particular, non-functional amino acid substitution.

The presence of similar patterns of mAb reactivity in divergent phylogenetic groups might be caused not only by amino acid substitutions within the nucleoprotein, but also by conformational changes of this protein, or changes to the structure of other gene fragments not examined in these studies. Antigenic epitopes for some Wistar mAbs were located near the C-terminus of the nucleoprotein, and an epitope for mAb 701 was found at position 75-90 of the phosphoprotein [2]. Epitopes for other "key" mAbs for Russian isolates are unknown.

Table 4: Comparison of phylogenetic groups and mAbs antigenic variants of rabies virus found in different regions of Russia.

Phylogenetic groups and their geographic distribution	**mAbs antigenic variants**								
	1	2	3	4	5	6	7	8	9
Arctic zone (A)*							✓		✓
South of East Siberia and Far East (B)		✓			✓				
Steepe zone from Black Sea to Tuva (C)		✓						✓	
Western area of Russia (D)	✓	✓							
North-west area near Baltics (E)				✓					

* Letters in parentheses correspond to genetic groups described by Kuzmin et al (2004).

Bourhy et al [6] examined positions 101 (fox isolates) and 115 (raccoon dogs isolates) of the nucleoprotein in relation to host adaptation of the RABV at the molecular level. Asp to Gly changes at position 115 (Gly_{115}) appeared to relate the raccoon dog isolates to the Arctic RABV. Indeed, this substitution was found in all Arctic isolates of polar origin, in arctic foxes, dogs, wolves and humans, and also in raccoon dogs from North East Europe, which did not belong to the Arctic or "Arctic-like" lineages. However, Gly_{115} was also detected in a steppe fox isolate from Eastern Siberia (RV248), which belonged to one of the "Arctic-like" lineages, and Gly_{115} was not found in the raccoon dog, or dog isolates from the Far East (RV303 and RV304) nor in the dog isolate from Japan (Komatsugawa) [23] belonging to another "Arctic-like" lineage. It appears that Gly_{115} may facilitate a positive reaction with mAb P-41, but the evolutionary or functional significance of this substitution is unclear. P-41-positive RABV isolates were significantly more frequently collected from animals than from humans [11].

Comparisons of antigenic and genetic data confirmed that most virus divergence was due to the different geographical origins of the isolates. Focal or clonal patterns of geographical distribution of the RABV variants were observed. In some cases, the distribution of the variants overlapped. The same patterns of distribution have been described in other parts of the world [3,6,22,24]. Some RABV variants were distributed within neighbouring areas of Russia and other states. Similar antigenic variants of Arctic RABV were described in North America and North East Asia [19,25]. Genetic analyses have confirmed that these isolates belonged to a common phylogenetic group [5,14]. This means that the Bering Strait is not an insurmountable barrier for polar foxes or for rabies.

Our data confirmed that wild canids contribute to the circulation of RABV in Russia. Two points should be underlined. Firstly, in contrast to western and central European countries where the red fox is the sole RABV reservoir, RABV in Russia circulates in six wild, canid species. Secondly, different virus lineages and antigenic variants can circulate in a particular host species (e.g. red fox, steppe fox, raccoon dog) across their distribution range.

We repeatedly tested the unique rodent RABV isolate because of its very unusual mAb reactivity pattern. No analogous antigenic patterns were found for other isolates of the panel. This isolate was recovered during active surveillance in the steppe valley within the high mountain region of Tuva, not far from the border with Mongolia. More than 700 wild animals, including 250 susliks, from this region were examined during 1983 – 1985, and only this unique isolate was recovered. However, isolates with similar antigenic profiles have been described in Madagascar [20]. No signs of specific adaptation were detected after experimental inoculation of rodents (*Citellus* or *Spermophyllus* genus) with different RABVs, including this one [26]. According to the entire N-gene sequence, this isolate belonged to the Arctic genetic group, and was apparently indistinguishable from the Arctic fox isolates (Fig. 1). All other RABV isolates (human, dog, wolf, cow) from the Tuva province had different antigenic patterns [19] and belonged to another phylogenetic group [11]. We have no satisfactory explanation for the origin of this isolate or of its unusual antigenic pattern.

Conclusions

RABV variants (serotype 1, genotype 1) can be discriminated on the basis of phenotype (epitopes of the nucleocapsid protein) and genetic analysis. Some antigenic variants were not strongly associated with one genetic group. Different antigenic patterns may be recognised in genetically related isolates. Divergence between genotypic and phenotypic diversity was seen in some instances. Despite the current popularity of genetic and phylogenetic methodologies in molecular epidemiology research, the application of inexpensive mAb typing can still be of great benefit to local diagnostic laboratories where resources are limited.

Acknowledgements

The study was supported by a grant from The Royal Society of Great Britain and the Department for Environment, Food and Rural Affairs (DEFRA), UK (Grant SE0417).

Preparations of mAbs were kindly supplied by Drs H. Koprowski (Wistar Institute of Anatomy and Biology, Philadelphia, USA), L. Schneider (Federal Research Centre for Animal Virus Diseases, Tübingen, Germany), A. King (CVL, Weybridge, UK). Drs M. Selimov and A. King provided invaluable assistance during the first steps of this research. Drs L. Gribanova (Research Institute for Natural Foci Infections, Omsk, Russia) and V. Khozinski (Institute of Polio and Viral Encephalidites, Moscow, Russia) took part in the creation of the RABV collection.

We would like to thank public health and veterinary specialists from Russia and the former Soviet Union (L. Antonova, N. Balanov, A. Barashkov, L. Barinova, V. Chernyavski, A. Chizh, P. Dolzhanov, P. Kolotvinova, S. Korneeva, A. Korzhenkova, S. Kravchenko, C. Machitidze, L. Petrenko, F. Rakhimova, R. Rozamova, U. Romanova, L. Shmatova, E. Toskar, R. Yastrebova) for their help in the collection of the samples.

References

1 Wiktor TJ, Koprowski H: Monoclonal Antibodies against Rabies Virus produced by Somatic Cell Hybridization: Detection of Antigenic Variants. Proc Natl Acad Sci (USA) 1978; 75: 3938-3942.

2 Dietzschold B, Rupprecht CE, Tollis M, Lafon M, Mattei J, Wiktor T, Koprowski H: Antigenic Diversity of the Glycoprotein and Nucleocapsid Proteins of Rabies and Rabies-Related Viruses: Implication for Epidemiology and Control of Rabies. Rev Infect Dis 1988; 10 (Suppl 4): S785-S798.

3 Smith JS: Rabies Virus Epitopic Variation: Use in Ecologic Studies. Adv Virus Res 1989; 36: 215-253.

4 Rupprecht CE, Deitzchold B, Wunner WH, Koprowski H: Antigenic Relationships of Lyssaviruses, in Baer GM (ed): The Natural History of Rabies, 2 nd. Boca Raton, CRC Press, 1991, pp 69-100.

5 Kissi B, Tordo N, Bourhy H: Genetic Polymorphism in the Rabies Virus Nucleoprotein Gene. Virology 1995; 209: 526-537.

6 Bourhy H, Kissi B, Audry L, Smreczak M, Sadkowska-Todys M, Kulonen K, Tordo N, Zmudzinski JF, Holmes ED: Ecology and Evolution of rabies virus in Europe. J Gen Virol 1999; 80: 2545-2557.

7 Johnson N, McElhinney LM, Smith J, Lowings P, Fooks AR: Phylogenetic comparison of the genus Lyssavirus using distal coding sequences of the glycoprotein and nucleoprotein genes. Arch Virol 2002; 147: 2111-2123.

8 Selimov MA, Botvinkin AD, Tatarov AG: Identification of the Strain of Sylvatic and Arctic Rabies Virus with the Help of Monoclonal Antibodies. Voprosi Virusologii 1983; 2: 243-244.

9 Selimov MA, Botvinkin AD, Khozinski VV Gribanova LY: New data about distribution of P-41 positive strains of rabies virus in arctic and non-arctic regions. J Microbiol Epidemiol Immunobiol 1994; 2: 53-56. (In Russian).

10 King A, Davies P, Lawrie A: The Rabies Viruses of Bats. Vet Microbiol 1990; 23: 165-174.

11 Botvinkin AD, Kuzmin IV, Khismatullina NA: A sum of Study of rabies virus diversity in the former Soviet Union with monoclonal antibodies. Vet Pathol 2004; 3 (10): 117-127. (In Russian).

12 McElhinney LM, Johnson N, Mansfield KL, Finnegan CJ, Smith J, Lowings JP, Fooks AR: Molecular Characterization of Rabies and Rabies Related Viruses, in Dodet B, Meslin FX (eds): Rabies Control in Asia. Paris, John Libbey Eurotext 2001, pp 178-184.

13 Vanaga S, van der Heide R, Joffe R, van der Poel WH: Rabies in Wildlife in Latvia. Vector Borne Zoonotic Dis 2003 Fall; 3 (3): 117-124.

14 Kuzmin IV, Botvinkin AD, McElhinney LM, Smith JS, Orciari LA, Clark J, Hughes GJ, Fooks AR, Rupprecht CE: Molecular Epidemiology of Terrestrial Rabies in the Former Soviet Union. J Wildl Dis 2004; 40 (4): 617-631.

15 Koprowski H: The Mouse Inoculation Test, in Kaplan MM, Koprowski H (eds): Laboratory techniques in Rabies, 3-d edn. Word Health Organization, Geneva 1973, pp 85-93.

16 Dean DJ, Abelseth MK: The fluorescent antibody test, in Kaplan MM, Koprowski H (eds): Laboratory Techniques in Rabies, 3nd. Geneva, Word Health Organization. 1973, pp 73-84.

17 Schneider LG, Odegaard OA, Muller J, Selimov M: Application of Monoclonal Antibodies for Epidemiological Investigation and Oral Vaccination Studies. II. Arctic Viruses, in Rabies in the Tropics. Proceedings of the International Conference on Rabies Control in the Tropics, Tunis, 1983, Berlin, Spring-Verlag, 1985, pp 47-59.

18 Heaton PR, Johnstone P, McElhinney LM, Cowley R, O'Sullivan E, Whitby JE: Hemi-nested PCR Assay for Detection of six Genotypes of rabies and rabies related viruses. J Clin Microbiol 1997; 35,1: 2762-2766.

19 Botvinkin AD, Selimov MA, Klueva EV, Gribanova LY, Khismatullina NA: Antigenic characteristic of field rabies virus isolates with the help of anti-nucleocapsid monoclonal antibodies from different regions of the URSS. J Microbiol Epidemiol Immunobiol 1990; 1: 50-54 (in Russian).

20 Sureau P, Rollin P, Wiktor TJ: Epidemiologic Analysis of Antigenic Variations of Street Rabies Virus: Detection by Monoclonal Antibodies. Am J Epidemiol 1983; 117: 605-609.

21 Kulonen K, Boldina I: Differentiation of Two Rabies strains in Estonia with Reference to recent Finnish Isolates. J Wildl Dis 1993; 29, 2: 209-213.

22 King AA, Meredith CD, Thomson GR: Canid and Viverrid Rabies Viruses in South Africa. Ondesterpoort J Vet Res (Special Issue) 1993; 60: 295-299.

23 Ito N, Kakemizu M, Ito KA, Yamamoto A, Yoshida Y, Sugiyama M, Minamoto N: A comparison of Complete Genome Sequences of the Attenuated RC-HL strain of Rabies Virus for production of Animal Vaccine in Japan, and the parental of Nishigahara strain. Microbiol Immunol 2001; 45, 1: 51-58.

24 Johnson N, Letshwenyo M, Maipoledi EK, Thobokwe G, Fooks AR: Molecular Epidemiology of Rabies in Botswana: a comparison between antibody typing and nucleotide sequence phylogeny. Vet Microbiol 2004; Jun 10; 101 (1): 31-38

25 Webster WA, Casey GA, Charlton KM, Wiktor TJ: Antigenic Variants of Rabies Virus of Rabies Virus in Isolates from Eastern, Central and Northern Canada. Can J Comp Med 1985; 49, 2: 186-188.

26 Malkov GB, Gribanova LY, Botvinkin AD, Sidorov GN, Fedorova TN, Vakhrushev AV, Nikiforova TA, Selezneva CK, Bachaev UP, Kolosov VM: Distribution and Epidemiological Significance of Rabies Natural Foci in Mountain Regions of South Siberia. Natural Foci Infections of Human: Omsk 1986: 84-94. (In Russian).

Dr. A. Botvinkin, Irkutsk State Medical University, 1, Krasnogo Vosstania, Irkutsk, RU-664003, Russia.
E-mail: botvinkin@irkutsk.ru

Dodet B, Schudel A, Pastoret PP, Lombard M (eds): Rabies in Europe.
Dev Biol (Basel). Basel, Karger, 2006, vol 125, pp 91-94.

Tools for Rabies Serology to Monitor the Effectiveness of Rabies Vaccination in Domestic and Wild Carnivores

A. Servat, M. Wasniewski, F. Cliquet

AFSSA Nancy, Laboratoire d'Etudes et de Recherches sur la Rage et la pathologie des Animaux Sauvages, WHO Collaborating Centre for Research and Management in Zoonoses Control, OIE Reference Laboratory for Rabies, Community Reference Laboratory for Rabies Serology, Malzéville, France

Key words: Rabies, serology, vaccination, standardisation.

Abstract: Serology remains the only way to monitor the effectiveness of vaccination of humans and animals against rabies. Many techniques for determining the level of rabies antibodies have been described, including seroneutralisation techniques such as tests for fluorescent antibody virus neutralisation (FAVN) and rapid fluorescent focus inhibition (RFFIT), enzyme-linked immunosorbent assay (ELISA), and in-vivo tests (the mouse neutralisation test, MNT).

The need to verify the effectiveness of rabies vaccination has become widespread, particularly in the context of international trading of domestic carnivores from infected to rabies-free territories. The standardisation of serological techniques, approval of laboratories and proficiency tests are key concepts to ensure the practicability of such systems.

Serological tests for rabies are also often used by laboratories in infected territories to assess the efficacy of campaigns aimed at the eradication of the disease via oral vaccination of wildlife. The adaptation of these methods should provide the means to titrate specific antibodies in dogs during mass parenteral vaccination in countries infected by canine rabies. However, in most cases these serological tests are carried without any standardised procedure.

On the basis of our experience in rabies serology and its harmonisation throughout laboratories worldwide, we propose here an adapted standard technique for the serological monitoring for rabies in wildlife at the European level. Such harmonisation would allow the monitoring of vaccination campaigns to be enhanced by increasing the exchange of epidemiological data, with the ultimate goal being the eradication of rabies in Europe.

INTRODUCTION

Serological methods are widely used to monitor the effectiveness of vaccination with parenteral or oral vaccines against rabies. These methods remain the only way to check the protection of domestic or wild carnivores, as well as humans, by measuring the level of protective antibodies against rabies. To give meaning to these serological controls, a protection threshold has been defined at 0.5 IU/ml. Above this value, animals and humans are considered to be protected against rabies. From a veterinary point of view, serological testing for rabies is mainly used in two fields: (i) the evaluation of the efficacy of vaccination in the context of the international trade in domestics carnivores; and (ii) the evaluation of the efficacy of vaccination campaigns in wild animals (in those countries conducting rabies eradication programmes). Currently, three main techniques are used to detect rabies antibodies in carnivores. The oldest method is an in vivo technique first described in 1935 [1] and consists of the neutralisation of rabies virus in a mouse model (Mouse Neutralisation Test, MNT). Several decades later, the Rapid Fluorescent Focus Inhibition Test (RFFIT) and the Fluorescent Antibody Virus Neutralisation (FAVN) test were described [2,3]. In these in-vitro techniques a fixed amount of rabies virus is seroneutralised and then inoculated to cells that are susceptible to infection by rabies virus. All of these methods are recommended by the World Organisation for Animal Health (OIE) [4]. The use of these tools to detect antibodies to rabies antibodies in carnivores is more or less subject to standardisation and harmonisation. The following review presents an update of the situation regarding the international trade in domestic carnivores and the evaluation of campaigns for the oral vaccination of wild carnivores.

International Trade in Domestic Carnivores

To prevent the introduction of rabies from infected into rabies-free territories, international trade in domestic carnivores was subject to strict legislation until recently. The quarantine measures widely adopted by rabies-free countries have proved to be an effective system. Quarantine was progressively abolished and replaced by a system linking the vaccination of pets with blood tests to check that the animals had seroconverted. At the present time, international trade in domestic carnivores must meet specific requirements. Pet owners must identify their animals (by tattoo number and/or microchip) and arrange for a rabies vaccination (with an inactivated vaccine) and a blood test. The blood test is performed 1-4 months after vaccination, depending on the country's legislation.

Laboratories performing the blood tests must use a technique approved by OIE (one of the two described in the fifth edition of the OIE *Manual of diagnostic tests and vaccines for terrestrial animals*). Laboratories must be also authorized and approved by an official authority (e.g. the European Commission) to perform rabies serological controls in the context of the international trade in pets. Approvals are granted provided that laboratories succeed in the proficiency tests. These tests are organized annually by the French agency for food safety (AFSSA) laboratory in Nancy, which was designated as the community reference institute (CRI) for rabies serology [5]. Once approved, laboratories are automatically involved in the proficiency test scheme that allows the CRI to check that their performance remains acceptable. The proficiency tests consist of a panel of several sera to be tested "blind" in three independent runs. The results obtained are analysed to determine specificity, reproducibility and consistency for each laboratory. On the basis of a technical report produced by the CRI, the European Commission grants, withdraws or maintains the approved status of the laboratories.

The proficiency test scheme was first initiated by AFSSA Nancy at the end of 1999. Fourteen laboratories were initially involved, and the number of participants increases yearly such that 5 years later, the CRI now assesses the performance of 44 laboratories. These laboratories are mainly located within the European Union, but also in the United States of America (USA), Asia, the Middle East and Australia. A list of approved laboratories is updated by the European Commission and is available at the following website: http://europa.eu.int/comm/food/animal/liveanimals/pets/approval_en.htm.

Evaluation of the Efficacy of Campaigns for Oral Vaccination Against Rabies

Rabies eradication programmes conducted in infected territories are based on vaccination of the rabies reservoir by distribution of oral vaccines in bait or by parenteral vaccination. Several target species exist depending on geographical area: in Europe, the main reservoir and vector of rabies is the fox (*Vulpes vulpes*); in the USA, several reservoirs maintain the disease (raccoon, skunk, fox, dog, and insectivorous bats); in South America, Africa and Asia, the dog represents the main reservoir and vector of rabies. In those countries using oral vaccination, assessment of the efficacy of vaccination campaigns is based on the evaluation of the uptake of baits (presence of tetracycline in the teeth of bait consumers) and on the evaluation of seroconversion (monitoring the level of rabies antibodies). Currently, and contrary to international trade contexts, there is no harmonisation of serological monitoring to assess humoral response after oral vaccination campaigns. Depending on the laboratory, seroconversion is monitored by FAVN test or adapted protocols thereof, RFFIT or adapted protocols thereof or in-house ELISA test. Sometimes seroconversion is not monitored at all. The serological techniques used at the present time are not always adapted to serological monitoring in wild carnivores. The MNT is very expensive, requires the use of animals, and several weeks are necessary to obtain the results. The FAVN test and RFFIT require the use of live rabies virus, the maintenance of cell cultures, and are potentially sensitive to cytotoxicity attributable to the poor quality of field samples (haemolysed serum, body fluids) and could lead to false-positive results. Consequently, these tests are not adapted to large-scale screening of field sera. This lack of validated methods for titrating rabies antibodies in poor quality sera, and lack of harmonization, make it difficult to survey and compare the efficacy of different vaccination protocols or strategies.

An ELISA test has been recently described for titrating rabies antibodies in foxes after oral vaccination [6,7]. This indirect ELISA test uses plates that have been pre-coated with purified G glycoprotein, and shows high correlation with an approved method (FAVN test). Moreover, this test has been validated for use with poor quality samples, such as body fluids and haemolysed samples. ELISA does not require the use of live virus and therefore high-containment laboratories, and has the advantage of being economical, rapid (a large number of samples can be sampled in only 4 hours), simple, and easily automated.

In October 2004, a workshop was organized at AFSSA Nancy to present this technique to those countries still conducting rabies eradication programmes. Many laboratories in Eastern Europe showed great interest in using the ELISA test to survey seroconversion after oral vaccination campaigns. Such a test would be better adapted to large-scale screening, especially in countries with large areas to be covered by vaccination campaigns and/or conducting their first campaigns.

Discussion and Conclusion

The last five years have demonstrated the importance of harmonisation in the monitoring of serology after the vaccination of domestic carnivores against rabies. Many countries have abandoned quarantine in favour of a system combining rabies vaccination and blood tests, as was done recently in Japan. The widespread adoption of this "rabies vaccination-blood test" scheme has increased the mobility of pets, and lead laboratories to apply in large numbers for approval and participation in proficiency testing. This has resulted in a large increase in the number of designated laboratories. The harmonisation of techniques to be used and the organisation of proficiency tests have allowed rabies serology activities in the pet trade to be perfectly managed at an international level. Standardisation for serological techniques of rabies in wildlife, at least at the European level, should be investigated in order to enhance the monitoring of vaccination campaigns and the exchange of epidemiological data. The use of techniques based on ELISA as proposed in this review should be encouraged as the beginning of such harmonisation, the ultimate goal being the eradication of rabies in Europe.

References

1 Webster LT, Dawson JR: Early diagnosis of rabies by mouse inoculation. Measurement of humoral immunity to rabies by mouse protection test. Proc Soc Exp Biol Med 1935; 32: 570-573.

2 Smith JS, Yager PA, Baer GM: A rapid reproducible test for determining rabies neutralizing antibody. Bull WHO 1973; 48 (5): 535-541.

3 Cliquet F, Aubert M, Sagné L: Development of a fluorescent antibody virus neutralisation test (FAVN test) for the quantification of rabies-neutralising antibody. J Immunol Meth 1998; 212: 79-87.

4 OIE (World organisation for animal health): Rabies. In OIE Manual of standards for diagnostic tests and vaccines, 5th Ed. OIE, Paris, 2004; pp 276-291.

5 Council decision 2000/258/CE, Official Journal of the European Communities.

6 Cliquet F, Sagne L, Schereffer JL, Aubert MF: ELISA test for rabies antibody titration in orally vaccinated foxes sampled in the field. Vaccine 2000; 18 (28): 3272-3279.

7 Cliquet F, Müller T, Mutinelli F, Geronutti S, Brochier B, Selhorst T, Schereffer JL, Kraft N, Burow J, Schameitat A, Schlüter H, Aubert M: Standardisation and Establishment of a rabies ELISA test in European laboratories for assessing the efficacy of oral fox vaccination campaigns. Vaccine 2003; 21: 2986-2993.

Dr. A. Servat, AFSSA Nancy, Laboratoire d'Etudes et de Recherches sur la Rage et la Pathologie des Animaux Sauvages, WHO Collaborating Centre for Research and Management in Zoonoses Control, OIE Reference Laboratory for Rabies, Community Reference Laboratory for Rabies Serology, Domaine de Pixérécourt, FR-54220 Malzéville, France.
E-mail: a.servat@nancy.afssa.fr

Dodet B, Schudel A, Pastoret PP, Lombard M (eds): Rabies in Europe.
Dev Biol (Basel). Basel, Karger, 2006, vol 125, pp 95-100.

Measures to Control an Imported Case of Canine Rabies in France

Information provided by the French Ministry of Agriculture & Ministry of Health
Presented by J. Barrat

Abstract: France has been free from terrestrial rabies since 2001. On 21 August 2004, a female dog aged 4 months died in Gironde (south-west France), after experiencing clinical symptoms suggestive of rabies for 3 days. On 26 August, a diagnosis of rabies was confirmed by the Pasteur Institute. This paper describes the measures that were taken to manage the risks to human and animal health, and analyses the alert raised in France as a result of this imported case of rabies, the third such case in 2004.

CASE DESCRIPTION

The last indigenous case of terrestrial rabies in France was detected in the Moselle department (north-east France) in December 1998, and France was officially declared free of terrestrial rabies in 2001 by the World Organisation for Animal Health (OIE). On 21 August 2004, a female dog aged 4 months in the Gironde department (south-west France) died after experiencing clinical symptoms suggestive of rabies for 3 days. The veterinarian in charge of the dog pound sent the head of the puppy to the Pasteur Institute for rabies diagnosis. On 26 August, the diagnosis of rabies was confirmed and Pasteur Institute alerted veterinary services across France.

EPIDEMIOLOGICAL INVESTIGATION

Preliminary results

The dog (named "Tikki") had come from near Agadir in Morocco. It was neither registered nor vaccinated and was introduced illegally into France via Spain on 11 July, thus entering European territory without any sanitary controls.

Between 2 and 21 August 2004, the animal and its owner visited many public places and attended several cultural events across three French departments (Gironde, Lot-et-Garonne, and Dordogne), as shown in Figure 1. During these travels, the infected animal had been in contact with other pets (mainly dogs) and with people (adults and children, locals and tourists). The risk of transmission was estimated using

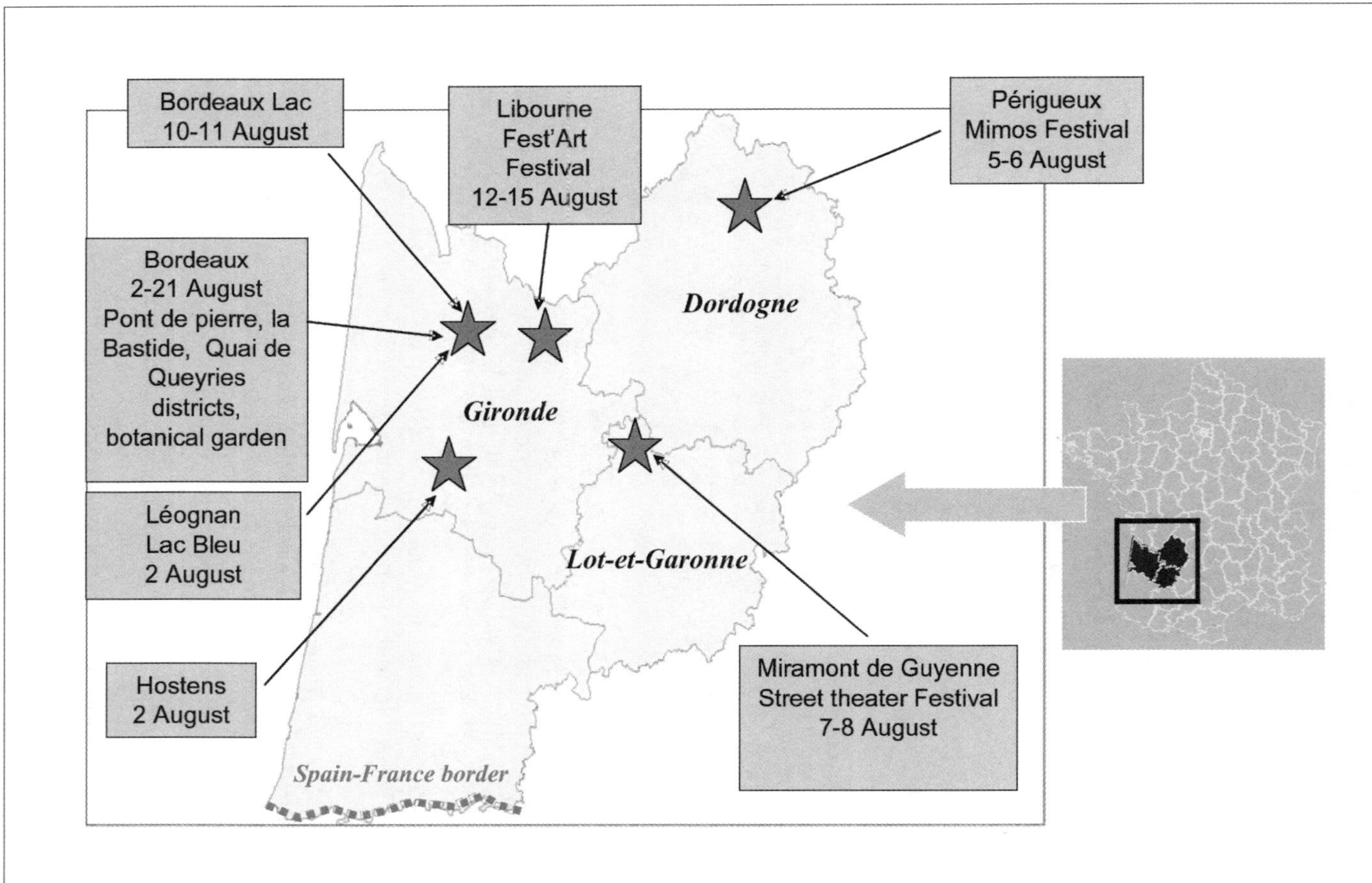

Fig. 1 : Movements of "Tikki", the infected dog, between 2 and 21 August, 2004.

a pre-defined model (see Fig. 2) that assumes that the "at risk" period begins 14 days before the onset of symptoms (as stipulated by French regulations) and that the closer the animal is to death, the higher the probability of virus shedding in saliva.

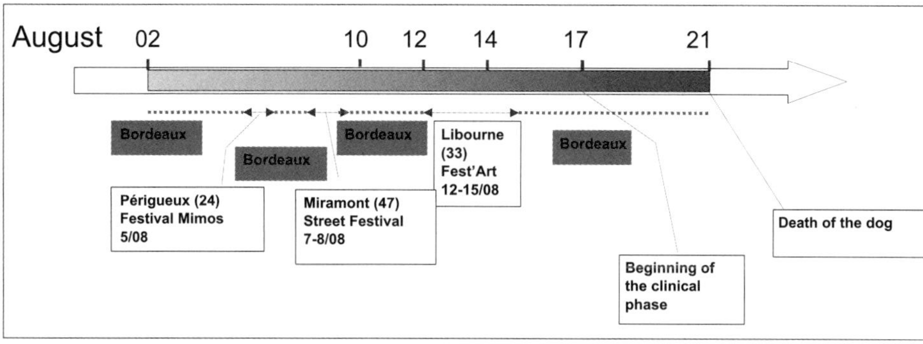

Fig. 2: Estimation of the risk of rabies transmission between 2 and 21 August, 2004.

Crisis structures

Various structures were involved in monitoring the crisis both locally and at a national level. At the local level, the prefecture (regional authority) of Bordeaux coordinated the activity of veterinary services, health services, police and gendarmerie. Health-service involvement included anti-rabies centres and first aid organisations. These services were on-call 24 hours per day. At the national level, the Ministries of Health and Agriculture were involved, along with an expert committee on rabies from the French Food Safety Agency (AFSSA), the Pasteur Institute and the National Reference Centre for Rabies. Decision-making and activities were coordinated at the local level through daily contacts between the participating services. The media were very helpful in informing the public of the risk and requesting that they look out for possibly infected people. Three national press releases were prepared, and there were many local press releases that were taken up by newspapers and television. During the surveillance phase, an electronic surveillance bulletin was sent out twice per month by AFSSA-LERRPAS (Laboratory for Study and Research on Rabies and Wildlife Diseases) to the participating services.

Regulations for the Prevention of Rabies

The French regulations on rabies include different case definitions and explain procedure to be followed in each circumstance.

- The "at risk" period begins 14 days before the onset of clinical signs and lasts until the death of the rabid animal.
- A domestic carnivore that has been in contact with a rabid animal of whatever species should be considered infected, even if it has not been bitten. Such animals must be euthanized unless they are regularly vaccinated (i.e. vaccinated and registered), in which case they must also receive a booster injection within 5 days of the contact.

- A suspect animal that exhibits abnormal behaviour and/or symptoms must be put under veterinary surveillance by order of the Prefect.
- A carnivore suspected of having been in contact with a suspected infected animal should be put under surveillance or euthanized depending upon the result of a veterinary services investigation.

Emergency Measures

The European Commission and the Chief Veterinary Officers of the 25 Member States were informed about this case on 27 August. OIE and the World Health Organization (WHO) were notified on 31 August. At the same time, a search was begun for potentially infected individuals. On 27 and 28 August, a prefectural order identified seven cities where the rabid animal had been staying during the "at risk" period; the movements of non-vaccinated animals were restricted and all gatherings of cats and dogs in these cities were prohibited.

Extension of the Measures

On 3 September, a national order from the Ministry of Agriculture extended the above measures to the three departments (i.e. the zone highlighted in Fig. 1) for a period of 6 months. This order also included other measures:

- Identified and correctly vaccinated dogs (i.e. both vaccinated and registered) could move freely in and out of the zone under the owner's supervision.
- Dogs and cats that were not "officially" vaccinated were to be kept on the leash or in confinement; dogs had to be leashed and muzzled, even if they were vaccinated.
- Pet owners could not givc away or sell their domestic carnivores if they were not vaccinated against rabies.
- Any sick or dead domestic carnivore had to be submitted for an epidemiological examination to the veterinary services

The three departments were not officially declared to be infected. This would have made anti-rabies vaccination of domestic carnivores compulsory. Cats and dogs captured and put in pounds from 2 August (i.e. during the "at risk" period) were treated as follows:

- Cats and dogs that were not identified or not vaccinated were euthanized.
- Cats and dogs that were identified with valid vaccination against rabies were given back to their owner if a vaccination certificate was provided.
- Pet shows and other gatherings of domestic carnivores in the zone were prohibited.
- Vaccinated cats and dogs were forbidden to participate in pet shows or other assemblies outside of the zone.

However, there were sometimes difficulties concerning the euthanasia of pets during the first months of the surveillance as the majority of animals were not vaccinated before the rabies alert. Reprieves were granted for psychological or humane reasons under supervision of the Prefect.

Activities of the Veterinary Services

During the alert, veterinary services made use of available regulatory tools along with the decentralised network of veterinary services and the network of official "sanitary veterinarians" (private practitioners allowed to intervene as state veterinarians). The surveillance of biting animals or those suspected to be infected was intensified as was the surveillance of pets introduced into France.

Final Evaluation: April 2005

Forty-nine dogs and eight cats were euthanized due to proven contact with "Tikki" during the "at risk" period or because of the probability of contact; laboratory diagnosis was performed on all of these animals. One-hundred-and-ten diagnostic tests for possible human contamination were carried out at the Pasteur Institute, Paris, and 1174 tests were carried out at AFSSA-LERRPAS-Nancy on domestic carnivores found dead or euthanized in pounds during the 6-month surveillance period. No secondary cases were identified. Epidemiological investigation was carried out for more than 300 people and 190 of these received post-exposure prophylaxis. In addition, twelve dogs, one cat and five persons that were implicated were not identified.

Other Rabies Cases Imported into France

Cases of rabies imported into France from Morocco between 1968 and 2004

Between 1968 and 2004, nine dogs illegally imported from Morocco became rabid in France (Fig. 3). In one case in the Nord (department in Northern France) in 1981, a secondary case was identified in a cat that had been infected by the rabid dog.

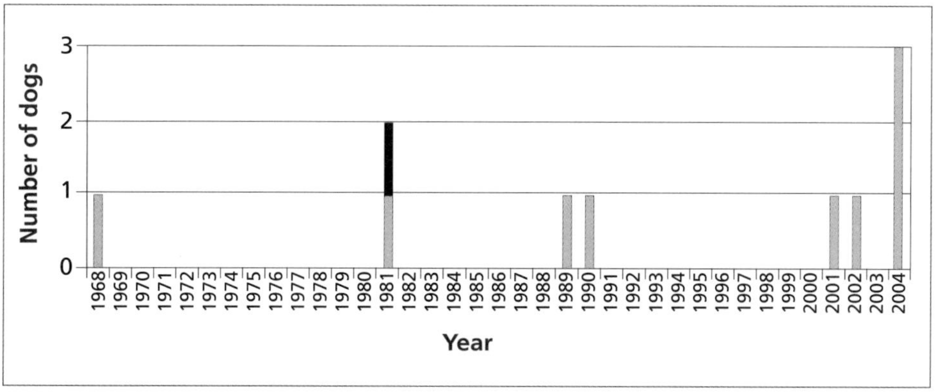

Fig. 3: Number of dogs illegally imported from Morocco to France in 1968 – 2004 that became rabid. The black bar corresponds to a secondary case on a cat.

February 2004: Morbihan, Brittany

An unidentified French dog, not correctly vaccinated (one injection 4 years previously) travelled by car to Morocco with its owner. While there, it fought with two stray dogs in the north of the country. The dog and owner returned via the Melilla enclave and Spain without any sanitary controls. Once back home, the dog was kept in the owner's house until its death.

- Two animals that had been in contact with the dog were euthanized; both tested negative for rabies. Thirty courses of post-exposure prophylaxis were administered, no cases in humans were recorded.

May 2004: Gironde

An unidentified, unvaccinated puppy, originating from northern Morocco entered France in a car via the Ceuta enclave and Spain without sanitary controls.

- Twenty animals that had been in contact were euthanized; all tested negative for rabies. Twenty courses of post-exposure prophylaxis were administered, no cases in humans were recorded.

Conclusions

Three main preventive measures should be taken to avoid such crises in the future:

- Travellers to countries where rabies is endemic should be informed of the dangers of illegal importation of animals and the risk of eventual human infection. This information should also be made available to tour operators to inform travellers.
- Sanitary and customs controls at European Union borders should be increased and the harmonised European Union regulation (Rule 998/2003) should be strictly enforced, especially in Member States neighbouring countries with enzootic rabies (Maghreb, Near and Middle East).
- Cooperative programmes with countries of the Maghreb for the prevention of rabies and control of dog populations should be developed and reinforced.

Dr. J. Barrat, AFSSA-LERRPAS, Domaine de Pixérécourt, BP 9, FR-54220 Malzéville, France.
E-mail: j.barrat@afssa.fr

Dodet B, Schudel A, Pastoret PP, Lombard M (eds): Rabies in Europe.
Dev Biol (Basel). Basel, Karger, 2006, vol 125, p 101.

SESSION III

Animal Rabies Control

Chairperson: *J. Zmudzinsky* (NVRI, Poland)
Rapporteur: *F. Cliquet* (AFSSA, France)

Dodet B, Schudel A, Pastoret PP, Lombard M (eds): Rabies in Europe.
Dev Biol (Basel). Basel, Karger, 2006, vol 125, pp 103-111.

Control and Prevention of Rabies in Animals: Paradigm Shifts

C.E. Rupprecht[1], *C.A. Hanlon*[1], *D. Slate*[2]

[1] Centers for Disease Control and Prevention, Atlanta, Georgia, USA

[2] United States Department of Agriculture, Animal and Plant Health Inspection Services, Wildlife Services, Concord, New Hampshire, USA

Key words: Rabies, disease prevention, population reduction, animal control.

Abstract: Animal management is the keystone of any modern programme for the prevention and control of rabies. Historically, "animal control" for local elimination of disease was largely equated with population reduction. However, with relatively few exceptions, culling alone has not led to effective control of rabies. In most documented examples of effective control of rabies in the 20th century, an integrated management approach was used that included public education, responsible stewardship of animal populations, manipulation of the population carrying capacity of the local habitat, and vaccination strategies.

Globally, the greatest burden on human health that is attributable to this zoonosis is caused by uncontrolled rabies in dogs. Where political willingness, biomedical infrastructure, and economic stability permit the sustained use of control measures (e.g. stray animal removal and mandatory parenteral vaccination), canine rabies has been significantly suppressed and even eliminated over large geographical areas. Examples include many island nations, most of North America, Europe, and increasingly in South America. Despite the effectiveness of such proven control techniques, however, their implementation in parts of Asia, Africa, and elsewhere has been limited, primarily because of a lack of dedicated resources and intersectoral cooperation, and also because of the burden of high-density populations of dogs. Implementation is often complicated by cultural and social factors, e.g. reluctance to cull apparently ownerless, nuisance animals that are suspected to have been exposed to rabies, partly on the basis of religious beliefs). Attempts to modify animal fertility (such as the encouragement of voluntary spay – neuter programmes or individual chemical contraception, and the extension of such actions to animals in the community) may provide ancillary support in line with other traditional methods of control of canine rabies. With the identification of complex situations in which wildlife rabies persists despite the elimination of canine rabies, e.g. in North America and Europe, cats can pose a significant public health risk requiring consideration of alternative approaches.

In any model system, the threat of translocation of infected animals, unintentional or otherwise, provides a strong rationale for the creation of barriers to prevent reintroduction or exacerbation of the disease, and the maintenance of a minimum body of expertise related to surveillance, diagnosis, and the enactment of mitigating measures. While control activities have traditionally focused upon certain Carnivora species, bats represent another worldwide rabies reservoir. Indiscriminate killing of bats and destruction of roosts was once the norm, but such activities are not sanctioned by reputable organizations today. Even vampire bats, responsible for substantial effects on health and agricultural losses in the New World (Mexico to Argentina), should be targeted only by specific control applications, rather than by more widespread, unconventional, non-specific methodology.

Bats should be excluded from human living quarters. Implementing measures to prevent bats from gaining access to homes should occur at an appropriate time when the bats are absent, especially to avoid sealing the non-flying young within a building. Although great progress has been made during the past four decades in the induction of herd immunity among free-ranging carnivores via oral vaccination against rabies, similar novel solutions have not been readily applied to bat populations. Given these challenges, new paradigm shifts are eagerly anticipated as additional biotechnological applications (including contraceptives and anticoagulants) are developed to deal with domestic animals and wildlife.

Introduction

Since the beginning of its history, *Homo sapiens* has existed as both predator and prey. With the development of direct manipulation of natural resources, and the early domestication of plants and animals, humans began to view other species as serious competitors in need of control. Not long after the direct adaptation and exploitation of domestic animals for food, fur, labour, and companionship, zoonotic disease became an additional element for consideration. As one of the oldest infectious diseases known, rabies has long been an important target for control, even before it was recognized as a virus.

Population reduction

An underlying premise of the use of population reduction as a control strategy is that the spread of rabies is density-dependent, or at least density-related. Therefore, reducing target populations in specific areas to below some theoretical threshold density should limit the opportunity for contact between susceptible animals, such that the disease cannot persist [1]. Social acceptability and economic costs are among several factors that preclude the broad-scale use of population reduction as a practical rabies control strategy. However, population reduction and vaccination are based upon the same theory, that is, that the effective reduction of the number of susceptible individuals in a population to a critical threshold will prevent disease spread, the greater proportion of that population being immunized, or removed, from access to virus.

Carnivores

Oral rabies vaccination has proved to be a powerful anti-rabies tool in Europe, Canada, and the USA [2]. Before the initiation of oral rabies vaccination technology for disease control in meso-carnivores, population reduction was often used as a rabies control strategy in wildlife, particularly in foxes [3] and skunks [4]. Trapping (e.g. using box traps, leg-hold traps, and snares) was often the preferred tactic, probably owing to familiarity with the effectiveness of traditional methods of harvesting fur [1]. Additional methods included shooting, gassing (e.g. sodium nitrate gas cartridge), and other "predacides" (e.g. sodium cyanide, strychnine, sodium fluoroacetate – "Compound 1080") [1,5-8].

Shooting, as well as trapping, was often used in bounty programmes targeting specific carnivores. Bounty programmes have historically produced questionable results and are rarely considered viable in rabies control owing to a myriad of social, technical and legal factors [1].

In the USA, the M44 (sodium cyanide ejector) is the only currently registered predacide that is labelled as being suitable for control of "vectors of...disease" according to the Environmental Protection Agency (EPA) (EPA Reg. No. 56228-15) [9]. This large gas cartridge may be used to target coyotes, foxes and skunks in some areas, but the label does not specify use for rabies or other disease control (EPA Reg. No. 56228-21). Gassing for rabies control has been used extensively in Europe; Wandeler [6] reported gassing to be the single most effective method against fox rabies (assessment before oral rabies vaccination).

Sodium fluoroacetate (Compound 1080) has been reported to be a successful method for the control of canine rabies in stray dogs and coyotes in Baja California [10] and to assist in the control of rabies in stray dogs and cats on Guam [11]. In the USA, use of Compound 1080 in "bait stations" to target coyotes on winter rangelands was banned by executive order in 1972, and its use is now restricted to livestock protection collars targeting specific coyotes (EPA Reg. No. 56228-22), a formulation of no value for population reduction in the USA [12].

In the 1960s, strychnine-tallow baits were used in some eastern states of the USA to reduce fox populations in areas where there had been outbreaks of rabies [13]. The relative success of this programme is not well documented. All above-ground use of strychnine was banned in the USA in 1986 [14]. However, strychnine was used with reported success in egg baits integrated with trapping to target striped skunks for rabies control in Alberta, Canada [4].

In Canada, population reduction of raccoons may be credited with contributing to the success in an integrated "point infection control" programme; this programme included intensive trapping and removal in a core outbreak area, surrounded by a contour treatment of trap – vaccinate – release, all overlaid with oral rabies vaccination [15]. However, as with any integrated programme, it is often difficult to isolate the weighted contribution of individual strategy components.

Bats

There are no published accounts of use of concerted, broad-scale efforts to suppress insectivorous bat populations as a rabies control strategy. Nevertheless, with special permission dichloro-diphenyl-dichloroethane (DDT) was approved as a toxicant for control of rabies in bats, in response to demonstrable public health hazards in the USA [16]. The EPA registration for this use was withdrawn in 1987 [16] in response to its debatable effectiveness, particularly when balanced against concerns about the environment and human exposure [17]. EPA registrations for special local needs were also in place for use of the anticoagulant chlorophacione for "nuisance bat control" in 17 states [16]. When used as a tracking powder, this formulation was ineffective in reducing populations, despite heavy applications in bat-occupied dwellings targeted for treatment, and the manufacturer withdrew all of its 24C registrations out of "concern" for endangered bat species in 1991 [16]. Judicious application of exclosure practices have historically been effective and remain the preferred alternative to population reduction to minimize contact between humans and bats.

The use of anticoagulants, either by systemic treatment of susceptible cattle with diphenadione, or topical application (chlorophacione or diphacinone [diphenadione]) to vampire bats (*Desmodus rotundus*) has been shown to be effective in reducing the threat of rabies transmission by vampire bats feeding on livestock in Mexico [18-20]. Methods involving anticoagulants are considered to be much more selective [21] than previously applied lethal methods that included dynamiting [22], gassing [23], placement of strychnine at vampire bat sites and mist netting/killing [24], cave entrance traps/killing [25], or fire arms and clubs [26]. Not only do these lethal methods indiscriminately jeopardize non-target species of bats that may roost in the same caves as vampire bats, but they may also not target the correct species of vampire bat. Although anticoagulants can be effective in reducing the threat of rabies associated with target populations of vampires [27], there has been no extensive, coordinated application of these approaches to measurably reduce the impact of rabies from vampire bats over broad geographical areas of Latin America [28].

Fertility control

Interest in oral contraception as a means to suppress populations of coyotes causing livestock depredations in the western USA and populations of red foxes responsible for the spread of rabies in the eastern USA can be traced to the early 1960s. An early candidate for testing was the reproductive inhibitor diethylstilbestrol, which was abandoned because it was not safe, effective, or long-lasting, and lacked effective delivery systems [29]. Today, contraception continues to receive attention as a prospective means of controlling wildlife populations, with much of the focus on immunocontraceptives and effective delivery systems [30]. If effective contraceptive vaccines become available, they may be applied in tandem with oral rabies vaccine in specific instances to achieve the objectives of population and rabies management.

Veterinary focus

Generations of domesticated animals have lived in the care of humans. Responsibility for these animals should not be abandoned, especially when considering the implications of disease. The following long-standing veterinary public health recommendations should be implemented in the prevention and control of rabies [31]. Primary rabies vaccination should be mandatory. Ideally, pets should be well supervised, to prevent exposure. Pets and livestock should be examined daily for obvious wounds. If wounds arc observed, appropriate first aid (i.e. cleansing with soap and water) is warranted, and the need for a rabies vaccine booster should be considered, depending upon circumstances. Although modern cell-culture vaccines are extremely potent, a vaccinated animal should receive a booster dose and be observed closely for 45 days after a potential exposure to a rabid or suspect animal. An unvaccinated animal should be euthanized or quarantined for six months after a potential exposure.

Dogs

The global burden of rabies arises from sustained transmission among domestic dogs, mainly in Asia and Africa. Historically, strong efforts directed towards the control and vaccination of stray dogs have eliminated the canine rabies virus variant in island nations such as Japan and the United Kingdom, and in broad geographical areas such as western Europe, North America and, more recently, throughout South America, where tremendous progress has been made [32]. In a subsequent juxtaposition, vaccination of dogs in the USA remains important, not as a means for rabies control among a reservoir population, but to prevent spill-over of rabies from the now predominant wildlife reservoirs (i.e. raccoons, skunks, foxes, bats) to individual dogs [33]. More importantly, maintaining the vaccination of dog populations, even with moderate rates of compliance, is an important safeguard against the re-introduction of a canine rabies virus variant by translocation.

In areas of the world where canine rabies remains uncontrolled, new measures are needed. Major hurdles to the control and elimination of canine rabies in these areas is the high density and rapid turnover of the dog population. Fertility control through traditional measures such as surgical or hormonal neutering is a powerful adjunct to vaccination. Novel methods are needed by which these principles can be applied to ownerless, free-ranging dogs, with greater community participation [34]. Research efforts are directed toward the development of combined potent, safe oral vaccines against rabies and oral immunocontraceptives that could be delivered in baits.

Cats

Cats are susceptible to rabies and capable of shedding rabies virus during the clinical period, although to date there has been no suggestion from laboratory or epizootiological studies that a rabies virus variant that is specifically adapted for successful sustained transmission among either domestic or wild felidae has emerged. In the USA, cases of rabies in domestic cats have consistently outnumbered cases in dogs since the early 1980s. During the past decade, more than twice as many rabid cats as rabid dogs have been reported in the USA [33]. Moreover, perhaps owing to the somewhat higher likelihood of a furious clinical presentation and possibly a lower index of suspicion of rabies, data from pilot studies of trends in humans after exposure suggest that rabid cats expose more humans to the risk of rabies per infected animal than do rabid dogs. Partly because of these considerations, the modern view of animal rabies control strongly supports the vaccination of cats, even those ostensibly maintained indoors. While continuing concerns about potential rabies vaccine-associated sarcomas in cats may discourage broad coverage of the domestic cat population, prevention of rabies provides a persuasive benefit [35]. Another complex issue is the maintenance of feral cat colonies through humane efforts to control disease and proliferation by trapping, vaccinating, and neutering. These efforts, while compassionate towards the colony population, do not directly address the problem of free-ranging feral domestic animals with regard to humane considerations for the individual cats, substantial effects of feline predation upon local wildlife, or long-term public health benefits.

International and Regional Translocation

Global travel increasingly includes domestic pets. Guidelines and regulations to prevent the introduction of exogenous infectious diseases exist, but vary according to country and region. Although health examination and certification are required for importation into the USA, this is insufficient to prevent a number of infectious diseases, including the potential introduction of a canine rabies virus variant or other exogenous variant, owing to naturally variable and potentially long incubation periods, as well as exemptions for rabies vaccination of young animals because of potentially inadequate responses if maternal antibodies are present. The threat of introduction is demonstrated by the example of a puppy that was imported in 2004 from Thailand and that became sick during travel and died of rabies within hours of arriving in the USA, and of another young dog imported from Puerto Rico that became rabid shortly after arrival in the USA. The importation of dogs from Puerto Rico continues as part of an organized dog rescue effort. Other international incidents have included the importation into France of a young dog that developed rabies associated with its country of origin, Morocco, as well as an infected North African bat from Belgium to France.

Local Translocation

Translocation of wildlife has contributed to one of the most intense rabies epizootics on record, the initiation of a mid-Atlantic focus of raccoon rabies caused by infected animals moved from a historical focus in the south-eastern USA [33]. Similar activities with coyotes and foxes from Texas that were released into enclosures for hunting have led to cases of rabies among hunting dogs. Even relatively local translocation of rabies reservoir species has the capacity to foil extensive control efforts if such translocation takes place in the vicinity of programmes for oral vaccination against rabies in wildlife. The international movement of wildlife is more highly regulated for some species than for others, but major oversights have occurred, such as the importation of raccoons from the USA into "rabies-free" Japan for the exotic pet trade, apparently leading to the establishment of free-ranging populations.

Infrastructure

The prevention and control of rabies is not just the function of a single government department, but increasingly requires the cooperation of community stakeholders [36]. As for many zoonoses, the control and prevention of rabies requires the cooperation of public health professionals, animal control personnel, veterinarians, laboratory personnel, physicians, and others. Responsibilities start locally and at the state level with health, animal control, law enforcement, and environmental conservation or natural resource agency personnel. Regulations for control are often antiquated. In the USA, for example, dog wardens or animal control officers were established locally in the 1950s and 1960s for the control of stray dogs and to check the compliance of registration and vaccination of owned dogs. With most cases now occurring in a range of wildlife species, locally-supported animal control officers should be trained and authorized to deal with situations involving a variety of domestic and wildlife species, not just dogs, or dogs and cats.

Surveillance Needs

Comprehensive prevention involves health education and access to data on contemporary cases. To this end, a real-time geographical information system (GIS) internet-based mapping tool (RabID) is being developed at the Centers for Disease Control and Prevention (CDC), to display rabies case data (and negative samples to reflect surveillance). With a GIS base, the spatiotemporal patterns of rabies may be analysed in relation to specific land features that affect the density and distribution of wildlife reservoir populations, to obtain a better understanding of environmental factors that would contribute to more effective prevention strategies. For example, such a tool may be used for designing the aerial distribution of vaccine-laden baits, taking account of potential barriers such as waterways and mountain ranges. It is also a powerful model for application to other infectious diseases and conditions that vary spatiotemporally and are influenced by particular environmental and geographical features.

Conclusions

Restricted and targeted population reduction or culling may have some role in rabies control, particularly when integrated into oral vaccination programmes in selective settings, such as parks and other green spaces, especially in a suburban – rural interface where high densities of some carnivores may exist [37-40]. Some researchers have suggested that local reduction may be an integral component in a variety of contingency actions to contain emerging rabies foci [15]. The judicious incorporation of population reduction into rabies oral vaccination efforts probably depends on many factors, but most important is the effectiveness of the vaccine and of baits for delivery to the target species. Access to highly effective parenteral and oral vaccines and baits may minimize the need for population reduction. Where practical, population reduction should be conducted in tandem with reduction of the local carrying capacity, to limit the potential of habitats to support high-density populations of the target carnivore. Most important among these tactics are reducing access to food subsidies through unintentional (e.g. household waste, outdoor or accessible pet feeders) or purposeful feeding. Contraception for free-ranging wildlife should not be discounted as a potential future tool for integration into rabies control strategies.

Acknowledgements

The authors thank the laboratory and field staff of their respective organizations, and their professional colleagues in the local, regional and international health and agricultural sectors for their expertise and continuing efforts. Thanks to these efforts, animal rabies prevention and control activities directly benefit public heath, and serve as realistic models for other zoonotic disease programmes.

References

1 Debbie JG: Rabies control of terrestrial wildlife by population reduction, in Baer GM (ed): The Natural History of Rabies. 2nd ed Boca Raton, FL CRC Press Inc, 1991, pp 477-489.

2 Slate D, Rupprecht CE, Rooney JA, Donovan D, Lein DH, Chipman RB: Status of oral rabies vaccination in wild carnivores in the United States. Virus Res 2005; 111 (1): 68-76.

3 Linhart SB: Rabies in wildlife and control methods in New York State. NY Fish Game J 1960; 7: 1.

4 Pybus MJ: Rabies and rabies control in striped skunks (*Mephitis mephitis*) in three prairie regions of western North America. J Wildl Dis 1988; 24: 434-449.

5 Trainer DO: Rabies and rabies control in Wisconsin, in Proc Natl Rabies Symp, Centers for Disease Control, Atlanta, GA, 1966, 121 p.

6 Wandeler A, Wachendorfer G, Schale G, Forster I, Steck F: Rabies in wild carnivores in central Europe. III. Ecology and biology of the fox in relation to control operations, Zentralbl Veterinaermed Reihe B 1974; 21: 765.

7 Aubert M. Epidemiology of Fox Rabies, in Bogel K, Meslin FX, Kaplan M (eds): Wildlife Rabies Control, Wells Medical Ltd, Kent, 1992, pp 9-18.

8 Hanlon CA, Childs JE, Nettles VF, the National Working Group on Rabies Prevention and Control: Recommendations of a national working group on prevention and control of rabies in the United States. Article III. Rabies in Wildlife. J Am Vet Med Assoc 1999; 215: 1612-1619.

9 Connolly G: A history of toxicant ejectors in coyote control, in Timm RM, Schmidt RH (eds): Proceedings of the 20th Vertebrate Pest Conference, Univ California, Davis, 2002, pp 201-218.

10 Cocozza J, Alba AM: Wildlife control project in Baja California. Public Health Reports 1962; 77: 147-151.

11 Glosser JW, Yarnell EP: Rabies control on Guam. Public Health Reports 1970; 85: 1113-1120.

12 Connolly G: Development and use of Compound 1080 in coyote control, 1944-1972, in Timm RM, Gorenzel WP (eds): Proceedings of the 21th Vertebrate Pest Conference, Univ. California, Davis, 2004, pp 221-239.

13 Gramlich FJ: Annual Report, Division of Wildlife Services, Maine. Bureau of Sport Fisheries and Wildlife, Augusta, ME, 1968, 11 p.

14 United States Environmental Protection Agency. Registration eligibility decision (RED) – Strychnine. EPA 738-R-96-33, July 1996, 135 p.

15 Rosatte RC, Donovan D, Allan M, Howes L, Silver A, Bennett K, MacInnes C, Davies C, Wandeler A, Radford B: Emergency response to raccoon rabies introduction in Ontario. J Wildl Dis 2001; 37: 265-279.

16 Brass DA: Rabies in bats, natural history and public health implications. Livia Press, Ridgefield, CT, 1994.

17 Trimarchi CV, Debbie JG: Report on the Northeastern Symposium on bat rabies management, in Wilson DE, Gardner AL (eds): Proceedings of the 5th International Bat Research Conference. Texas Tech Press, Lubbock, TX, 1980, pp 213-216.

18 Greenhall AM: Vampire bat control: A review and proposed research programme for Latin America. Proc. 4th Vert Pest Conf 1970; 4: 41-54.

19 Thompson RD, Mitchell GC, Burns RJ: Vampire bat control by systemic treatment of livestock with an anticoagulant. Science 1972; 177: 806-808.

20 Linhart SB, Crespo RF, Mitchell GC: Control of vampire bats by topical application of an anticoagulant, chlorophacinone. Bol of Sant Panam 1972; 6: 31-38.

21 Mitchell GC: Vampire bat control in Latin America. In Committee on the Applications of Ecological Theory to Environmental Problems, Commission on Life Sciences, National Research Council, editor. Ecological Knowledge and Environmental Problem-Solving, Concepts and Case Studies. Washington, DC, National Academy Press, 1986, pp 151-164.

22 Villa RB: The ecology and biology of vampire bats and their relationship to paralytic rabies. Report to the Government of Brazil. Rep. No. TA 2656. U.N. Development Programme/Food and Agriculture Organization. Rome, 1969.

23 Arteche E: Rabia en Rio Grande do Sul Brazil. Zoonosis 1969; 11: 34-35.

24 Greenhall AM: Use of mist nets and strychnine for vampire bat control in Trinidad. J Mammal 1963; 44: 396-399.

25 Constantine DG: Portable trap for vampire bats used in rabies control campaigns. Bol of Sant Panam 1969; 67: 39-42.

26 Constantine DG: Bats in relation to health, welfare, and economy of man, in Wimsatt WA (ed): Biology of Bats. Academic Press, 1970, vol 2, pp 319-449.

27 Piccinini RS: The use of diphenadione (2-diphenylacetyl-1,3 indandione) for vampire bat control in endemic rabies areas, Northeastern Brazil. MS Thesis, Univ CA, Davis, 1977.

28 Lord RD: Control of vampire bats, in Greenhall AM, Schmidt U (eds): Natural History of Vampire Bats. Boca Raton, FL, CRC Press Inc, 1988, pp 215-226.

29 Linhart SB: Acceptance by wild foxes of certain baits for administering antifertility agents. NY Fish Game J 1964; 11: 69-77.

30 United States Department of Agriculture: Contraception in wildlife. Animal and Plant Health Inspection Service. Technical Bulletin 1853, 1997, 272 p.

31 Centers for Disease Control: Compendium of animal rabies prevention and control, 2005: National Association of State Public Health Veterinarians, Inc (NASPHV). MMWR 2005; 54 (N°RR-3): 1-7.

32 Belotto A, Leanes LF, Schneider MC, Tamayo H, Correa E: Overview of rabies in the Americas. Virus Res 2005; 111 (1): 5-12.

33 Krebs JW, Mandel EJ, Swerdlow DL, Rupprecht CE: Rabies surveillance in the United States during 2003. J Am Vet Med Assoc 2004; 225 (12): 1837-1849.

34 Wilde H, Khawplod P, Khamoltham T, Hemachudha T, Tepsumethanon V, Lumlerdacha B, Mitmoonpitak C, Sitprija V: Rabies control in South and Southeast Asia. Vaccine 2005; 23 (17-18): 2284-2289.

35 Hauck M: Feline injection site sarcomas. Vet Clin North Am Small Anim Pract 2003; 33 (3): 553-557, vii.

36 Sintunawa C, Wacharapluesadee S, Wilde H, Hemachudha T: Paradigm shift in rabies control: a system approach. J Med Assoc Thai 2004; 87 (12): 1530-1538.

37 Schinner and Cauley: The ecology of urban raccoons in Cincinnati, Ohio, in Noyes JH, Progulske DR (eds): Wildlife in an Urbanizing Environment. Planning and Resource Development Series No. 28, Holdsworth Natural Resource Center, Amherst, MA, 1974, pp 125-130.

38 Hoffman CO, Gottschang JL: Numbers, distribution, and movements of a raccoon population in a suburban residential community. J Mammal 1997; 58: 623-336.

39 Riley SPD, Hadidian J, Manski DA: Population density, survival, and rabies in raccoons in an urban national park. Can J Zoology 1998; 76: 1153-1164.

40 Prange S, Gehrt SD, Wiggers EP: Demographic factors contributing to high raccoon densities in urban landscapes. J Wildl Manage 2003; 67: 324-333.

Dr. C.E. Rupprecht, Centers for Disease Control & Prevention, 1600 Clifton Rd., MS G33, Atlanta, GA 30333, USA.
E-mail: cyr5@cdc.gov

Dodet B, Schudel A, Pastoret PP, Lombard M (eds): Rabies in Europe.
Dev Biol (Basel). Basel, Karger, 2006, vol 125, pp 113-118.

Wildlife Rabies Control Policy in Great Britain

G.C. Smith[1], *A.R. Fooks*[2]

1 Central Science Laboratory, Sand Hutton, York, UK
2 Veterinary Laboratory Agency, New Haw, Addlestone, Surrey, UK

Abstract: Following the outbreak of foot-and-mouth disease in the United Kingdom (UK) in 2001, the British government initiated a review and update of the Rabies Contingency Plan to ensure that the implementation of control policies was proportionate and based on operational efficiency and appropriate command structures (see http://www.defra.gov.uk/animalh/rabies/default.htm). Control of classical rabies in wildlife will primarily be based on emergency oral vaccination around the focal outbreak, in line with European recommended practice. However, theoretical and practical experience suggests that vaccination may not be the most effective means of control in high-density populations of foxes. In this scenario, and when the primary case has been identified, vaccination may be supplemented by culling in some circumstances. The theoretical basis for this will be discussed. In the event of an outbreak of rabies in wildlife, the government's control strategy will be supported by output from computer models, which will simulate various control strategies to optimise methods and areas of control, and human resources.

INTRODUCTION

Diseases with symptoms suggestive of rabies have been recorded since antiquity, and legal texts dealing with the control of domestic dogs existed in the Mesopotamian and Persian empires [1]. However, references to cases of rabies in wildlife are more recent – in the 1st century AD in Greece and the 5th century AD in Turkey [1]. The earliest reference to a wildlife reservoir host in Europe is in the 18th century in wolves and in the early 19th century in foxes in Germany and Switzerland [1]. In Russia, given the low density of the human and thus the dog population, the presence of a wildlife reservoir for rabies during the Middle Ages seems more certain [2].

Within Great Britain (GB), laws authorising "rabid" dogs to be killed date back about 1000 years [1]. There are frequent records of urban (dog) rabies over the centuries, but there are only two records of human rabies caused by foxes (one in the late 17th century and another in the early 18th century [3]) and both may be attributable to foxes kept as pets. Two outbreaks of rabies were also recorded in deer parks in the 19th century [4]. This appears to be the extent of the evidence for wildlife rabies in Britain.

GB Government Policy

After an increase in the number of recorded cases of rabies in the late 19th century, a "General Rabies Order" was passed in 1897. Powers to muzzle dogs were enforced and a quarantine of 3 (later 6) months was established for imported dogs [1]. Since 1901, GB has relied on the quarantine of imported dogs, cats and other mammals to protect the country from rabies. GB became free of rabies in 1902 and remained free until servicemen returning after the First World War smuggled infected dogs into the country in 1918. The disease was eradicated in 1922 after the imposition of rigorous restrictions and the destruction of stray dogs. Between 1922 and 1969, 27 cases of rabies occurred in quarantine [4]. In 1969, and again in 1970, dogs suffered from rabies after being released from quarantine [5,6]. In the case in 1969, the dog had shown initial signs 10 days after release from quarantine, it had been exercised on public land and was known to have been rabid while at large. Subsequently, all susceptible wildlife in the immediate area were shot or poisoned. A government report recommended the continuation of quarantine and the use of "intensive control by gassing, trapping or poisoning", but not shooting, within 12 miles (19 km) of an outbreak in wildlife, and additional reduction of the fox population in a further 12 miles radius.

Rabies may only be controlled if the authorities responsible have the necessary statutory powers to effect control measures. Powers to control rabies are set out in the Rabies Control Order 1974 made under the Animal Health Act 1981, the enabling legislation. The definition of "animal" in the Control Order brings a wide range of species within its ambit and has the following powers, outlined below:

1. Statutory notification to the authorities if disease is suspected.
2. Seizure, investigation, isolation or destruction of suspect cases.
3. Confirmation of disease.
4. Declaration of an infected place (IP) and control movements into and out of it.
5. Confining, control, seizure, isolation, or destruction of contact animals.
6. The leashing of cats, and leashing and muzzling of dogs during exercise in a public place.
7. Vaccination.
8. Declaration of an infected area (IA).
9. Control animal movements into and out of the IA.
10. Prohibition or placing of conditions on gatherings of animals in an IA.
11. Prohibition of any form of hunting or shooting in an IA.
12. Seizure of stray animals and destruction of unclaimed stray animals in the IA
13. Control of wildlife by destruction in the IA.
14. Vaccination and identification of vaccinated dogs and cats in the IA.
15. Control of deliberate feeding of wildlife and access of wildlife to waste food.

In the unlikely event that powers to exercise control are found to be insufficient in a future outbreak, additional powers will be sought under the Animal Health Act 1981 (as amended). Consequently, the Rabies Control Order 1974 authorises an IA to be declared within which foxes, and other wildlife as required, could be destroyed.

Since this period, the British government has maintained a contingency plan for rabies in wildlife, which has been regularly reviewed and updated. It details the strategy for the eradication of rabies in wildlife by the distribution of poison baits and gassing of fox dens. The British government planned to control foxes by the distribution of poison baits within alternate 1 km National Grid squares from an Ordnance Survey map within a radius of 19 km from the point of infection, as described by Meldrum [7]. Bait-points would be identified on a circular walk within each chosen square kilometre and pre-baited chicken heads lightly buried under turf or soil. Each day, baits that had been removed would be replaced and after 7-10 days, all baits would be replaced by 1-day-old chicks containing strychnine sulphate [7]. After a maximum of 4 days, remaining poison baits would be recovered; the poison-baiting operation may be repeated two to three times. By the early 1990s, gassing was withdrawn from the plan and vaccination was to be considered if the focal outbreak was not contained.

During the 1980s, the widespread distribution of vaccine baits for foxes began in Europe [8], and by the mid 1990s it was evident that this strategy was successful and that vaccination could eradicate endemic rabies in wildlife [9]. These events catalysed a need for change. Another government report [10] recommended the use of microchips and vaccination of domestic animals to replace quarantine for importation from specified countries. This was enacted in February 2000, initially under the Pet Travel Scheme (Pilot Arrangements) (England) Order 1999, with the creation of the Pet Travel Scheme Non-Commercial Movement of Pet Animals (PETS) for a limited number of qualifying countries – 22 at that time. The European Community regulation on the Non-Commercial Movement of Pet Animals, July 1998/2003 is directly applicable in the UK and has been applied since 2004. The list of qualifying countries and territories has since increased to 89 [11].

Following the outbreak of foot-and-mouth disease in Britain in 2001, the British government initiated a review and update of the Rabies Contingency Plan to ensure that the implementation of control policies was proportionate and based on operational efficiency and appropriate command structures. Control of rabies in wildlife will now primarily be based on emergency vaccination around the focal outbreak, in line with European recommended practice [12]. However, focal control using poisons may still be recommended in limited circumstances when the location and timing of the index case is known. A replacement, carbamate-based poison bait formulation, which is more humane than strychnine sulphate, has been developed and tested in the field. It has been shown that neither compound interferes with the diagnosis of rabies [13].

Current GB plans were made available on the Internet in late 2004 [14] and were subject to a period of public consultation. These plans detail the local and national operational structures that will be adopted in a disease-related emergency, the actions to be taken on finding a suspect case, and the resources that will be called upon if the plan is extended as the outbreak develops. A computer simulation of the spread and control of rabies was produced to help define an infected area within which wildlife control would take place. The program has been maintained and updated by the Central Science Laboratory since 1990. The disease control strategy

[15] includes up-to-date details about laboratory confirmation of infection with rabies virus, the virus being genotyped and the strain determined. The response will then depend on the strain of rabies (i.e. whether it is wildlife-adapted), the potential involvement of other species (e.g. badger *Meles meles* or bats) and the history of the case. Available evidence suggests that the badger does not respond as well as foxes to oral rabies vaccine [16], so should control of badgers be required, it would at the present time be restricted to poisoning. Control of bats is only likely if the rabies virus involved is not a European bat lyssavirus (EBLV), the disease outbreak is spatially restricted and eradication is a realistic possibility.

Scientific Support for Policy

In the years before the widespread use and success of oral rabies vaccines in Europe, culling was the only means of fox control. Although in general unable to substantially affect endemic rabies, culling has been shown to control the spread of rabies when such spread is restricted in area [17-19]. The main potential problem for the eradication of rabies in the UK was perceived to be the high density of the fox population in some urban areas [20] combined with the low level of bait uptake [21], which would necessitate repeated baiting operations. A computer simulation model was constructed to investigate fox control in urban areas [20,22]. This predicted that the high density of the fox population in urban areas would lead to an enhanced epizootic, potentially killing about 99 % of all foxes locally, but also that insufficient control would lead to a longer, smouldering enzootic outbreak [22]. This effect on disease dynamics may be responsible for the poor control of rabies achieved in parts of Europe [23].

In the early 1990s, the fox/rabies model was used to investigate poisoning, vaccination and ring vaccination (central poisoning with a ring of vaccine baits) around focal outbreaks. This determined that vaccination could replace poisoning when the density of the fox population was low, and that ring vaccination could replace poisoning at higher fox-population densities [24]. A later analysis demonstrated that as the density of the fox population increased, the use of vaccination became less and less successful when compared with culling, and that the efficacy of vaccination varied seasonally [25]. There may also be a seasonal variability in the efficacy of vaccination due to the presence of maternal antibodies to rabies in fox cubs [26]. By using the simulation model described above and a simple mathematical model [27], it was shown that the main reason for this reduction in the efficacy of vaccination as host population density increased was the seasonal birth of young, which sufficiently increased the density of animals susceptible to infection such that the epizootic was allowed to continue.

There is concern in Europe that after the recent increase in fox density, vaccination may be insufficient to eradicate rabies [28] and focal culling may be beneficial [29]. Focal trap-and-cull techniques, with a ring of trap-and-vaccinate, have been used successfully to control rabies in raccoons [30].

The badger *Meles meles* was the only other wildlife species to be substantially affected by the rabies epizootic in Europe; badger density in some parts of the UK may be an order of magnitude higher than that in Europe, so it may be necessary to control the badger in these regions [16]. Since the available evidence suggests that badgers do not respond as well as foxes to oral rabies vaccine [16], if control of badgers were required, it would at the present time be restricted to poisoning.

Reduction of bat populations has been carried out extensively in South America because of the economic losses attributable to rabies transmitted by vampire bats; however, this has not led to any sustained reduction in the incidence of rabies in cattle [31]. Despite this, a reduction in the population of vampire bats is still recommended by some scientists [32]. Although not yet employed in the field, the use of vaccines to protect bats against rabies is possible [33]. However, the only currently available means of control is still population reduction, and this may be warranted in limited circumstances if a focal outbreak of an exotic (non-EBLV) lyssavirus was discovered.

Conclusion

Although the UK government has been considering the use of vaccination to eradicate outbreaks of rabies for 10 years, vaccination is now stated as the main method of control in the revised and updated contingency plan of 2005. The use of focal culling has been shown to have advantages where the density of the host population is high, and when the cause of a focal infection is known; focal culling of foxes could thus be recommended at high population densities. This may have implications for rabies control in European countries as a result of an increase in fox population densities following eradication of rabies.

Acknowledgements

The authors would like to thank the UK Department for Food Environment and Rural Affairs (Defra) for funding and John Woods for comments on the manuscript.

References

1 Blancou J: Rabies in Europe and the Mediterranean basin: from antiquity to the 19th Century, in King AA, Fooks AR, Aubert M, Wandeler AI (eds): Historical perspectives of rabies in Europe and the Mediterranean basin. Paris, OIE, 2004, pp 15-24.

2 Botvinkin A, Kosenko M: Rabies in the European parts of Russia, Belarus and Ukraine, in King AA, Fooks AR, Aubert M, Wandeler AI (eds): Historical perspectives of rabies in Europe and the Mediterranean basin. Paris, OIE, 2004, pp 47-63.

3 Lloyd HG: The red fox. London, Batsford, 1980.

4 Fooks AR, Roberts DH, Lynch M, Hersteinsson P, Runolfsson H: Rabies in the United Kingdom, Ireland and Iceland, in King AA, Fooks AR, Aubert M, Wandeler AI (eds): Historical perspectives of rabies in Europe and the Mediterranean basin. Paris, OIE, 2004, pp 25-32.

5 Loxam JG: A case of canine rabies in Newmarket. State Vet J 1970; 25: 195-199.

6 Hendrie EW, Westcott EJ: The Camberley case of rabies. State Veterinary Journal 1970; 25: 186-192.

7 Meldrum KC: Rabies contingency plans in the United Kingdom. Parassitologia 1988; 30: 97-103.

8 Flamand A, Coulon P, Lafay F, Kappeler A, Artois M, Blancou J, et al: Eradication of rabies in Europe. Nature 1992; 360: 115-116.

9 Stöhr K, Meslin FX: Progress and setbacks in the oral immunisation of foxes against rabies in Europe. Vet Rec 1996; 139 (2): 32-35.

10 Kennedy I, Aubert M, Bannister B, DeVile P, Dye C, Higgins A, et al: Quarantine & Rabies: A reappraisal. London, MAFF Publications, 1998.

11 http://www.defra.gov.uk/animalh/quarantine/pets/territory.htm.

12 European Commission. The oral vaccination of foxes against rabies, 23 October 2002. Report No.: Report of the Scientific Committee on Animal Health and Animal Welfare, 2002.

13 McElhinney LM, Parsons G, Nadian A, Lowings JP, Fooks AR: Rabies diagnosis in the presence of strychnine and carbamate. Vet Rec 2004; 155: 303-304.

14 http://www.defra.gov.uk/corporate/consult/rabies-plan/index.htm.

15 http://www.defra.gov.uk/corporate/consult/rabies-plan/discontrolstrat.pdf.

16 Smith GC: The role of the badger (*Meles meles*) in rabies epizootiology and the implications for Great Britain. Mammal Review 2002; 32 (1): 13-26.

17 Irsara A, Ruatti A, Gagliardi G, Orfei Z, Bellani L, Mantouani A: Control of wildlife rabies in north-eastern Italy. Comp Immunol Microbiol Infect Dis1982; 5: 327-335.

18 Müller J: The effect of fox reduction on the occurrence of rabies. Observations from two outbreaks of rabies in Denmark. Bulletin. l'Office International des Épizooties 1971; 75 (9-10): 7673-7776.

19 Westergaard JM: Measures applied in Denmark to control the rabies epizootic in 1977-1980. Comp Immunol Microbiol Infect Dis 1982; 5: 383-387.

20 Smith GC, Harris S: Rabies in urban foxes (*Vulpes vulpes*) in Britain: the use of a spatial stochastic simulation model to examine the pattern of spread and evaluate the efficacy of different control regimes. Philosophical Transactions of the Royal Society of London B 1991; 334: 459-479.

21 Trewhella WJ, Harris S, Smith GC, Nadian AK: A field trial evaluating bait uptake by an urban fox (*Vulpes vulpes*) population. J Appl Ecology 1991; 28 (2): 454-466.

22 Smith GC, Harris S: The control of rabies in urban fox populations, in Putman RJ (ed): Mammals as Pests. London, Chapman & Hall, 1989, pp 209-224.

23 Aubert M: Control of rabies in foxes: what are the appropriate measures? Veterinary Record 1994; 134: 55-59.

24 Smith GC: Modelling rabies control in the U.K.: the inclusion of vaccination. Mammalia 1995; 59: 629-637.

25 Smith GC, Wilkinson D: Modelling control of rabies outbreaks in red fox populations to evaluate culling, vaccination, and vaccination combined with fertility control. Journal of Wildlife Diseases 2003; 39 (2): 278-286.

26 Vos A, Muller T, Selhorst T, Schuster P, Neubert A, Schluter H: Optimising spring oral vaccination campaigns of foxes against rabies. Deutsche Tieräztliche Wochenschrift 2001; 108 (2): 55-59.

27 Smith GC, Cheeseman CL: The control of diseases in wildlife populations: culling, vaccine and fertility control. Ecological Modelling 2002; 150 (1-2): 45-53.

28 Chautan M, Pontier D, Artois M: Role of rabies in recent demographic changes in red fox (*Vulpes vulpes*) populations in Europe. Mammalia 2000; 64 (4): 391-410.

29 Johnston DH, Tinline RR: Rabies control in wildlife, in Jackson AC, Wunner WH (eds): Rabies. Boston, Academic Press, 2002, pp 445-471.

30 Rosatte RC, Donovan D, Allan M, Howes LA, Silver A, Bennett K, et al: Emergency response to raccoon rabies introduction into Ontario. J Wildl Diseases 2001; 37 (2): 265-279.

31 Mayen F: Haematophagous bats in Brazil, their role in rabies transmission, impact on public health, livestock industry and alternatives to an indiscriminate reduction of bat population. Journal of Veterinary Medicine B 2003; 50: 469-472.

32 Delpietro HA, Russo RG: Ecological and epidemiological aspects of attacks by vampire bats in relation to paralytic rabies in Argentina, and an analysis of proposals for control. Revue Scientifique et Technique de l'Office International des Epizooties 1996; 15 (3): 971-984.

33 Aguilar-Setién A, Campos YL, Cruz ET, Kretschmer R, Brochier B, Pastoret PP: Vaccination of vampire bats using recombinant Vaccinia-rabies virus. Journal of Wildlife Diseases 2002; 38 (3): 539-544.

Dr. G.C. Smith, Central Science Laboratory, Sand Hutton, York, YO41 1LZ, UK
E-mail: g.smith@csl.gov.uk

Dodet B, Schudel A, Pastoret PP, Lombard M (eds): Rabies in Europe.
Dev Biol (Basel). Basel, Karger, 2006, vol 125, pp 119-126.

Means Used for Terrestrial Rabies Elimination in France and Policy for Rabies Surveillance in Case of Re-emergence

F. Cliquet[1], B. Combes[2], J. Barrat[1]

[1] WHO Collaborating Centre for Research and Management in Zoonoses Control, OIE Reference Laboratory for Rabies, Community Reference Laboratory for Rabies Serology, AFSSA, Malzéville, France

[2] Entente interdépartementale de lutte contre la rage et autres zoonoses, Malzéville, France

The authors wish to thank several people who were or still are involved in rabies control in France: M. Aubert from AFSSA Sophia Antipolis, France, J. Blancou, L. Andral†, E. Masson†, P. Vuillaume from Entente Interdépartementale de Lutte contre la Rage et autres Zoonoses, Malzéville, France, Marc Artois from the Ecole Nationale Vétérinaire de Lyon, Marcy l'Etoile.

Abstract: In France, the first case of wildlife rabies was detected in 1968, with the red fox (Vulpes vulpes) as reservoir and vector of terrestrial rabies. The last case was reported at the end of 1998. The maximum infected area amounted to 140,000 km² in 1989 with a record number of 4,213 infected wild and domestic animals. The contaminated areas included various landscapes such as low populated farming areas and low mountainous areas as well as very densely populated areas and industrial areas contiguously urbanised.
Oral vaccination of wildlife against rabies was implemented in 1986 and 1987 on limited areas treated by hand distribution and then helicopter distribution was implemented in 1988. The control of wildlife rabies was centralised at the country level in one institute for elaboration of baiting strategies, rabies surveillance network, laboratory investigations such as tetracycline and serological testing, vaccine titration and rabies diagnosis.
Oral vaccination campaigns were organised in spring and in autumn by dropping annually 40 baits/km². The following vaccine baits were used: SAD B19 from 1986 to 1992, SAG1/SAG2 from 1990 to 2003 and VRG from 1989 to 2003.

This paper is dedicated to the memory of Drs Louis Andral and Eric Masson. Dr Andral was the first director of the laboratory of research on rabies and wildlife diseases in Malzéville (France) and he initiated the first studies for the development of oral vaccines against rabies. Dr Masson was in charge of oral vaccination program organisation and implementation during the 1990's.

A cost analysis study of the system of oral vaccination implemented in France demonstrated that it is beneficial compared to the traditional expenses of rabies control.
Animal rabies prophylaxis has been progressively adapted to the disease free status of the country; the surveillance network for rabies is still working and an emergency procedure is in place in the event of a re-emergence of the disease in the context of high density fox populations.

INTRODUCTION

As in other European countries, canine rabies predominated in France until the 20th century. France became free of canine rabies in 1960.

The first terrestrial case of rabies was recorded in a red fox (*Vulpes vulpes*) in March 1968 near the German border. The same year, the entire administrative department of Moselle, 6216 km^2, concerned by this case was infected and a total of 58 foxes were diagnosed positive for rabies by the end of 1968. In 1969, 5 neighbouring departments were infected; in 1972, this number was 12, in 1978 it was 25 and in 1986, at the time of the first field trial of oral vaccination, rabies cases were founded in 29 departments. A total of 42 departments located in the Northeast of the country (which comprises 96 Metropolitan departments) have been infected and 58 "translocated" cases have been reported. Since 1968, a total number of 49,771 terrestrial cases have been diagnosed and the infected area reached its maximum (140,000 km^2) in 1989. The progression of the disease was evaluated at an annual rate of 30 to 60 km, even though rivers and canals delayed its advance (see [1] for map details).

It should be noted that, like several Western European countries, the contaminated areas included varied landscapes such as low populated farming areas and low mountainous areas as well as very densely populated areas (surroundings of Paris and big cities) and industrial areas contiguously urbanised.

This paper is intended to briefly review the means used in France for rabies control in wildlife which has allowed for the elimination of elimination.

First prophylactic measures

Thanks to coordinated actions of public health administrations, several measures were organized regarding both animals and humans: limitation of the fox population, prevention of the disease by anti-rabies vaccination of domestic animals and post exposure prophylaxis in humans.

Destruction of foxes did not halt the spread of the disease [2] whereas rabies vaccination of domestic animals, in particular vaccination of cattle, was more efficient. However, drastic reduction of the fox population by different means (gassing or shooting) was encouraged in France until the end of 1991 as a complement to the other methods.

Oral vaccination programs

Oral vaccination of wildlife was implemented in 1986 as a joint vaccination program with Luxembourg and Belgium on a very limited area (720 km^2) and using the only available baits (SAD B19). From 1986 to 1989 limited trials were conducted by hand distribution in areas of vaccination located mainly near the borders with Luxembourg, Belgium, and Switzerland.

VRG was used for the first time in 1989 on a small area (724 km^2) in order to assess its efficacy whereas SAD B19 was used on larger territories (14,882 km^2).

The vaccinated areas were not contiguous and not sufficiently large to stop the progression of the rabies wave. In 1989, the highest number of rabies cases were recorded (4,213 cases) [3]. Therefore, in autumn of 1990 the strategy was changed with the establishment of a continuous immunological barrier 50 km wide from the English Channel to the Swiss border to protect the Southwest of the country. The SAG1 vaccine baits were used for the first time in 1990, to complement VRG and SAD B19 baits. From 1992 to 1997 the whole contaminated area was vaccinated. As a result, rabies incidence decreased significantly during the following years (27 % in 1991, 41 % in 1992, 80 % in 1993, 65 % in 1994, and 60 % in 1996) [4]. The last cases of vulpine rabies were recorded in 1998 with one fox and one cat. However, oral vaccination campaigns were still carried out twice a year (except in 2003, where only one campaign was carried out in autumn) until the end of 2003 along the German border over an area of 5 500 km^2 to prevent any rabies re-infection.

Technical specifications required for oral vaccination programs have strictly followed the EC recommendations and WHO requirements [5,6].

Oral vaccination campaigns were conducted in spring and autumn by helicopter only (no additional manual bait distribution) and with one passage, hence a total of 40 baits per km^2 were distributed annually. Dropping of baits was achieved by two trained technicians. Hand dropping from the helicopter was preferred in place of automatic dropping as it allows more flexible adaptation of bait distribution to the different fox habitats (the dropping was stopped when flying over lakes, persons, and densely urbanized areas). The bait density used for many years was 18 to 20 baits/km^2 per campaign.

Despite the fact that SAG2 and VRG baits have proved their high thermostability [7], a refrigerated lorry containing a sufficient number of baits followed the vaccination team to different airports. (SAD B19 use was abandoned in 1993 because of lower efficacy [8] and safety concerns [6]; those questions are still with us as Austria has recently related [9] a case of vaccine-induced rabies in a young fox and there has been a recent report of three similar cases in Germany [10]).

Since 1990, the overall organisation of the oral vaccination campaigns has been centralised: one structure (AFSSA Nancy) was requested by the Ministry of Agriculture to organise, in close and constant collaboration with its delegates, and implement oral vaccination campaigns of foxes (OVF). AFSSA Nancy was also in charge of planning surveillance at the national level (all animals that did not contaminate humans were analyzed for rabies diagnosis at AFSSA Nancy) and evaluating the efficacy of OVF (assessment of tetracycline in foxes culled at night and testing of fox sera for rabies virus antibodies).

Several field and experimental trials were conducted to improve the efficiency of oral vaccination campaigns, particularly to improve contact of baits with cubs (which constitute 65 % of fox population) and also to counterbalance the increase in fox populations (see Fig. 1 representing evolution of fox populations in Eastern France (Lorraine region); depending upon the area examined, the night counting index is three to eight fold higher than in the 1980's).

Vaccination in the summer using VRG baits

Vaccinating with highly thermostable baits in summer could allow for an increase of bait uptake by older cubs which have started to disperse, and hence an improvement in protection against rabies. Results of a field trial demonstrated that a first vaccination conducted in the summer is less efficient than a first vaccination conducted in autumn [11].

Additional distribution of baits at the entrance of dens

Results of several field trials showed that this vaccination method had nearly no effect on the adult fox population [12,13]. However, vaccination at den entrances induces a significant increase of bait uptake by and seroconversion in cubs.

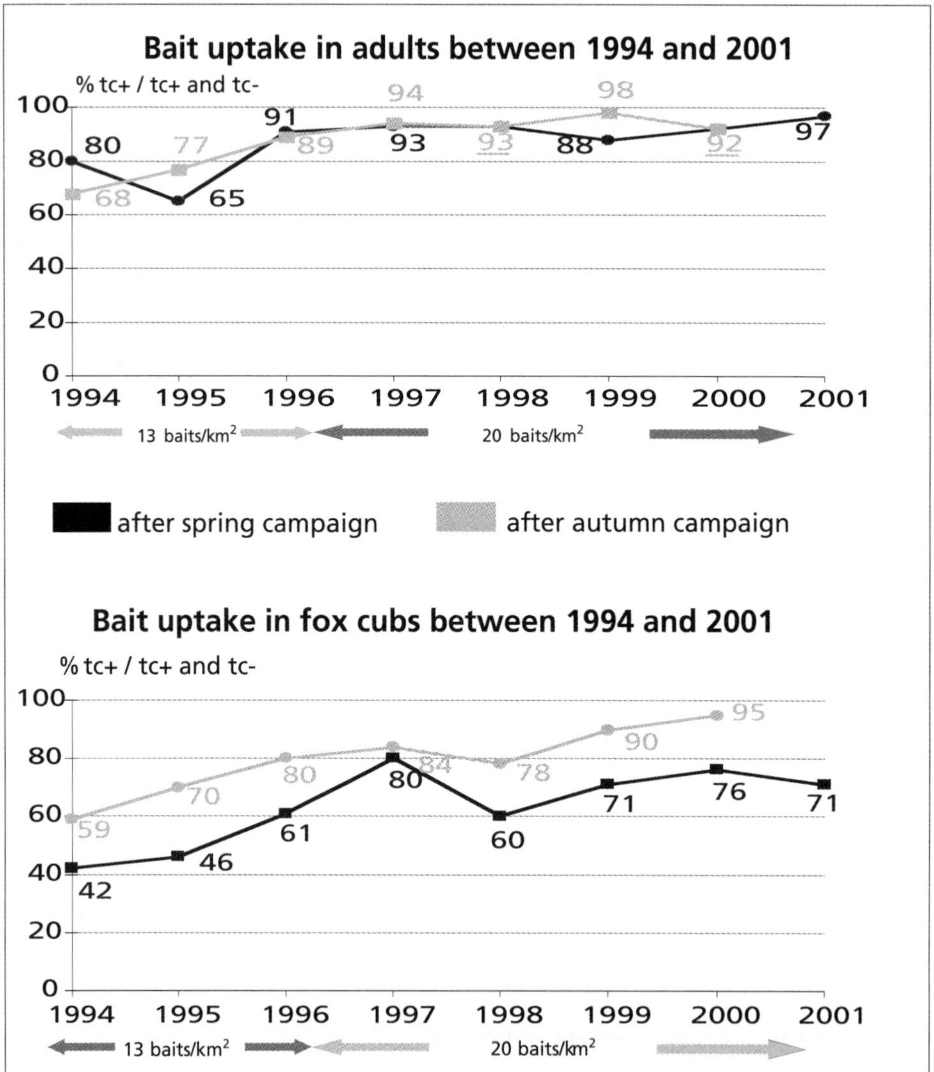

Fig. 1: Bait uptake by assessment of tetracycline in adult foxes and cubs from 1994 to 2001.

It is a useful means for eliminating rabies in remnant foci as a complement to the aerial distribution of baits. However, in view of the costs of terrestrial vaccination (the cost of hand distribution is 3.5 times higher than classical aerial distribution) and the fact that this method is cumbersome (it takes 63.5 time longer) it cannot be easily and consistently used on large areas.

Increase of bait density to compensate for increases in fox density

The most efficient bait density for routine campaigns, under conditions in France, has proven to be 18-20 baits/km^2 with homogeneous distribution by helicopter (see the section Monitoring of vaccination).

Double bait distribution

Bait distribution was doubled at two to four week intervals to act as a booster as well as to increase bait uptake rate. No significant effect on a double, compared to single, vaccination strategy has been demonstrated in the field either in adults or in cubs [14].

Determination of the optimal period of vaccination in spring in order to enhance consumption of baits by cubs

In spring, cubs comprise the largest group of the fox population. If not appropriately chosen, the time of oral vaccination may coincide with the period of fox whelping. In Western European countries, this period takes place in March. Vaccinating during the suckling period will not result in the uptake of baits by, even if adult foxes carry baits into the dens. We have demonstrated that a single vaccination at the end of May instead of in April induced higher bait uptake and better serological response in adults and cubs. Furthermore, with VRG [15] and SAG2 baits (manuscript in preparation), passively acquired antibodies do not significantly interfere with active immunization.

Monitoring of vaccination

The surveillance of animal rabies was centralized at AFSSA-Nancy:

- Incidence of rabies in animals. Diagnosis of rabies was performed using the WHO/OIE recommended techniques [5,16]. Analysis was performed on animals suspected of having rabies or found dead, and road kills, to determine the incidence of rabies. It should be noted that several thousands of samples from foxes culled at night for the follow up of OVF were never detected as rabid.
- Assessment of bait uptake by testing the target species for tetracycline. Tetracycline was searched for in the lower jaw and inferior canine of foxes and detected by UV light examination of a section of the canine by inverse microscopy. We studied bait uptake in fox cubs (less than 12 months of age) and adult foxes separately and differentiated both age categories on the basis of histological dental examination [17]. Figure 2 shows the percentage of foxes marked by tetracycline in the vaccinated areas after spring and autumn campaigns from 1994 to 2001. In adult foxes, this mean percentage reached 86 % after spring and autumn campaigns. In fox cubs, the mean percentages were 63 % and 79 % after spring and autumn campaigns, respectively. This regular follow up of bait consumption

allows to improve the bait density: an increase of 13 to 20 baits per square kilometre demonstrated a significant increase of bait uptake in fox cubs (the mean percentage of marked cubs was 50 % with 13 baits/km^2, and reached 72 % with 20 baits/km^2 after spring campaign) and also in adult foxes (from 78 % with 13 baits/km^2 to 93 % with 20 baits/km^2).

- Assessment of rabies antibodies in target species from vaccinated areas by ELISA.
- An ELISA test was developed for testing even highly haemolysed field samples [18] (as the FAVN test and other cell culture-based techniques were too heavy for large scale screening of field sera and too sensitive to cytotoxicity that occurs with poor quality samples). With a bait density of 20 baits/km^2, the percentage of adult foxes with rabies antibodies was approximately 70 % in spring and 90 % in autumn; for fox cubs these percentages were 35 % in spring and 65 % in autumn.

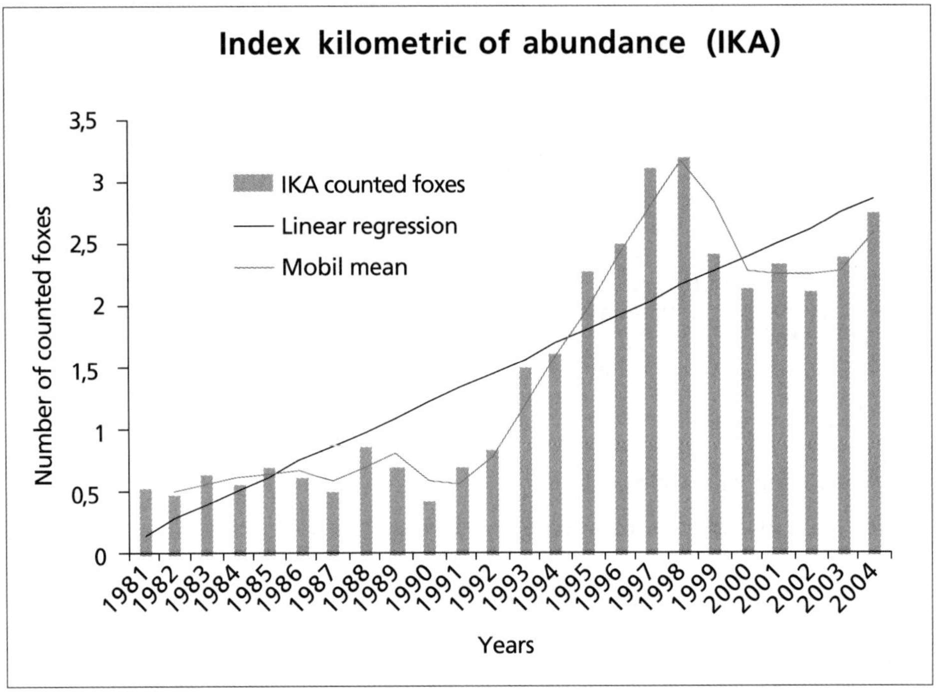

Fig. 2: Evolution of fox populations in East of France (Lorraine).

Although vaccine companies produced batch release certificates, each vaccine batch was checked for viral rabies titre at reception and samples randomly chosen "in the helicopter" during and after oral vaccination campaigns were titrated as well, in order to check the stability of the viral suspension (and therefore stability of bait casing). A minimal titre of $10^8 TCID_{50}$/dose is required before dropping.

Typing of field isolates was performed (either by using monoclonal antibodies or, more recently, by sequencing) on samples from areas where SAG2 was distributed in order to distinguish vaccine and field virus strains and no vaccine-induced case has been recorded among the tested samples.

Animal rabies prophylaxis in the event of an emergency

Control of wildlife rabies requires long-term financial support to maintain implementation, as several years are required for reaching rabies elimination.

These authors have evaluated the cost-effectiveness of rabies eradication by oral vaccination of wildlife [19]. The costs of vaccine baits, their delivery and monitoring of vaccination have been compared to the costs associated with rabies epizootics: vaccination of domestic animals, reinforcement of epidemiological surveillance networks, support for rabies diagnosis, animal and economic losses, clinical observation of animals which have bitten humans, prophylactic vaccination and post exposure treatment of humans.

The benefit of OVF was obtained after the fourth consecutive year of the programme. In view of this analysis, and based on the fact that rabies elimination has not been achieved in all Western European countries, we have implemented a plan of rabies prophylaxis in the event of the re-emergence of rabies. Since 2000, AFSSA Nancy has been responsible for the organisation and storage of an emergency stock of 100,000 baits.

Furthermore, a dedicated budget for aerial distribution is scheduled annually; persons involved in oral bait dropping are continuously trained. This emergency plan could allow for the possible rapid implementation of two oral vaccination campaigns over an area of 5000 km^2.

This emergency procedure was tested in 2005, as it was decided, in February 2005, to use oral vaccination to immunize foxes in a case of re-emergence (no oral vaccination was carried out in 2004). Indeed, an outbreak of rabies has occurred after January 2005 in Rhineland-Palatinate which had been rabies free since 1998, and Germany recorded 25 cases of rabies during the first quarter (18 cases in Rhineland-Palatinate) [20]. The vaccine baits from the emergency stock were used, administrative delays and procedures were respected (in particular the delay for aerial system tendering) and oral vaccination was carried out from May 16 to 25, 2005. An additional autumn vaccination campaign will be carried out from September 26 to October 6, 2005.

Conclusion

The oral vaccination of foxes over large areas (> 5000 km^2) by homogeneous distribution of baits as recently recommended by WHO [21], twice per year from 1988 to 1998 with an annual density of 40 baits/km^2 has allowed for the elimination of rabies.

In the recent past, cross-border meetings were organized annually in France gathering specialists from Belgium, Luxembourg, Germany and Switzerland to exchange epidemiological data and to discuss cross-border strategies of vaccination. The authors stress the importance of the rapid exchange of epidemiological data between neighbouring countries to facilitate the timely implementation of oral vaccination programmes in those countries free of rabies: these programmes are difficult to organize from the technical and administrative point of view, sufficient time is required for all procedures, and if possible the best period for bait dropping (spring and autumn) should be respected.

Acknowledgements

The authors wish to thank the European Commission, the French Ministry of Agriculture, the WHO and OIE, the French Directions of Veterinary Services, and all the colleagues of AFSSA Nancy involved in rabies epidemiology.

References

1 Cliquet F, Aubert M: Elimination of Terrestrial Rabies in Western European Countries, in Schudel A, Lombard M (eds): Control of Infectious Diseases by Vaccination, Dev Biol, Basel, Karger, 2004, vol 119, pp 185-204.

2 Aubert M: Epidemiology of fox rabies, in Bögel L, Meslin FX, Kaplan M (eds): Wildlife Rabies Control, Kent, Wells Medical Ltd, 1992, pp 9-18.

3 Aubert MFA, Masson E, Artois M, Barrat J: Oral wildlife rabies vaccination field trials in Europe, with recent emphasis on France, in Rupprecht CE, Dietzschold B, Koprowski E (eds): "*Lyssaviruses*". Berlin, Springer Verlag, 1994, pp 219-243.

4 Aubert M: Epidémiologie et lutte contre la rage en France et en Europe. Bull Acad Natl Méd 1995; 179 (5): 1033-1054, séance du 23 mai 1995.

5 WHO: Eight Report of WHO Expert Committee on rabies, Geneva, 1992.

6 Anonymous: The oral vaccination of foxes against rabies. Report of the Scientific Committee on Animal Health and Animal Welfare, October 2002, European Commission, 55 pages.

7 Anonymous FAIR Project CT 97-3515: Wildlife vaccination against rabies in difficult and emergency situations and its potential impact on the environment, Final Report, 2002.

8 Masson E, Aubert MFA, Barrat J, Vuillaume P: Comparison of the efficacy of the antirabies vaccines used for foxes in France. Vet Res 1996; 27: 255-266.

9 Vanek E, Wodak E, Revilla-Fernandez S, Bago Z, Schildorfer H, Hoeflechner A, Schoenbauer M: Fox rabies in Carinthia, Austria: A case report. Rabies Bulletin Europe 2004; 2: 9.

10 Anonymous: Report on the inspection visit of the food and Veterinary Office to Germany from 22 to 26 November 2004 to assess the rabies eradication plan, DG Sanco/7216/2004, European Commission, Health and Consumer Protection Directorate General, Directorate F, Food and Veterinary Office, 22 pages (http://europa.eu.int/comm/food/fvo).

11 Masson E, Bruyère-Masson V, Vuillaume P, Lemoyne S, Aubert M: Rabies oral vaccination of foxes during summer with the VRG vaccine bait. Vet Res 1999; 30: 595-605.

12 Vuillaume P, Aubert M, Demerson JM, Cliquet F, Barrat J, Breitenmoser U: Vaccination des renards contre la rage par dépôt d'appâts vaccinaux à l'entrée des terriers. Ann Méd Vét 1997; 141: 55-62.

13 Vuillaume P, Bruyère V, Aubert M: Comparison of the effectiveness of two protocols of antirabies bait distribution for foxes (*Vulpes vulpes*). Vet Res 1998; 29 (6): 537-546.

14 Bruyère V, Vuillaume P, Cliquet F, Aubert M: Oral rabies vaccination of foxes with one or two delayed distributions of SAG2 baits during the spring. Vet Res 2000; 31: 339-345.

15 Blasco E, Lambot M, Barrat J, Cliquet F, Brochier B, Renders C, Krafft N, Bailly J, Munier M, Pastoret P-P, Aubert MFA: Kinetics of humoral immune response after rabies VR-G oral vaccination of captive fox cubs (*Vulpes vulpes*) with or without maternally derived antibodies against the vaccine. Vaccine 2001; 19: 4816-4823.

16 Cliquet F, Barrat J: Rabies, in Manual of Diagnostic Tests and Vaccines for Terrestrial Animals. World Organisation for Animal Health, Fifth Edition, 2004, pp 328-346.

17 Johnston DH, Watt IDA: Rapid method for sectioning undecalcified carnivore teeth for aging, in Chapman JA, Pursley D (eds): Proceedings Worldwide Furbearer Conference. Maryland, USA, Frosburg, 3-11 August 1980, pp 407-422.

18 Cliquet F, Sagne L, Schereffer JL, Aubert MFA: ELISA test for rabies antibody titration in orally vaccinated foxes sampled in the fields. Vaccine 2000; 18: 3272-3279.

19 Aubert M: Costs and benefits of rabies control in wildlife in France, Rev Sci Tech 1999; 18 (2): 533-543.

20 Anonymous: Rabies Bulletin Europe, 2005, first quarter, 30 pages.

21 WHO: WHO expert consultation on rabies, first report, WHO Technical Report Series 931, 2005, 121 pages.

Dr. F. Cliquet, WHO Collaborating Centre for Research and Management in Zoonoses Control, OIE Reference Laboratory for Rabies, Community Reference Laboratory for Rabies Serology, AFSSA, Domaine de Pixérécourt, BP 9, FR-54220 Malzéville, France.
E-mail: f.cliquet@afssa.fr

Dodet B, Schudel A, Pastoret PP, Lombard M (eds): Rabies in Europe.
Dev Biol (Basel). Basel, Karger, 2006, vol 125, pp 127-132.

Epidemiological Analysis of Setbacks in Oral Vaccination in the Final Stage of Fox Rabies Elimination in Densely Populated Areas in Germany

T. Selhorst[1], *T. Müller*[1], *H.-J. Bätza*[2]

[1] Federal Res. Inst. for Animal Health, Institute of Epidemiology, Wusterhausen, Germany

[2] Ministry of Consumer Protection Food and Agriculture, Bonn, Germany

Abstract: Despite a long history of oral vaccination of foxes (OVF) against rabies, in a few restricted areas of Germany rabies is still endemic, posing a continuous risk of re-introduction of rabies into adjacent, rabies-free areas. The endemic area is characterized by a high density population.

It is hypothesized that the degree of urbanization in the area under consideration influences the number of rabies cases via the mode of bait distribution. In urban areas vaccine baits are distributed by hand, whereas in non-urban areas baits can be distributed aerially with the help of fixed-winged aircraft.

Statistical analysis of the effect of the mode of bait distribution upon the number of rabies cases shows a significant influence. In areas where baits are distributed by hand the number of rabies cases is significantly higher than the expected number.

This finding forces managers to reassess the procedure of bait distribution by hand in urban areas, taking into account the ecologically and biologically different dynamics of urban fox populations. If the oral vaccination of foxes in urban areas can be refined, rabies eradication in Germany is expected to succeed in due course.

INTRODUCTION

Rabies is the most important viral zoonosis from a global perspective [1]. In the 1990s most European countries showed considerable numbers of rabies cases, predominantly in the main host, the red fox (*Vulpes vulpes*). However, with the widespread application of oral vaccination of red fox populations against rabies, the number of cases has declined considerably and today, in 2005, nearly all Western European countries are free from the disease, and in the Eastern European countries the situation has improved considerably.

As already mentioned, the method of control is oral vaccination of the rabies host population which decreases the number of susceptible animals below a threshold density at which the chain of infection breaks down. Vaccines are administered using baits attractive to the target population. The baits contain a vaccine capsule which has to be broken by the animals for vaccination to occur. Vaccine baits are distributed by hand or by aircraft (fixed-wing aircraft or helicopter). Aerial distribution is superior to hand distribution of baits because large areas can be covered readily at low cost, while bait distribution by hand is usually more costly because human resources are needed for distribution. Clearly, hand vaccination is usually done on a smaller scale.

In Germany, oral vaccination of foxes (OVF) against rabies has been established as the method of choice since 1983. As a consequence the number of rabies cases dropped from 10,484 cases in 1983 to 33 cases in 2004 (bat, dog and cat rabies excluded). Nevertheless, in a small pocket of Germany, rabies is still endemic despite long-term oral vaccination. This area is characterized by an extremely high population density (400-500 inhabitants per square kilometre) and it is hypothesised that the structure of the rabies endemic area influences the rabies incidence via the mode of bait distribution.

Material and Methods

The hypothesis tested in this paper is whether the spatial distribution of rabies cases (bat, dog and cat rabies cases excluded) observed between 2003 and 2005 (as of June 8th 2005) is influenced by the mode of bait distribution. Two modes are compared: (i) distribution of baits by hand versus (ii) the aerial distribution of baits. The categorization of an area into urban and non-urban areas determines the mode of bait distribution.

A total of 90 fox rabies cases were officially confirmed from 2003 to 2005 (as of June 8th 2005); their spatial distribution is shown in Figure 1.

Each rabies case depicted in Figure 1 is geographically referenced by the GPS system. The rabies cases under consideration are grouped into four different clusters and the analysis is done for each of the clusters separately. From figure 1 it is obvious that two rabies cases (one being a vaccine associated one) are dislodged from the clusters. These two cases (outliers) are excluded form the statistical analysis.

To characterize the geographical structure in each cluster, a circle with a 15 kilometre radius is drawn around each rabies case and the unification of all circles defines the four areas (clusters) for investigation. Within each cluster, the geographical structure can be analysed and in this analysis the geographical structure is categorized into urban and non-urban areas. These two groups determine the mode of bait distribution. In urban areas baits are distributed by hand while in non-urban areas, aerial distribution of baits is conducted.

Within each cluster the size of the area baited by hand and baited aerially can readily be calculated with the help of a Geographical Information System.

Because all rabies cases used in this analysis are geographically referenced, it is possible to determine whether a case originates from an area where hand or aerial distribution of baits had been conducted. The observed number of rabies cases originating from areas baited by hand or aerially are compared with the expected numbers. The expected numbers are calculated as follows. If there is no effect of the mode of bait distribution on the number of rabies cases, the cases should be randomly distributed within the areas of investigation and their classification into cases coming from areas baited aerially or by hand should be proportional to the percentage of hand and aerial baited areas to the total area of each cluster.

A one-way Chi square test is performed to test for a significant difference between the observed and the expected number of rabies cases within the two groups (i.e. modes) of bait distribution. Because expected cell counts are low, p-values are computed by Monte Carlo simulation with 10,000 replicates. The statistical calculations are done in R (www.cran.r-project.org) with the Chi square test routine.

A p-value lower than 0.05 indicates a significant effect of the mode of bait distribution upon the number of rabies cases.

Results

In Table 1, for each cluster, the size and proportion (in brackets) of urban and non-urban areas and the number of rabies cases officially confirmed from 2003 to 8th June 2005 is given.

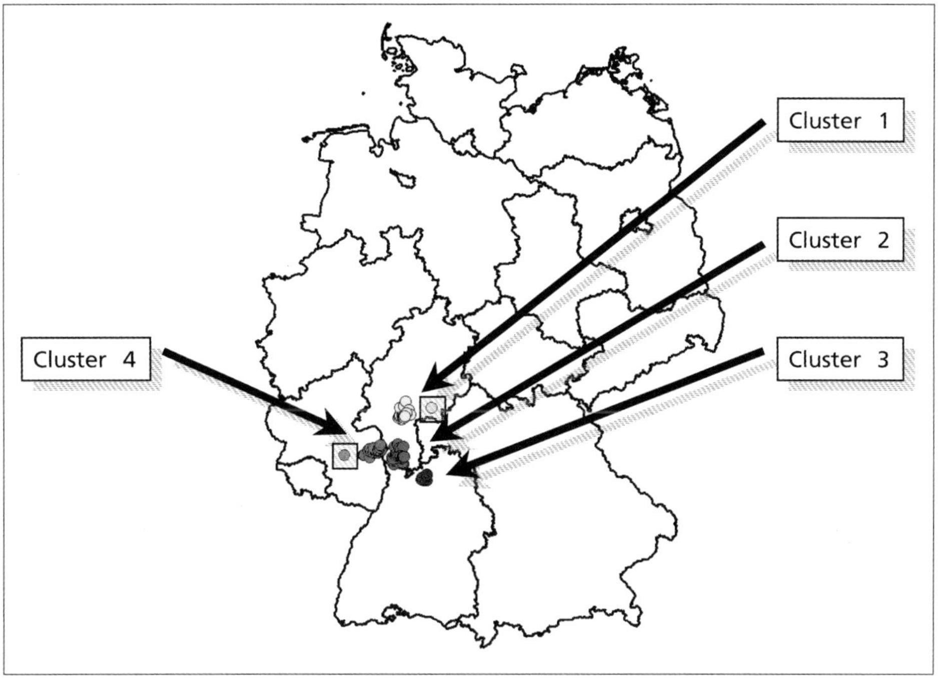

Fig. 1: Geographical location of fox rabies cases officially confirmed within the period from 2003 until 8th June 2005. The cases are confined to four separated clusters. Two cases are marked with grey squares and are not included in the statistical analysis.

Table 1: Size and proportion (given in brackets) of urban and non-urban areas and the number of rabies cases officially confirmed from 2003 until 8th June 2005.

Size in [sqkm]	**Cluster**			
Area category	1	2	3	4
Urban	431.72 (0.28)	255.52 (0.14)	72.92 (0.06)	113.28 (0.08)
Non-urban	1,094.31 (0.72)	1,536.47 (0.86)	1,165.27 (0.94)	1,357.30 (0.92)
Total	1,526.03	1,791.99	1,238.19	1,496.96
Rabies cases	23	32	9	24

Table 2 gives the observed and the expected numbers of rabies cases in urban and non-urban areas together with the calculated Chi-square figure and the level of significance.

According to Table 2 the number of observed rabies cases in urban and non-urban areas significantly differs from that expected with respect to Cluster 2 and Cluster 4. In both clusters the number of observed rabies cases in urban areas is significantly higher than expected.

Table 2: Observed and expected numbers of rabies cases in urban and non-urban areas together with the calculated Chi-square figure and the level of significance in four different cluster.

	Cluster							
	1		**2**		**3**		**4**	
	Obs.	Exp.	Obs.	Exp.	Obs.	Exp.	Obs.	Exp.
Urban	9	6.44	9	4.48	0	0.54	5	1.85
Non-urban	14	16.56	23	27.52	9	8.46	19	22.15
Chi-square	1.3322		5.0324		0.5632		5.8198	
Level of significance	0.36		0.04		0.67		0.03	

Discussion

In this paper the hypothesis of an influence of the degree of urbanization on the number of rabies cases in densely populated areas of Germany via its influence on the mode of bait distribution is tested. A total number of 90 officially confirmed fox rabies cases for the period 2003 to 2005 (status June 8th 2005) are used in the analysis. Two rabies cases are excluded as outliers. The remaining 88 rabies cases are distributed among four clusters located in the federal states Hesse (2 clusters), Baden-Wurttemberg and Rhineland-Palatinate.

Statistical analysis indicates that the degree of urbanization has a significant influence on the number of rabies cases in two out of four clusters (one in Hesse and one in Rhineland-Palatinate). In both clusters the number of observed rabies cases significantly exceeds what would be expected.

One explanation for the significantly higher number of rabies cases in urban areas might be the effect of the mode of bait distribution. In urban areas, vaccine baits are distributed solely by hand, while in non-urban areas baits can be distributed by aircraft. Because in urban and non-urban areas the type of baits (SAD B19) as well as the number of baits distributed per square kilometre is the same, other factors must have influenced the effect of vaccination upon the number of rabies cases. If the mode of bait distribution does not mask other influential factors, it can be stated that in two out of four areas investigated in this analysis, bait distribution by hand is inferior to distribution by aircraft.

It is well known that fox biology and ecology differ with respect to urban and non-urban foxes. As already mentioned by Hegglin [2], urban areas provide plentiful food resources, and are well suited to sustain high fox population densities [3], up to 10 adult foxes per square kilometre [4,5]. Urban foxes tend to have small home ranges and low dispersing distances [6,7]. Additionally urban fox populations are organized in family groups, in which young vixens remain in their parental home range and help to rear fox cubs [7,8]. As a consequence, offspring frequently inherit the parental territory and do not have to disperse. Furthermore a low urban immigration rate [9] and low hunting pressure [2] contribute to the moderate spatial dynamics of urban fox populations.

Small home ranges and moderate spatial population dynamics create small areas of discovery (i.e. the area that is searched by a fox for food and other resources).

Therefore the task of facilitating contact between the fox and the vaccine bait is much more challenging, because the distance between the vaccine baits and the target (the fox) has to be as close as possible. Deficient spatial distribution of baits in urban areas would lead to inferior bait uptake and, as a consequence, to inferior vaccination coverage. Unfortunately, in Germany, bait uptake can no longer be assessed, because vaccine baits are no longer allowed to contain the biomarker tetracycline. On account of this abolition it is now impossible to trace the bait intake preceding immunization, and it becomes more important to determine the seroprevalence accurately in order to asses the vaccination coverage. Nevertheless, because this study also shows that the number of observed rabies cases in non-urban areas is lower that expected, the possibility of vaccinating foxes against rabies is supported and the focus of possible improvements of oral vaccination of urban foxes against rabies should be directed to the refinement of bait distribution in urban areas.

First of all, habitats attractive for urban foxes need to be identified, i.e. public and private parks, private gardens, graveyards, factory sites (abandoned or operating), areas beside railways and roads, and airports, etc. Within these habitats, distribution of baits by hand must be well organized, especially including giving information to the public and guidance of the personnel distributing the baits. Another important factor influencing the success of oral vaccination in urban areas is access to private property, which has to be facilitated.

Furthermore, because urban fox population densities might be very high, bait density has to be adapted accordingly. When calculating the bait density, the abundance of bait competitors (hedgehogs, dogs, rodents and other animals) has to be taken into account. Unpublished data ascertained by Hegglin et al show that 50 % of the baits distributed in urban areas are taken by other animals.

Additionally, the number and the timing of vaccination campaigns need to be discussed. Usually, in non-urban areas, the vaccine baits are distributed twice per year, in spring and in autumn. These periods coincide with a low abundance of the food supply of foxes, but, in urban areas, where manifold food resources are available, the timing of vaccination campaigns should reflect other dependencies.

Because of the high densities of foxes and bait competitors and the distribution of baits in attractive, small areas, the retention period of baits possibly decreases, resulting in a lower number of foxes which have access to the baits. To counterbalance this possible effect, baits could be distributed at shorter intervals, for example, every six weeks. This schedule could also include the distribution of baits in the late spring, when many adolescent foxes are present [2]. Simulation studies conducted by Selhorst et al [10] allude to a possible beneficial effect of vaccination campaigns conducted during this period.

Conclusion

This epidemiological analysis was intended to identify influential effects on the number of rabies cases in residual areas of Germany. The results of the investigation indicate that the mode of bait distribution, either by hand or by aircraft, has a statistically significant effect on the number of rabies cases in some areas.

In areas where vaccine baits are distributed by hand (urban areas), a higher number of rabies cases than expected appears, whereas in areas where vaccine bait can be aerially distributed (non-urban areas) the number of rabies cases is lower than expected.

This finding forces managers to pay more attention to the bait distribution by hand in urban areas to eradicate rabies completely in Germany in due course.

Acknowledgement

The authors wish to thank Anke Kliemt for her assistance in preparing the data used in this analysis and for her assistance in the maintenance of the rabies database run at the Friedrich-Loeffler-Institute in Wusterhausen/Germany.

References

1 Eisinger D, Thulke HH, Selhorst T, Müller T: Emergency vaccination of rabies under limited resources – combating or containing? BMC Infect Dis 2005; 5: 10.

2 Hegglin D, Ward PI, Deplazes P: Anthelmintic baiting of foxes against urban contamination with Echinococcus multilocularis. Emerg Infect Dis 2003; 9: 1266-1272.

3 Saunders G, White PCL, Harris S, Rayner JMV: Urban foxes (*Vulpes vulpes*): food acquisition, time and energy budgeting of a generalized predator, in Dunstone N, Gorman ML (eds): Mammals as predators. London, Oxford University Press, 1993, pp 215-234.

4 Contesse P, Hegglin D, Gloor S, Bontadida F, Deplazes P: The diet of urban foxes (*Vulpes vulpes*) and the availability of anthropogenic food in the city of Zurich, Switzerland. Mammalian Biology 2004; 69: 81-95.

5 Gloor S: The rise of urban foxes (*Vulpes vulpes*) in Switzerland and ecological and parasitological aspects of a population in the recently colonised city of Zurich [Dissertation]. Zurich: University of Zurich, 2002.

6 Trewhella WJ, Harris S, McAllister FE: Dispersal distance, home-range size and population density in the red fox (*Vulpes vulpes*): a quantitative analysis. Journal of Applied Ecology 1988; 25: 423-434.

7 Baker PJ, Funk SM, Harris S, White PCL: Flexible spatial organization of urban foxes, *Vulpes vulpes*, before and during an outbreak of sarcoptic mange. Anim Behav 2000; 59: 127-146.

8 Macdonal DW: Resource dispersion and social organization of the red fox, Vulpes vulpes, in Chapman A, Pursley D (eds): Proceedings of the Worldwide Furbearer Conference 1980 Aug 3-11; Forstburg, Maryland. Falls Church (VA), RR Donnelly and Sons Company, 1981, pp 918-949.

9 Wanderler P, Funk SM, Largiadèr R, Gloor S, Breitenmoser U: The city-fox phenomenon: genetic consequences of a recent colonization of urban habitat. Mol Ecol 2003; 12: 647-656.

10 Selhorst T, Thulke HH, Müller T: Cost efficient vaccination of foxes (*Vulpes vulpes*) against rabies and the need of a new baiting strategy. Prev Vet Med 2001; 51 (1-2): 95-105.

Dr. T. Selhorst, Friedrich–Loeffler–Institute, Institute of Epidemiology, Seestrasse 55, DE-16868 Wusterhausen, Germany.
E-mail: thomas.selhorst@fli.bund.de

Dodet B, Schudel A, Pastoret PP, Lombard M (eds): Rabies in Europe.
Dev Biol (Basel). Basel, Karger, 2006, vol 125, pp 133-140.

Rabies Vaccination Programme for Red Foxes (*Vulpes vulpes*) and Golden Jackals (*Canis aureus*) in Israel (1999-2004)

B.A. Yakobson[1], R. King[2], S. Amir[2], N. Devers[1], N. Sheichat[1], D. Rutenberg[1], Z. Mildenberg[1], D. David[1]

[1] Kimron Veterinary Institute, Bet Dagan, Israel

[2] Nature & Parks Authority, Israel

Abstract: Since 1956, red foxes (Vulpes vulpes) and, to a lesser extent, golden jackals (Canis aureus), have been the primary vectors maintaining endemic wildlife rabies in Israel. Starting in the autumn of 1998, oral rabies vaccination campaigns have been conducted in Israel targeting these two wildlife species, with increasing yearly geographical extension. Significant data have been accumulated from an area of approximately 5,200 km^2 in Northern Israel. In the spring of 2003 the project was extended to 14,000 km^2 and in the autumn to 21,000 km^2, covering almost all inhabited areas in Israel and the West Bank. A total of two million RABORAL V-RG® (Merial) vaccine-filled baits were distributed bi-annually by plane or helicopter at 14-19 baits km^2. Since the onset of oral vaccination activities in 1998, annual bait acceptance in the vaccination zones has been demonstrated by biomarker detection (with tetracycline) in 55 % (429/783) of bone samples of target animals submitted for diagnosis. In 1999 to 2004, vaccine contact and induction of immunity in animals collected from the vaccination zones were reflected by seroconversion in 66 of 284 animals (23 %). By the year 2004, rabies cases declined sharply in all progressively vaccinated areas.

Introduction

The epidemiology of rabies in Israel is complex, involving a range of interacting animal species that differ in behaviour, ecology, and in the potential for contact with humans [1,2]. Three cases of human rabies in 1996 and 1997 (the first for many years) and an increase in wild and domestic animal rabies cases have accelerated interest in Israel to identify the underlying epizootiology and apply modern rabies virus control methods such as oral vaccination. Urbanization and agricultural development of rural areas have contributed to more accessible food sources, resulting in an increased carrying capacity of the area for wild canids. This increase in canid populations and the decrease in suitable habitats have been responsible for an increased vector population density. The proximity of the jackals' and foxes' home ranges to populated areas, coupled with high population densities, increases the contact rate between wildlife and domestic animals. These variables are major factors in the transmission of the disease.

Rabies used to occur in almost all parts of Israel with an apparent clustering in the north and, up to 1958, mainly in urban areas. Since the mid 1970s, sylvatic rabies has become the dominant form, and rabid foxes accounted for 49 % of all cases between 1988 and 1997, establishing the fox population as the principal current reservoir of rabies virus in Israel. Despite the implementation over the years of rabies control measures such as compulsory dog vaccination, elimination of stray dogs and cats, and quarantine of suspected rabid animals, the prevalence of rabies has remained stable over the past 30 years. In 1996, the decision was made to apply oral rabies vaccination for wildlife as an additional method of rabies control. The programme was initiated in 1996 with bait acceptance trials in the field [3,4]. RABORAL V-RG® vaccine efficacy and safety trials in captive foxes and safety trials in non-target species were conducted according to WHO recommendations [5]. Efficacy trials in caged golden jackals were deemed necessary, as there was no previous experience with oral vaccination in this species. Groups of nine and 11 jackals were given a single oral dose of RABORAL V-RG® and SAG-2 (Virbac), respectively, while an additional 10 jackals served as non-vaccinated controls [6]. The thermal and mechanical stability of both vaccines were tested under field conditions [7].

Bi-annual vaccination trials were carried out from 1998 to 2004 starting in the heavily infected northern region and progressing to eventually include the majority of Israel as well as the West Bank.

Materials and Methods

The vaccination team responsible for carrying out the project consisted of Veterinary Services and personnel from the Nature and Parks Authority of Israel trained in field surveys and validated methods for rabies diagnosis, as well as other laboratory techniques [7]. Before beginning the vaccination campaign, background levels of the tetracycline biomarker were analysed in fox and jackal populations. The baiting strategy was designed according to the epidemiological situation of rabies cases and a previous molecular analysis of rabies isolates [8]. Recombinant vaccinia-rabies RABORAL V-RG® vaccine-filled baits produced by Merial were used. The RABORAL V-RG® vaccine was incorporated into fishmeal polymer baits containing a polyethylene sachet with at least 1.5 ml of vaccine containing a minimum of $10^{8.0}$ $TCID_{50}$/dose. The aerial field trials started in 1998 within an area of 500 km^2. In the following years (1999-2000), the vaccinated area was progressively widened in the north to 5,500 km^2, while an additional area of 1,000 km^2 was added in the south in the Negev desert (Table 1 and Fig. 1). In 2003, the project was again expanded to cover nearly the entire country as well as the entire West Bank in 2004 (in total 21,000 km^2).

Baits were distributed in the spring and autumn according to maps with pre-defined bait quantity for each marked polygon. Aerial distribution took place over uninhabited areas by plane and helicopter at a density of approximately 14-19 baits/km^2, in parallel lines 300m apart, using GPS (global positioning system) guidance. Additional manual distribution (approximately 5 % of total baits) was applied in close proximity to urban areas.

Bait acceptance was measured by uptake at baiting stations within the vaccination zones. Bait consumption was confirmed by biomarker detection and seroconversion in animals sampled two to four months after each distribution. Rabies prevalence was used to determine vaccination campaign efficacy.

Biomarker detection was expedited by examination of the lower mandibles of all the animals collected for surveillance or submitted for rabies diagnosis, from vaccinated and adjacent unvaccinated areas. The presence of the tetracycline hydrochloride-specific fluorescence in the calciphilic tissues was recorded [9].

For serology, serum samples were obtained from foxes and jackals sampled for surveillance from the vaccination areas. Blood samples were drawn by intra-cardiac puncture and the sera were stored at -20^{0}C, until tested by rapid fluorescent focus inhibition test (RFFIT) [10].

Rabies diagnosis was made in the brains of all the animals submitted for routine rabies diagnosis or collected actively from vaccinated and non-vaccinated areas, by direct fluorescence analysis. Each positive sample was confirmed by virus isolation and by PCR analysis. Viral sequencing determined the genotype of local strains and confirmed molecular epidemiology. The sequences were compared to sequences of viruses that were present in Israel before the start of oral vaccination (ORV) [8].

Table 1 : Vaccination areas in Israel, 1998-2004.

Year	Area vaccinated	Number of baits	Area (km^2)
Autumn 1998	A North	7.250	450
Spring 1999	A North	6.950	450
Autumn 1999	A North	0	0
Spring 2000	A North	61.500	3.750
Autumn 2000	A North	100.000	5.210
Total 2000		**161.500**	6.000
Spring 2001	A North & A South	110.000	
Autumn 2001	A North & A South	110.000	6.000
Total 2001[a]		**220.000**	
Spring 2002	A North & A South	110.000	6.600
Autumn 2002	A North & A South	110.000	6.600
Total 2002[b]		**220.000**	
Spring 2003	A (North & South), B (North, Central & South)	240.000	14.000
Autumn 2003	A (North & South), B (North, Central & South)	295.000	17.000
Total 2003[c]		**535.000**	
Spring 2004	A (North & South), B (North, Central & South)	260.000	14.000
Autumn 2004	A (North & South), B (North, Central & South) and Area C	350.000	20.000
Total 2004[d]		**610.000**	

a In 2001, a 1,000 km^2 arid area was added in the South.

b In 2002, a 600 km^2 area was added in the Jordan Valley.

c In 2003, the vaccination zones were extended to include Zone B : North, Central, and South.

d In 2004, the vaccination zones were expanded (see Fig. 1).

Results

Captive animal trials

The survival rate of the jackals challenged 180 days after receiving a single vaccine filled bait of RABORAL V-RG® was 77.7 % (7/9). The serological response at day 30 was 30 % (3/9) and 44 % (4/9) at day 150. The survival rate of jackals receiving one Virbac vaccine (SAG-2) bait was 85 % (12/14). The serology results were 57 % 8/14 positive at day 30 and 78 % 11/14 at day 150.

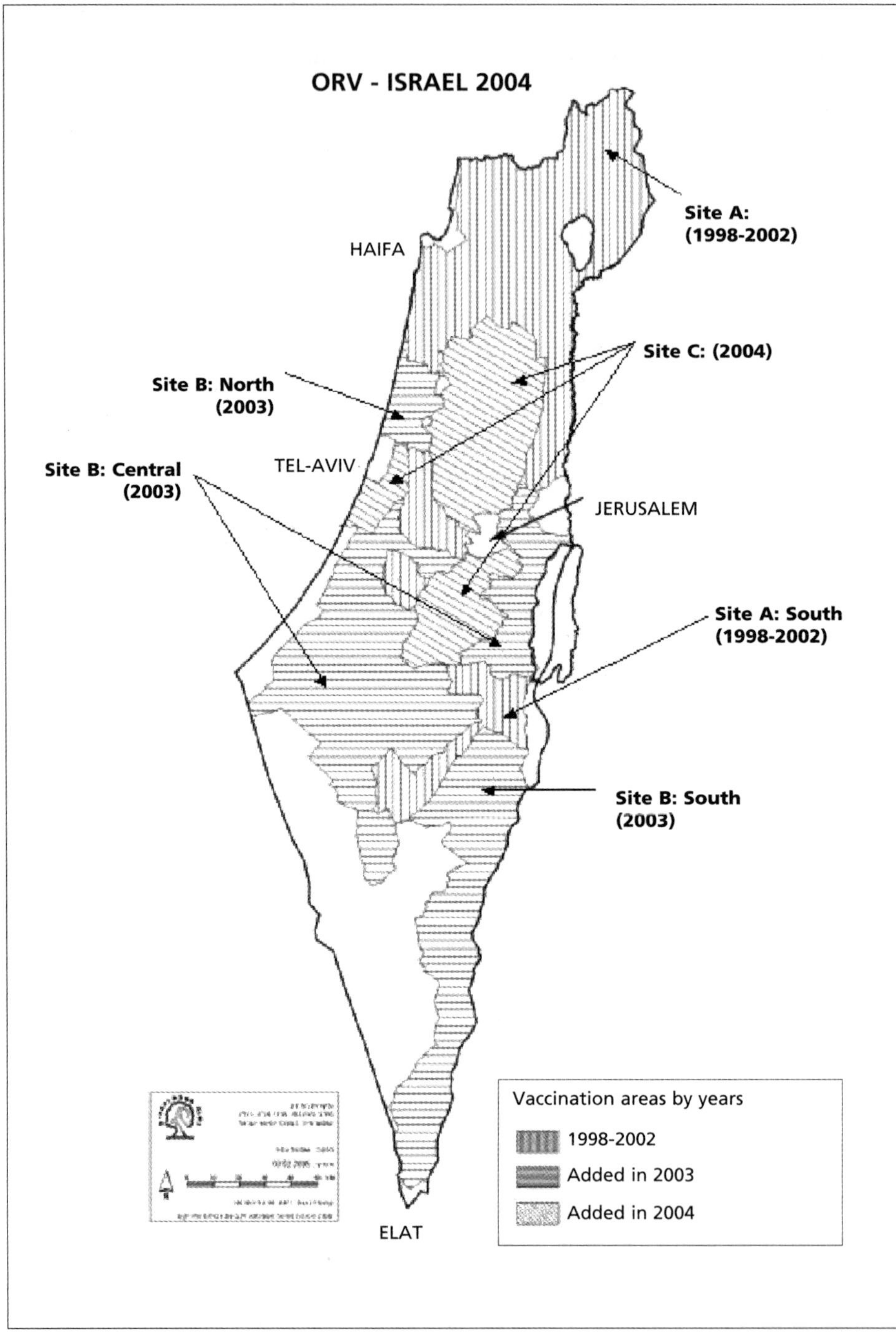

Fig. 1: Vaccination areas in Israel in 2004.

Comparative field trials showed that the V-RG vaccine bait was suitable, while the SAG-2 vaccine bait failed the performance requirements for use under local conditions (i.e. bait matrix melted in direct sun exposure).

Bait acceptance

Acceptance rate of baits in the target species was evaluated by the use of tracking stations (70-120 baits per location) within vaccination zones. Analysis of over 2,500 bait-uptake events revealed an acceptance rate of 40-90 % during the first night.

Biomarker

One to three months after bait dispersal, a total of 783 jackals and foxes were sampled (1998-2004) for identification of bone tetracycline, the biomarker for bait ingestion (Table 2). The average percent of positive samples was 55 % for the entire period. A decrease in percentage of positive biomarker samples in 2003, compared to previous years, was due to the inclusion of bone samples collected before the initiation of baiting from the expanded vaccination zone. This same sample set included 45 rabies-infected cases, of which all were negative for biomarker.

Table 2 : Tetracycline and antibody detection in jackals and foxes collected from vaccination zones.

Year	Tetracycline		Seroconversion	
	positive/tested	% positive	positive/tested	% positive
1999	11/20	55.0	12/18	66.6
2000	35/77	45.0	13/51	25.5
2001	56/74	75.7	10/37	27.0
2002	57/90	63.3	4/28	14.0
2003	116/269	43.1	11/63	17.5
2004	123/275	44.7	28/106	26.6
Total	440/803	54.4	78/302	29.5

Rabies antibodies

A subset of the total animals collected provided sera for rabies antibody analysis (n = 284). The average percent positive was 29.5 % for the years 1999-2004 (Table 3).

Rabies incidence

In the northern rural part of Israel (Site A North), and in the southern desert part (Site B South) rabies incidence decreased sharply after the first year of baiting. All the rabies cases reported from these areas from 2002 to 2004 were located on the edges of the vaccinated area. In 2002, five foxes were found in the Jordan valley,

Table 3: Number of baiting events and rabies diagnosed cases over time, in expanding vaccination zones.

Year	Site A (1998) 500 km²		Site A (2000) 6.500 km²		Site B (2003) 14.000 km²		Total positive cases
	Baiting events	Positive cases	Baiting events	Positive cases	Baiting events	Positive cases	
1998	0	34	0	36	0	27	97
1999	2	0	0	57	0	19	76
2000	3	0	1	3	0	29	32
2001	4	0	2	1	0	5	6
2002	5	0	3	5	0	59	64
2003	6	0	4	3*	2	66	69
2004	7	0	6	3**	4	25	28

* Three fox cases just within the vaccinated area (a distance < 1 km inside vaccinated zone).

** Two cattle cases adjacent to the border with Lebanon and one cow from the Golan Heights adjacent to the Syrian border.

between the unvaccinated West Bank and Jordan. In 2003, three foxes were found just within the vaccinated area (a distance < 1 km inside the zone). In 2004, two cows adjacent to the border with Lebanon and one cow from the Golan Heights adjacent to the Syrian border were found to be positive.

In contrast, in Site B North, two years of baitings (four campaigns) were required to obtain a decrease in rabies incidence. This area is a narrow urban zone, located along the central coastal part of Israel adjacent to the West Bank (average width of ~30 km). In 2004 zone C (West Bank) was included in the ORV project (Fig. 1).

Refer to (http://agri3.huji.ac.il/~yakobson/rabheb/mapa2005.html) for maps of rabies incidence in Israel.

Discussion

The use of a number of oral rabies vaccines most suitable for the hot Israeli climate was considered. The SAG-2 and RABORAL V-RG® vaccines were chosen for further evaluation, based on their favourable safety data and WHO and EU recommendations [11]. While both vaccines fared comparably well in captive animal studies, the SAG-2 bait was excluded due to its incompatibility with the local high summer heat conditions (melting in direct sun).

The baiting strategy rationale was based on previous experience and red fox data in France. Selection of 300m flight lines spacing and bait densities were in accordance with conclusions reached after 15 years of ORV campaigns in Europe [12]. This approach resulted in the expected bait uptake in target species populations after several baiting campaigns.

Serology results were in accordance with the results obtained in caged animals and the immunological response (humoral and cellular) characteristic for vaccinia recombinant rabies vaccine [13]. The percentage of tetracycline marked animals recorded after 2003 was lower because it included data from animals collected for rabies diagnosis from the entire country. The samples were collected from areas that were baited at variable times, as well as from untreated areas. After 2005 we expect tetracycline and serology levels to increase again once the entire country is homogeneously vaccinated. Our work showed that tetracycline results and serology are only indicators of bait uptake and vaccine contact, and may be confounded by multiple variables. Biomarker sero-antibody levels cannot serve as reliable indicators of the ORV success. Therefore, we consider the rapid decline of rabies incidence as observed in Israel, which is the goal of the project, as the ultimate sign of campaign success. This result is significant and specific for vaccine use and efficacy, as similar results were not observed in unvaccinated areas.

Favourable results first observed in the northern region (Site A) were gradually obtained in other progressively vaccinated areas. While new outbreaks from residual foci are unlikely to occur in the treated areas, there will be re-introductions of rabies from neighbouring countries where no systematic rabies control measures are applied. To avoid future outbreaks we should maintain wildlife immunity with annual ORV campaigns, unless a regional approach for rabies control is adopted.

Conclusions

RABORAL VRG® vaccine was found to be efficacious when used in jackals in captivity and in the field. Bait acceptance, as witnessed by > 50 % cumulative presence of a bone biomarker in both target species, was satisfactory. Rabies incidence in Israel has dropped dramatically in the vaccinated areas in comparison to the non-vaccinated areas since the beginning of the ORV programme.

After successful reduction of rabies cases in vaccinated areas, bi-annual ORV campaigns may be replaced by annual baiting, if all variables remain the same.

Re-introduction of rabies cases across international frontiers (by dogs and foxes), remains a serious threat until a comprehensive regional approach is adopted.

References

1 Yakobson B, Manalo DL, Bader K, Perl S, Haber A, Shahimov B, Shechat N: An epidemiological retrospective study of rabies diagnosis and control in Israel 1948-1997. Isr J Vet Med 1998; 53: 114-127.

2 Yakobson BA, David D, Aldomy F: in King et al (eds): Historical perspective of rabies in Europe and the Mediterranean basin. OIE 2004; 13: 171-183.

3 Linhart SB, King R, Zamir S, Naveh S, Davidson M, Perl S: Oral rabies vaccination of red foxes and golden jackals in Israel: preliminary bait evaluation. Rev Sci Tech 1997:16: 874-880.

4 Katz D, Zamir S, King R, Fuchs P, Freeman E, Davidson M: Pilot project for wildlife rabies control on Israel and neighbouring countries. Trinational Fourth Scientific Workshop and Symposium of Trinational Animal Health Project, Tiberias, Israel, 1995.

5 Report of a WHO Consultation on Requirements and Criteria for Field Trials on Oral Rabies Vaccination of Dogs and Wild Carnivores, World Health Organization, Geneva, 1989 (WHO/Rab. Res./89.32).

6 Yakobson BA, King RJ, David D, Sheichat N, Rotenberg D, Devers N, Samina I, Zaharin Y, Perl S, Orgad U: Comparative efficacy of two oral vaccines in captive jackals (*Canis aureus*) The 10th Annual Rabies in the Americas meeting, San Diego, California, USA, 1999.

7 Yakobson BA, King R, David D, Sheichat N, Devers N, Rotenberg D: Captivity and field trails of Raboral VRG rabies vaccine in Israel 1998-2000. XII International Meeting on advances in rabies research and control in the Americas, Peterborough. Ontario, Canada, 2001.

8 David D, Yakobson B, Smith JS, Stram Y: Molecular epidemiology of rabies virus isolates from Israel and other middle- and near-eastern countries. J Clin Microbiol 2000; 38: 755-762.

9 Johnston DH, Tinline RR: Rabies control in wildlife, in Jackson AC, Wunner WH (eds): Academic Press, an Elsevier Science Imprint, CA, USA, 2002, pp 445-471.

10 Manual of Diagnostic Tests and Vaccines for Terrestrial Animals, Rabies (http://www.oie.int/eng/normes/mmanual/A_00044.htm, accessed 27-June-2005.

11 The oral vaccination of foxes against rabies. Report of the Scientific Committee on Animal Health and Animal Wildlife. Adopted on 23 October 2002. European Commission (http://europa.eu.int/comm/food/fs/sc/scah/outcome_en.html, accessed 15 April 2005.

12 Cliquet F, Aubert M: Elimination of terrestrial rabies in Western European countries, in Schudel A, Lombard M (eds): Control of Infectious Animal Diseases by Vaccination. Dev Biol. Basel, Karger, 2004, vol 119, pp 185-204.

13 Brochier B, Dechamps P, Costy F, Hallet L, Leuris J, Villers M, Peharpre D, Mosselmans F, Beier R, Lecomte L, Mullier P, Roland H, Bauduin B, Kervyn T, Renders C, Escutenaire S, Pastoret PP: Eradication of rabies in Belgium by oral vaccination of red fox (*Vulpes vulpes).* Ann Med Vet 2001; 145: 293-305.

Dr. B.A. Yakobson, Kimron Veterinary Institute, P.O.B 12, IL-50250 Bet Dagan, Israel.
E-mail: dir-kimron@moag.gov.il

Dodet B, Schudel A, Pastoret PP, Lombard M (eds): Rabies in Europe.
Dev Biol (Basel). Basel, Karger, 2006, vol 125, pp 141-143.

Elimination of Rabies in the Czech Republic

O. Matouch[1], *J. Vitasek*[2], *Z. Semerad*[2], *M. Malena*[2]

[1] State Veterinary Institute, Liberec, Czech Republic
[2] State Veterinary Administration, Prague, Czech Republic

Abstract: Rabies in foxes was widespread in the territory of the Czech Republic after the Second World War. The first three cases of fox rabies appeared in North and South Bohemia in 1947.
In the following year, a considerable increase in rabies incidence was reported and of the 146 cases, 106 (74 %) of the 117 wildlife cases were in foxes. Rabies in foxes and other wild animals was verified in many border Czech and Moravian districts. Sylvatic rabies was established in the Czech Republic and persisted there enzootically for many years as a continuing problem. The red fox (*Vulpes vulpes*) became the principal vector and reservoir.
Averaging rabies cases over the long term, foxes account for about 90 % of all positive cases. The highest incidence of rabies was recorded in 1984, reaching 2,232 reported cases. Since then a continual decline in the number of cases has been visible, especially since 1992 when the positive effect of oral vaccination became evident.

Rabies Control in Wild Animals

In previous decades, rabies control was based, as in other European countries, on the numerical reduction of foxes. Several methods, including widespread gassing of fox dens, were used. The intensive culling of foxes only had a local and time-restricted effect, and did not stop the spread of the disease. Therefore, oral vaccination was introduced as a basic method of rabies control in foxes.

Oral Vaccination of Foxes

The field trial of oral immunization of foxes began in the Czech Republic in the spring of 1989. The first application of the oral rabies vaccine was carried out in the Klatovy, Domazlice, and Tachov districts adjacent to the German border. In the course of the following campaigns the treated area was extended to cover 44 districts in the autumn of 1992. In the autumn of 1993, the whole territory of the Czech Republic, with exception of rabies free districts bordering Germany, was included. The imported vaccine, of German origin, type Tübingen, prepared from attenuated strain SAD-B19, was used at the beginning of the rabies elimination programme.

Since 1992, this vaccine has been replaced by the Czech made vaccine LYSVULPEN, manufactured by BIOVETA Ivanovice, based on the SAD Bern.

The "Bavarian model" was applied during all vaccination campaigns. Volunteer hunters manually placed the vaccine baits in their hunting preserves. The strategy of distributing vaccine baits twice per year, in spring and autumn, was applied. Veterinary authorities were responsible for coordination and supervision of the campaigns at the district level. The original baiting density of 15 doses per $km^{2,}$ was gradually increased, mainly in the areas with an inconvenient epidemiological situation. After 1996, aerial distribution of the vaccine baits was selectively used on a restricted territory (4-6 districts). Aerial distribution has proven to be more efficient compared to hand distribution and the area of aerial distribution has been continuously enlarged to cover the whole treated area. Almost 25 million vaccine baits were used from 1989 through autumn of 2004.

The oral vaccination strategy was not always optimal. Vaccinated areas included only rabies infected administrative units (districts) because of limited financial resources. For this reason, oral vaccination was finished prematurely in some districts and untreated holes were created in the middle of vaccinated areas. These were the source of new outbreaks of disease, requiring the launch of additional vaccination campaigns. This complicated the whole process of rabies elimination, prolonged it, and increased the overall cost. The reduced epidemiological awareness and ineffective monitoring in originally free areas outside vaccination zones often led to re-occurrence of rabies. This was facilitated by a high population density of unvaccinated red foxes, and by an adverse disease situation near the Czech border on the territory of neighbouring states. A typical example was rabies re-occurrence in the district of Rychnov nad Kněžnou in 2001.

Monitoring of Oral Vaccination Effectiveness 1989-2004

Laboratory control examination

Follow-up investigations were aimed at the National Reference Laboratory for Rabies and were directed towards bait uptake, tetracycline marking, antibody formation, rabies diagnosis and characterisation of isolated strains by monoclonal antibodies.

Bait uptake was assessed by hunters and reached about 88 %. The indirect, but more precise, measurement of bait uptake was performed by testing fox bones for tetracycline incorporation. Tetracycline was found in 65 % to 80 % of examined samples, with an average of 75.5 %, and with considerable differences in particular areas. Antibody formation was tested in fox body fluids by the rapid fluorescent focus inhibition test (RFFIT). Specific rabies virus neutralising antibodies were detected in 61 % of examined samples.

As recommended by WHO, after each campaign, wildlife specimens were collected within vaccination areas for examination. Over 50,000 animals were examined for rabies during all campaigns. Two thousand one hundred and forty-eight rabies isolates were tested with monoclonal antibodies. All isolates were found to be street virus strains.

Epidemiology

Since the launch of the vaccination programme in 1989, the incidence of rabies in the Czech Republic has exhibited a pronounced decline. By the year 1995, the overall count of positive findings had decreased by 88 %. This positive trend has continued with minor variations. In 2001 only 35 rabies cases were registered and in 2002 only three cases were registered. The last rabies case was found in April of 2002 in a red fox in the district of Trutnov. Since that time there has not been a single case of rabies diagnosed. The Czech Republic thereby fulfilled the criteria for recognition as a rabies-free state. This event was documented in the OIE journal, Disease Information No. 30, 23 June 2004. Also, the Czech Republic has remained rabies-free for 2004. This undisputed success forces the Czech Republic to fulfill the strict criteria for maintaining this status. Proper surveillance in all areas is part of the criteria and it is focused on examination of any suspected cases or new infection foci. Continual rabies-free status has to be documented by proper monitoring.

Planning for the Future

For the coming years it is planned that oral vaccination will be restricted to the 60 km wide protective belts that border countries to the north and east, where there is still an infectious rabies situation.

Eight hundred thousand vaccine doses were applied over a territory of 31,900 km^2 in the spring campaign of 2005. The same extent of oral vaccination should be performed in the autumn and in both campaings next year.

Furthermore, we must continue to cooperate with hunters, since fox hunting remains the primary population density regulation mechanism, and an important source of laboratory samples. In order to declare the absence of rabies in the Czech Republic, about six hundred foxes per year must be examined.

Conclusions

- Oral vaccination was efficacious and brought about the elimination of rabies in the Czech Republic, which is undoubtedly a significant achievement.
- For inland countries, the oral vaccination method requires many years of application and a permanent coordination strategy with neighbouring countries.
- The oral vaccination method is a very expensive undertaking, and this can restrain its application.
- Re-infection of areas with an increasing population density of foxes called for alternative strategies using a higher number of vaccine doses and aerial distribution.

Dr. O. Matouch, State Veterinary Institute, National Reference Laboratories for Rabies, U Sila 1139, CZ-46311, Liberec 30, Czech Republic.
E-mail: matouch@volny.cz

Dodet B, Schudel A, Pastoret PP, Lombard M (eds): Rabies in Europe.
Dev Biol (Basel). Basel, Karger, 2006, vol 125, pp 145-147.

First Oral Vaccination of Wildlife Against Rabies in Estonia

E. Niin[1], *J. Barrat*[2], *M. Kristian*[1], *J.M. Demerson*[2], *F. Cliquet*[2]

[1] Veterinary and Food Board of Estonia, Tallinn, Estonia

[2] WHO Coll Cent for Research and Management in Zoonoses Control, Malzéville, France

Abstract: Estonia is a small country, with many islands, that covers a total area of 45,000 km^2 in the Baltic region. Rabies is widely distributed all over the country, even on some islands. The disease is maintained by two species: red foxes and raccoon dogs. In 2003, 813 cases of rabies were recorded with 315 cases in foxes and 362 cases in raccoon dogs; since 2002 the latter species has had the highest level of rabies infection among all animal species in Estonia. The measure used to control rabies is vaccination of dogs and cats, as they are the source on infection of humans.
In Spring 2004, a limited trial of oral vaccination of wildlife was conducted. The goal of this was to train the actors who will be implicated in larger future campaigns.
This trial was conducted on Vormsi island (92 km^2), located 10 km away from the west coast. Oral vaccination was performed manually over three days with SAG2 baits (Virbac company, France), by three teams.

INTRODUCTION

During the 1950's most rabies cases in Estonia were recorded in stray dogs. After 1953, control measures were based on the culling of stray dogs and compulsory vaccination of pets. These measures were successful, with no case recorded between 1960 and 1969. In 1969 wildlife rabies entered Estonia and has since been a constant problem.

The pattern of infected species has been relatively constant over time. Between 1968 and 2004, farm animals accounted for 5 % of cases, dogs and cats for 20 % and wildlife for 75 %. Figure 1 shows the evolution of rabies cases between 1968 and 2003.

The method used thus far to prevent human rabies has been the vaccination of dogs and cats, as these species are the main source of human contamination. The cost of the vaccine is covered by the State Budget. The last human case was recorded in 1986 in Estonia.

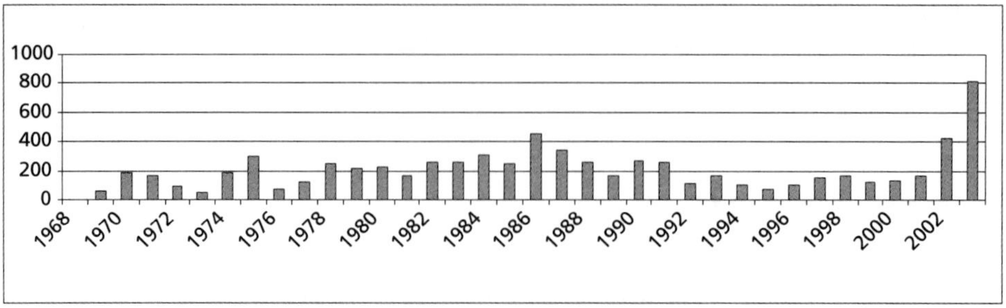

Fig. 1 : Terrestrial rabies cases from 1968 to 2003.

The aim of the Republic of Estonia is to achieve rabies free status. To reach this goal, the present control measures are not sufficient, as vaccination of pets protects humans with no impact on the the virus reservoirs, the red fox and racoon dog.

Towards this end, a small-scale field trial was conducted on a small island (Vormsi island, 92 km^2), situated 10 km away from the west coast. On that island, two rabies cases were diagnosed in 2003, with no case identified for the previous 6 years. The goal of the trial was to assess, on a limited scale, the feasibility of oral vaccination in Estonia.

Materials and Methods

The trial was included in the frames of the Twining light project PHARE "Minimalisation of number of rabies cases among wild and domestic animals in Estonia". Two campaigns were conducted in the spring (02-04 June) and autumn (20-22 September).

Vormsi is a group of islands comprised of one main island and 30 smaller ones. Half of the area is covered by forest. The western part is a landscape of meadows and junipers forests. The eastern side is comprised of marshlands. Human density in this region is very low as well as the density of agricultural animals. Wildlife is abundant; there are 25 different species of mammals, 211 species of birds, including the white tailed eagle and the crane; the fox population is estimated at 45 adults, the raccoon dog population at 50 adults; there are 3 lynxes, 30 martens and lots of wild boars.

Before the beginning of the study, the Veterinary and Food Board (VFB) informed the Ministries involved and the Press, and posters were installed in shops, schools including kindergarden, and bus stops across the island. Local government and hunters associations were informed in order to obtain their participation.

Three thousand five hundred doses of SAG_2 were received from France and stored at – 20° C until distribution. Maps at a scale of 1/50,000 were used to precisely define the areas to be treated daily.

Three groups were constituted to distribute baits. Each one was comprised of three to four volunteers (veterinarians, veterinary officers, and students). Each group was assisted by a local hunter functioning as a specialist of the local environment. Three cars and auxiliaries (baits, gloves, maps, storage boxes, forms…) were provided by VFB. Overall coordination was performed by VFB and WHO Collaborative Centre in Nancy, France.

Vaccination was implemented within 3 working days. Each working day began with a general meeting where distribution areas and the distribution scheme were exposed. Baits were then delivered to the head of the group. After vaccination, treated areas were identified to assess that is the entire area was treated. The baiting density was 20 baits/km^2, two to five baits were identified in the field per group and per day to monitor bait uptake. At the end of each day, another meeting was held to fill-in the monitoring form, define the area actually treated and compare it to the planned treatment area, and collect global data on control baits, dens found in the area, animals seen, etc.A the end of the trial, a final meeting was held to summarize the campaign and highlight the need for monitoring rabies (suspect animals sent for diagnosis) and oral vaccination (seroconversion rate and tetracycline examination for bait uptake).

Results

Bait consumption was controlled with 20 control baits in the spring and 22 in autumn. Five of the 20 spring control baits were eaten within two days, 14 within one week and 17 within three weeks. Two remained untouched and in one case the casing alone was eaten. In autumn, among the 22 control baits, seven baits were consumed in two days, 21 in one week and all 22 baits were consumed within three weeks.

The viral titre of vaccine baits was controlled in eight baits in the spring and six in autumn. These baits were collected at the end of the working day and brought back to France. All measured titres were over 10^8 $TCID_{50}$ per dose which is more than 10 times the 100 % protection dose.

Eight raccoon dogs and three foxes were sacrificed on Vormsi island between 2004 and May 2005 and tested by fluorescent antibody test (FAT) at the Veterinary and Food Laboratory. They were all found negative for rabies.

The teeth of these animals were examined for tetracycline: nine were positive, two were negative.

Conclusions

This first field trial of oral vaccination of wildlife in Estonia conducted with a small budget showed the feasibility of the method. It should be followed by a larger, aerial campaign.

Acknowledgements

This work was conducted with the help of Estonian volunteers, hunters associations in Vormsi, and the Veterinary and Food Board.

Dr. E. Niin, Veterinary and Food Board of Estonia, Väike Paala str. 3, 11415 Tallinn, Estonia.
E-mail: enel.niin@vet.agri.ee

Dodet B, Schudel A, Pastoret PP, Lombard M (eds): Rabies in Europe.
Dev Biol (Basel). Basel, Karger, 2006, vol 125, pp 149-151.

Teaching Rabies: A CD Rom for Training Students and Veterinarians

M. Artois[1], M. Drouet[1], I.F. Ravier[2], S. Thomas-Touze[1]

[1] Ecole Nationale Vétérinaire de Lyon, Marcy l'Etoile, France
[2] Mérial, Villeurbanne, France

Abstract: This brief note justifies the need for updated information for the education of veterinarians; it introduces a pedagogic CD Rom which is dedicated for this purpose in the field of rabies prevention.

INTRODUCTION

Rabies is a typical example of a veterinary public health concern, where preservation of a person's life at the individual level requires the organised participation of the veterinary profession. Any success in this field is based on close cooperation between veterinary officers and practitioners who are at the interface of risk of transmission by potentially infected pets and exposed owners. Unacceptable consequences can result from the failure of this strategic approach, which is based on individual protection, when potential rabies vectors are exposed to an uncontrolled reservoir.

Rabies was originally described in dogs more than 2,500 years ago [1] but disappeared in the so-called "industrial" world during the first years of the 20th century. Nevertheless, in the Northern Hemisphere, large epizootics of rabies began to be reported in wildlife from the end of the 19th century onward, to the extent that infection in dogs has been controlled by sanitary and medical measures. Fox rabies is thought to have emerged in Europe around the time of the Second World War [2,3]. After five decades, this outbreak seems to be under control in most Western European countries where oral vaccination of foxes appears as a success story (see articles in this volume). For European citizens, however, the risk of being infected by the rabies virus still exists due to either indigenous bats or the introduction of a companion animal incubating the virus, coming from a neighbouring infected country.

For example, in 2004, three dogs were introduced into France, in spite of regulations banning the importation of non-vaccinated animals, and were subsequently recognised as rabid [4]; they were the cause of a great number of human post exposure treatments.

Veterinary surgeons are consequently on the front line of preventing human contamination, supplying appropriate information to pet owners, regarding vaccination, and travellers, regarding the risk of exposure in enzootic countries.

In Western Europe, most practising veterinarians used to receive extensive information on rabies in foxes and clinical diagnosis in domestic animals, the victims of virus spill-over from wild reservoirs. Actually, most of the teaching support has been based on this main form of the disease [5]. This knowledge needs to be updated. Current veterinary students as well as veterinarians must be precisely informed about the new dangers presented by rabies introduction and the available methods of prevention.

A pedagogic CD Rom has been created to deliver exactly this type of information using text, photographs and videos in an easy access and interactive format. All information is solely available in French. This CD has been prepared [6] with the financial support of the Merial Company and the technical support of the new technologies department (pole Aventi) at the veterinary school of Lyon.

Pedagogic aims of this material are summarised as follows, after use of this CD rom, the user should be able to:

- Give information to clients about the history of rabies and the countries affected by the disease.
- Identify a case presenting clinical and epidemiological evidence of recent exposure to the rabies virus.
- Develop the best comportment regarding the risk that an animal presented in consultation may be infected.
- Justify this comportment with the most recent scientific arguments.
- Present the main aspects of the international regulation for the movement of pet animals accompanying their owner.

Chapter headings of the CD are divided into: history, teaching course, Quiz, documents, and links. By clicking on a menu, the user can access charts explaining virus transmission, disease incubation, salivary excretion of virus, virus replication and immune response to infection and vaccination. Clinical signs are introduced with photographs and videos, and laboratory diagnostic tests are presented and illustrated with original slides.

A quiz allows the user to verify if he manages to adopt the correct behaviour when facing situations inspired by real cases. More than four hours of reading are expected for comprehensive use of the material which includes a recent version of the hand-out on rabies dedicated to veterinary students in France [5]. Most of the material is also available for consultation on line at http://fr.merial.com/.

It is infrequent that innovation in the area of teaching and training is documented in a scientific support. The authors believe it is important to put to use knowledge of appropriate media for educational purposes. Since animal health is now a global concern, improvement in this field must be brought to the attention of managers and officers worldwide, or at least in French speaking countries, which can use this learning tool.

Acknowledgements

The authors thank Yves MONLIEN, Pôle AVENTI, who prepared the CD Rom and carried out the computer animation. Contributions of experts at the Veterinary School of Maisons Alfort: Professor B. TOMA, Laboratoire d'Etudes et de Recherches sur la Rage et la Pathologie des Animaux Sauvages (AFSSA): Dr Florence CLIQUET and her colleagues, Ministry of Agriculture (Veterinary Services): Dr Nathalie MELIK and her colleagues, Pasteur Institute in Paris: Dr Hervé BOURHY and "Entente interdépartementale de lutte contre la rage et autres zoonoses": M. Benoît COMBES must be acknowledged for their highly relevant contribution to this CD Rom.

References

1 Blancou J: Histoire de la surveillance et du contrôle des maladies animales transmissibles. Office International des Epizooties, Paris, 2000, 366 p.

2 Pitzschke H: Epizootologische Betrachtungen über den Verlauf des Tollwut 1945-1958 in Europa mit besonderer Berücksichtigung Deutschlands. Arch Exp Veterinarmed 1959; 23: 992-1017.

3 Schaaf J: Die wichtigeren Tierseuchen im früheren Polen. Dtsch Tierarztl Wochenschr 1940; 45: 540-543.

4 French Ministry of Agriculture and Ministry of Health: Measures to Control an Imported Case of Canine Rabies in France, in Dodet B, Schudel A, Pastoret PP, Lombard M (eds): Rabies in Europe. Dev Biol (Basel). Basel, Karger, 2006, vol 125, pp 95-100.

5 Toma B (ed): La rage. Polycopiés de maladies contagieuses. Lyon, Merial, 2004, 69 p.

6 Drouet M: La rage animale, revue de la littérature: réalisation d'un document pédagogique interactif. Thèse de Médecine vétérinaire. Lyon, 2004, 37 p (+ CD Rom).

Prof. M. Artois, Ecole nationale vétérinaire de Lyon, Unité de Pathologie infectieuse et épidémiologie, 1, avenue Bourgelat, FR-69280 Marcy l'Etoile, France.
E-mail: m.artois@vet-lyon.fr

Dodet B, Schudel A, Pastoret PP, Lombard M (eds): Rabies in Europe.
Dev Biol (Basel). Basel, Karger, 2006, vol 125, p 153.

SESSION IV

Human Rabies Prevention

Chairperson: *Y. Rotivel* (Institut Pasteur, France)
Rapporteur: *M. Warrel* (CTM, United Kingdom)

Dodet B, Schudel A, Pastoret PP, Lombard M (eds): Rabies in Europe.
Dev Biol (Basel). Basel, Karger, 2006, vol 125, pp 155-164.

Human Rabies Prevention

M.E. Miranda[1], F.X. Meslin[2], the WHO Rabies Expert Consultation Members

[1] World Health Organization Regional Office for the Western Pacific, Manila, Philippines

[2] World Health Organization, Food Safety and Veterinary Public Health, Geneva, Switzerland

Rabies control suffers from neglect brought about by the perceived small number of cases from poor disease surveillance. This in turn leads to a lack of incentive and funding for effective control and elimination efforts. Given that a major factor in the low level of commitment to rabies control is the lack of accurate data on the true public health and economic impact of the disease, WHO initiated a re-evaluation of the burden of rabies in Asia and Africa. Output of this study was published in the Bulletin of WHO in May 2005 [1].

A data-driven assessment could result in better and more studies on cost-effectiveness and the impact of intervention, and better policy decisions. Human mortality from endemic canine rabies was estimated to be 55,000 deaths per year globally. In Africa the mortality was estimated to be 24,000 deaths per year with less than 500,000 post-exposure prophylaxis (PEP) administered, and in Asia 31,000 deaths per year with more than 8,000,000 PEPs provided. Deaths due to rabies are responsible for 1.74 million disability adjusted life years (DALYs) lost each year. The estimated annual cost of rabies is US$ 584 million with Asia representing 96 % of this cost (primarily due to the cost of human treatment). Children aged less than 15 years represent an average of 40 % of those seeking PEP.

In comparison, Europe, North America and the Latin Americas collectively report less than 80 human deaths and less than 450,000 PEPs per year yet the estimated total annual expenditure for rabies prevention amounts to more than US$ 300 million [2].

The following Chapter and Annex on **Human Rabies Prevention** is taken in toto from the **WHO Expert Consultation on Rabies Report**, WHO Technical Report Series No. 931, June 2005 [2]. The readers are kindly referred to the full document on www.who.int/rabies

Chapter 6. Prevention of rabies in humans

Vaccines used for the prevention of rabies in humans, including both pre- and post-exposure prophylaxis, should always meet WHO recommendations for production and control. Treatment for the prevention of rabies in humans exposed to rabies should begin as soon as possible after the exposure occurs. Treatment consists of thorough wound cleansing for a minimum of 15 minutes using water, soap and a virucidal antiseptic (e.g. povidone iodine or ethanol) followed by the administration of rabies passive immunization and cell-culture or purified embryonated egg rabies vaccine of proven efficacy. The initial treatment of severely exposed (category III) subjects must include injection of rabies immunoglobulin according to WHO recommendations (see Annex 1). The Consultation strongly advocates the use of cell-culture or purified embryonated egg rabies vaccines that comply with WHO criteria for potency, immunogenicity, innocuity, and safety that have been satisfactorily assessed in well-designed clinical trials.

6.1 Pre-exposure vaccination

National authorities should provide guidance as to who should receive pre-exposure vaccination. Generally pre-exposure vaccination should be offered to people at high risk of exposure such as those working in rabies diagnostic or research laboratories, veterinarians, animal handlers (including bat handlers), animal rehabilitators and wildlife officers, as well as other people (especially children) living in or travelling to high-risk areas. Children under 15 years of age are the most frequently exposed age group, representing approximately 50 % of human exposures in canine rabies-infected areas. Vaccines produced in cell culture or from embryonated eggs should be used for pre-exposure vaccination of humans. Pre-exposure vaccination is administered as one full dose of vaccine intramuscularly or 0.1 ml intradermally on days 0, 7 and either day 21 or 28. A few days' variation is acceptable. Vaccine is administered into the upper arm (deltoid region) of adults and into the anterolateral thigh region of young children. Vaccine should never be administered into the gluteal region as absorption is unpredictable. Rabies vaccines having a potency of at least 2.5 IU per single intramuscular dose (NIH test) will induce long-lasting memory cells causing an accelerated immune response when a booster dose of vaccine is administered. People currently receiving malaria prophylaxis or who are unable to complete the entire three-dose pre-exposure series prior to initiation of malarial prophylaxis should receive pre-exposure vaccination by the intramuscular route. If the immune status of a patient is questionable at the time of vaccination, his or her immune response to the vaccine should be assessed after the three-dose pre-exposure series has been administered.

Periodic booster injections are recommended for people who are at continual risk of rabies exposure. The following guidelines are recommended for determining when boosters should be administered.

- All people who work with live rabies virus in a diagnostic or research laboratory or in vaccine production should have periodic antibody determinations to avoid unnecessary boosters.
- People at continuous risk, e.g. rabies researchers, diagnostic laboratory workers (where virus is present continuously, often in high concentrations, and where specific exposures are likely to go unrecognized) should have serological test-

ing every 6 months. Judging the relative risk of exposure and the monitoring of vaccination status is the responsibility of the laboratory supervisor. A booster is recommended if the titre falls below 0.5 IU/ml.

- Responsible authorities should ensure that all people at risk are vaccinated and that serological status is monitored.
  A rabies pre-exposure certificate should be completed and given to the vaccinee indicating the type of vaccine and vaccine regimen used, lot number of vaccine, and any adverse reactions that occurred during vaccination.

6.2 Post-exposure prophylaxis

6.2.1 General considerations

All people exposed to rabies should promptly and thoroughly cleanse their wound(s) and apply appropriate antiseptics. Professional assistance is advised. This should be followed, if careful medical assessment requires it, by a complete vaccine series using a potent and effective vaccine that meets WHO criteria and passive immunization in category III exposure. A complete guide to post-exposure prophylaxis can be found in Annex 1. Strict adherence to the WHO-recommended guidelines for optimal post-exposure rabies prophylaxis virtually guarantees protection from the disease. Rabies vaccines for human use that meet WHO requirements for production and control are safe and effective and are free from the neuroparalytic adverse reactions associated with nerve tissue-derived products. Pregnancy, infancy, old age and concurrent illness are not contraindications for rabies post-exposure prophylaxis in the event of an exposure. Prolonged incubation periods have been associated with human rabies; therefore people who present for treatment even months after a possible rabies exposure should be evaluated and treated as if the event had occurred recently.

Factors that should be considered in deciding whether or not to initiate post-exposure prophylaxis include:

- nature of the contact or injury;
- presence of rabies in the area where the contact occurred or where the animal responsible originated;
- availability of the animal for laboratory examination or observation;
- species of the animal;
- clinical status of the animal responsible;
- vaccination history of the animal, and type and timing of vaccine used.

The decision to administer post-exposure prophylaxis after an exposure to an apparently healthy animal should be based on a careful risk assessment by a qualified medical professional. The risk assessment should consider the criteria outlined above. A history of rabies vaccination in an animal is not always a guarantee that the biting animal is not rabid. Animal vaccine failures may occur because of improper administration or poor quality of the vaccine, poor health status of the animal, and the fact that one vaccine dose does not always provide long-lasting protection against infection in dogs. Whether a dog bite was provoked rather than unprovoked should not be considered a guarantee that the animal is not rabid as it can be difficult to understand what an attacking dog considers provocation for an attack. If the animal involved in the exposure is a potential rabies vector in a rabies-endemic region, initiation of post-exposure prophylaxis should never await the results of laboratory examination, nor should the responsible animal be observed for signs of rabies prior to starting post-exposure prophylaxis. Wound treatment and administration of rabies biologicals, including a passive immunization product, when required, and vaccine, should be started as soon as possible after exposure. Immediate humane killing of the animal and examination of the brain at a reliable laboratory should be performed whenever possible. If the species involved is unlikely to be infected with rabies, treatment may be deferred pending the outcome of laboratory testing, providing that results can be obtained within 48 hours.

If the attacking animal is a pet dog or cat that is available, it should be kept under observation for 10 days, preferably under the supervision of a veterinarian. Prophylaxis can be discontinued if the dog or cat remains healthy for at least 10 days after the exposure occurred. The natural history of rabies in mammals other than dogs or cats is not fully understood and therefore the 10-day observation period may not be applicable. Humans exposed to other species of mammals suspected to be rabid, including bats and other wild animals involved in the transmission of rabies should therefore receive post-exposure prophylaxis unless the animal can be captured, humanely killed and immediately examined at a reliable laboratory.

6.2.2 Certificate of post-exposure prophylaxis

A certificate of post-exposure prophylaxis should be filled in and given to each vaccinee.

6.2.3 Complications of post-exposure prophylaxis

Rabies immunoglobulins

Early local injection-site reactions consisting of erythema and itching are not uncommon with both human and purified equine immunoglobulins. Published data indicate that immunoglobulins can be safely injected into already infected animal bite wounds following proper wound cleansing and the administration of appropriate antibiotics.

Equine rabies immunoglobulin (ERIG)

Most ERIGs that are manufactured presently are highly purified and the occurrence of adverse events has been significantly reduced. Unlike the original unpurified rabies antisera which resulted in adverse reactions in as many as 40 % of recipients, the adverse-reaction rate of patients receiving highly purified ERIGs has been reduced to < 1 – 2 %. Serious adverse reactions, including anaphylaxis, may occur in spite of a negative skin test. ERIG should only be used by medical staff trained and equipped to manage such an adverse reaction. Unpurified rabies antisera are not recommended.

F(ab´)2 products

F(ab´)2 fragments are obtained by cleavage of the immunoglobulin by a proteolytic enzyme, pepsin, followed by separation of the F (ab´) 2 fragments from the Fc fragment. Many of the ERIGs now available are produced in this way.

F(ab´)2 fragments are cleared more rapidly in vivo than intact immunoglobulins. Undesirable side-effects are rare and are similar to those listed above for ERIGs.

Human rabies immunoglobulin

HRIG produced under good manufacturing practices is virtually devoid of serious adverse reactions. It is purified from carefully selected donors, and processing eliminates viral contaminants including those of the human immunodeficiency and hepatitis viruses.

Purified cell-culture and embryonated egg rabies vaccines

These vaccines have not been causally associated with serious adverse effects. Mild serum sickness-like and urticarial reactions have been occasionally been observed following booster doses of human diploid cell vaccine.

ANNEX 1

GUIDE FOR POST-EXPOSURE PROPHYLAXIS

A1. General considerations

The recommendations given here are intended as a general guide. It is understood that, in certain situations, modifications of these recommendations may be warranted. Such situations include, but are not limited to: exposure of infants or mentally disabled people to a suspect or confirmed rabid animal; and when a reliable exposure history cannot be ascertained, particularly in areas where rabies is enzootic, even when the animal is considered to be healthy at the time of exposure. A careful risk assessment should be conducted by a qualified medical professional on every patient exposed to a potentially rabid animal (see section 6.2).

Post-exposure prophylaxis consists of local treatment of the wound, initiated as soon as possible after an exposure, followed by the administration of passive immunization, if indicated, and a potent and effective rabies vaccine that meets WHO criteria [2]. Post-exposure prophylaxis may be discontinued if the animal involved is a dog or cat that remains healthy for an observation period of 10 days after the exposure occurred; or if the animal is humanely killed and proven to be negative for rabies by a reliable diagnostic laboratory using a prescribed test. If the animal inflicting the wound is suspected of being rabid and is not apprehended, post-exposure prophylaxis should be instituted immediately. When animal bites occur in a rabies-free area where adequate rabies surveillance is in effect, post-exposure prophylaxis may not be required depending upon the outcome of a risk assessment conducted by a medical expert knowledgeable in the epidemiology of rabies in the area and the proper requirements for assessing the risk involved (see section 6.2). In areas where canine or wildlife rabies is enzootic, adequate laboratory surveillance is in place, and data from laboratory and field experience indicate that there is no infection in the species involved, local health authorities may not recommend antirabies prophylaxis.

A2. Local treatment of wounds

Elimination of rabies virus at the site of the infection by chemical or physical means is an effective mechanism of protection. Therefore, the Consultation emphasized the importance of prompt local treatment of all bite wounds and scratches that might be contaminated with rabies virus. Recommended first-aid procedures include immediate and thorough flushing and washing of the wound for a minimum of 15 minutes with soap and water, detergent, povidone iodine or other substances of proven lethal effect on rabies virus. If soap or an antiviral agent is not available, the wound should be thoroughly and extensively washed with water. People who live in rabies-infected areas should be educated in simple local wound treatment and warned not to use procedures that may further contaminate the wounds. Most severe bite wounds are best treated by daily dressing followed by secondary suturing where necessary. If suturing after wound cleansing cannot be avoided, the wound should first be infiltrated with passive rabies immunization products and suturing delayed for several hours. This will allow diffusion of the antibody to occur through the tissues before suturing is performed. Other treatments, such as the administration of antibiotics and tetanus prophylaxis, should be applied as appropriate for other bite wounds.

A3. Administration of rabies biologicals for passive immunization

The role of passive rabies immunization products is to provide the immediate availability of neutralizing antibodies at the site of the exposure before it is physiologically possible for the patient to begin producing his or her own antibodies after vaccination. Therefore, passive immunization products should be administered to all patients presenting with exposure to rabies-infected material onto mucous membranes or into transdermal wounds.

A3.1 Classes of rabies biologicals and precautions for their use

There are three classes of rabies biological products for passive immunization available at present: human rabies immunoglobulin (HRIG); equine rabies immunoglobulin (ERIG), and highly purified F(ab´)2 products produced from ERIG. Most ERIG products currently being manufactured are highly purified and the occurrence of adverse events has been significantly reduced. Given that the clearance of F(ab´)2 fragments is more rapid than intact immunoglobulins, the Consultation recommended that in cases of multiple severe exposures, HRIG should be used for passive immunization. Most of the new ERIG preparations are potent, highly purified, safe and considerably less expensive than HRIG. However, they are of heterologous origin and carry a small risk of hypersensitivity reactions and therefore a skin test should be conducted prior to administration of ERIG and F(ab´)2 products according to the guidelines of the manufacturer. Serum sickness, using a highly purified ERIG product, appears among < 1 – 2 % of recipients and usually develops 1 week after administration. In the event of a positive skin test to ERIG or an F(ab´)2 product, HRIG should be administered. If HRIG is not available, ERIG or F(ab´)2 products should still be used but should be administered under the close supervision of competent staff located in adequate medical facilities.

A3.2 Dosage and administration

The dose for HRIG is 20 IU/kg body weight, and for ERIG and F (ab´) 2 products is 40 IU/kg body weight. As much of the recommended dose of passive immunization products as is anatomically feasible should be infiltrated into and around the wounds. Multiple needle injections into the wound should be avoided. If a finger or toe needs to be infiltrated, care must be taken not to cause a compartment syndrome, which can occur when an excessive volume is infiltrated under pressure and blood circulation is impaired. In the event that a remainder of passive rabies immunization product is left after all wounds have been infiltrated, it should be administered by deep intramuscular injection at an injection site distant from the vaccine injection site. Animal bite wounds inflicted can be severe and multiple, especially in small children. In such cases, the calculated dose of the passive rabies immunization product may not be sufficient to infiltrate all wounds. In these circumstances, it is advisable to dilute the passive immunization product in normal saline to a sufficient volume to be able to inject all wounds. A full course of vaccine should follow thorough wound cleansing and passive immunization.

A4. Vaccine administration for active immunization

Intramuscular regimens

Cell-culture or purified embryonated egg rabies vaccines having a potency of at least 2.5 IU per single intramuscular immunizing dose should be applied according to one of the following regimens.

Five-dose intramuscular regimen (Essen regimen)

One dose of vaccine is administered intramuscularly on days 0, 3, 7, 14 and 28. Injections must be given in the upper arm (deltoid region) or, in small children, into the anterolateral thigh muscle. *Vaccine should never be administered into the gluteal region, where absorption is unpredictable.*

Abbreviated multisite intramuscular regimen ("2–1–1" or Zagreb regimen)

One dose of vaccine is administered intramuscularly into the left and one into the right upper arm (deltoid region) on day 0 followed by one dose into the upper arm (deltoid region) on days 7 and 21. This schedule saves two clinic visits and one vaccine dose.

Intradermal regimens

A limited number of rabies vaccines has been recognized to date by WHO as safe and efficacious for post-exposure prophylaxis when administered by the intradermal route in two different regimens. Local manufacturers in rabies-endemic countries are beginning to produce rabies vaccines. The intradermal use of these vaccines should be based on adherence to WHO requirements for that route and approval by national health authorities (see section 5). New vaccine manufacturers should provide clinical evidence that their products are immunogenic and safe when used intradermally. Clinical evidence should include clinical trials involving a vaccine of known immunogenicity and efficacy when used by this route as control, serological testing with rapid fluorescent focus inhibition test, and publication in internationally peer-reviewed journals.

Updated Thai Red Cross intradermal regimen ("2–2–2–0–2" regimen)

Sufficient clinical evidence was presented to the Consultation indicating that a single dose of vaccine given on day 90 of the original Thai Red Cross regimen ("2–2–2–0–1–1" regimen) can be replaced if two doses of vaccine are given on day 28 ("2–2–2–0–2" regimen). The Thai Red Cross regimen considerably lowers the cost of vaccination as the total volume of vaccine required is much less than that needed for intramuscular regimens.

The schedule for the updated Thai Red Cross intradermal regimen is as follows: one dose of vaccine, in a volume of 0.1 ml is given intradermally at two different lymphatic drainage sites, usually the left and right upper arm, on days 0, 3, 7 and 28. Vaccine administered intradermally must raise a visible and palpable "bleb" in the skin. In the event that a dose of vaccine is inadvertently given subcutaneously or intramuscularly, a new dose should be administered intradermally. Currently there are two vaccines that have been proven to be efficacious in the Thai Red Cross regimen: purified Vero cell rabies vaccine produced by Aventis Pasteur and purified chick embryo cell rabies vaccine produced by Chiron Vaccines.

Eight-site intradermal regimen ("8–0–4–0–1–1" regimen)

One dose of 0.1 ml is administered intradermally at eight different sites (upper arms, lateral thighs, suprascapular region, and lower quadrant of abdomen) on day 0. On day 7, four 0.1 ml injections are administered intradermally into each upper arm (deltoid region) and each lateral thigh. Following these injections, one additional 0.1 ml dose is administered on days 28 and 90. This regimen lowers the cost of vaccine administered by intramuscular regimens and generally produces a higher antibody response than the other recommended schedules by day 14. It does not result in a significantly earlier antibody response and in order to ensure optimal treatment, a passive immune product must be administered to patients presenting with severe exposures. Only two commercial products are today considered safe and efficacious when administered according to this regimen. They include a human diploid cell vaccine produced by Aventis Pasteur and a purified chick embryo cell rabies vaccine produced by Chiron Vaccines.

Intradermal injections must be administered by staff trained in this technique. Vaccine vials should be stored between 2 °C and 8 °C after reconstitution and the total content should be used as soon as possible, but at least within 8 hours. Rabies vaccines formulated with an adjuvant should not be administered intradermally.

A5. Post-exposure prophylaxis of previously vaccinated people

Individuals who are not immunocompromised and who have been previously vaccinated with a potent and effective rabies vaccine that meets WHO criteria for vaccine production and have adequate documentation should receive a two-booster series consisting of one intramuscular or intradermal dose on days 0 and 3. The administration of passive immunization is not required.

Local wound treatment should be completed as noted above. People who have received pre-exposure or post-exposure vaccination using a vaccine of unproven potency, should receive a full post-exposure vaccination series including passive immunization.

A6. Post-exposure prophylaxis of HIV-infected people and HIV/AIDS patients

Several studies of patients with HIV/AIDS have reported that those with very low CD4 counts will mount a significantly lower or no detectable neutralizing antibody response to rabies. In such patients and those in whom the presence of immunological memory is no longer assured as a result of other causes, proper and thorough wound treatment as described above and antisepsis accompanied by local infiltration of a passive immunization product are of utmost importance.

Immunocompromised patients with category II exposures should receive rabies immunoglobulin in addition to a full post-exposure vaccination series as listed above. An infectious disease specialist with expert knowledge of rabies prevention should be consulted.

A7. Type of contact, exposure and recommended post-exposure prophylaxis

Table A1 should serve as a guide for post-exposure prophylaxis. In cases where exposure is questionable or a patient has a concurrent medical condition that may complicate post-exposure prophylaxis, an expert in the administration of rabies prophylaxis should be consulted.

Table A1: Type of contact, exposure and recommended post-exposure prophylaxis.

Category	Type of contact with a suspect or confirmed rabid domestic or wild[a] animal, or animal unavailable for testing	Type of exposure	Recommended post-exposure prophylaxis
I	Touching or feeding of animals Licks on intact skin	None	None, if reliable case history is available
II	Nibbling of uncovered skin Minor scratches or abrasions without bleeding	Minor	Administer vaccine immediately[b] Stop treatment if animal remains healthy throughout an observation period of 10 days[c] or if animal is proven to be negative for rabies by a reliable laboratory using appropriate diagnostic techniques
III	Single or multiple transdermal bites or scratches, licks on broken skin Contamination of mucous membrane with saliva (i.e. licks) Exposures to bats[d]	Severe	Administer rabies immunoglobulin and vaccine immediately. Stop treatment if animal remains healthy throughout an observation period of 10 days or if animal is found to be negative for rabies by a reliable laboratory using appropriate diagnostic techniques

[a] Exposure to rodents, rabbits and hares seldom, if ever, requires specific anti-rabies post-exposure prophylaxis.

[b] If an apparently healthy dog or cat in or from a low-risk area is placed under observation, the situation may warrant delaying initiation of treatment.

[c] This observation period applies only to dogs and cats. Except in the case of threatened or endangered species, other domestic and wild animals suspected as rabid should be humanely killed and their tissues examined for the presence of rabies antigen using appropriate laboratory techniques.

[d] Post-exposure prophylaxis should be considered when contact between a human and a bat has occurred unless the exposed person can rule out a bite or scratch, or exposure to a mucous membrane.

References

1 Knobel DL, Cleaveland S, Coleman PG, Fevre EM, Meltzer MI, Miranda MEG, Shaw A, Zinsstag J, Meslin FX: Re-evaluating the burden of rabies in Africa and Asia. Bull WHO, May 2005; 83 (5): 360-368.

2 WHO Expert Consultation on Rabies, First Report, WHO Technical Report Series 931, Geneva, World Health Organization, 2005

Dr. M.E. Miranda, World Health Organization Regional Office for the Western Pacific, P.O. Box 2932, 1000 Manila, Philippines.
E-mail: rhysmiranda@yahoo.com; rabnet@who.int

Dodet B, Schudel A, Pastoret PP, Lombard M (eds): Rabies in Europe.
Dev Biol (Basel). Basel, Karger, 2006, vol 125, pp 165-173.

Occupational Lyssavirus Risks and Post-Vaccination Monitoring

S.M. Brookes, A.R. Fooks

Rabies and Wildlife Zoonoses Group, Veterinary Laboratories Agency (VLA), WHO Collaborating Centre for the Characterisation of Rabies and Rabies-Related Viruses, Addlestone, Surrey, United Kingdom

Key words: Rabies virus, lyssaviruses, vaccine, occupational risk.

Abstract: In the UK, rabies pre-exposure vaccination involves a 3-dose course (D0, 7 & 28) and reinforcing doses at a 2-3 year intervals. This booster schedule had been implemented following scientific evidence indicating that a reduction in the previous regime interval of 3-5 years was warranted. The regime changes were particularly relevant to high risk groups that may encounter rabies virus. Those at known high risk of exposure to rabies and other Lyssaviruses include laboratory staff and a diverse group of animal handlers. Since the detection of EBLV-2 in the UK in four Daubenton's bats between 1996-2004 and a human case in 2002, those who now come into contact with bats are also considered at risk. Prior to 2002, data indicated that less than 50 % ($n = 193$) of all bat handlers had been vaccinated against rabies and 25 % of this group had exceeded the recommended booster interval. Following the human fatality, the vaccine became free to all UK bat handlers and all licensed and the majority of unlicensed bat handlers were vaccinated.
Vaccinated laboratory workers are serologically monitored and boosted following a blood test of < 1.0 IU/ml of neutralising antibodies (FAVN-CVS). An analysis of laboratory staff ($n = 25$) indicated that 28 % ($n = 7$) maintained a suitable antibody level for greater than 5 years after their final boost, but 16 % ($n = 4$) had a titre of 1.0 IU/ml for < 12 months. Of the 25 individuals, 70 % required a booster in 2.5 years. In 2002, internal VLA policy was amended to increase antibody monitoring from 2 to 4 times per annum and to insist that all laboratory workers maintained a RABV titre of > 5.0 IU/ml for those in contact with non-RABV lyssaviruses in order to ensure that all individuals had antibody levels capable of neutralising the phylogroup I lyssaviruses.

INTRODUCTION

In the UK there are currently two-licensed rabies vaccines: rabies human diploid vaccine (HDCV, Aventis Pasteur Ltd) and purified chick embryo cell rabies vaccine (PCECV, Chiron Vaccines). These vaccines are mainly used in the occupational health setting, as the UK is 'rabies free' according to the World Organisation for Animal Health (OIE) definition. There is no indigenous terrestrial rabies in the UK, however, there have been five cases of European bat lyssavirus type 2 (EBLV-2) since 1996; four cases in Daubenton's bats and one human case in 2002 [1]. Pre-exposure (prophylactic) immunisation with rabies vaccine is offered to laboratory workers, and animal handlers, especially those dealing with imported animals and bat handlers, and some health workers (those about to deal with probable or confirmed human rabies cases). Vaccination is also recommended for travellers to rabies endemic areas [2].

Post-exposure prophylaxis (PEP) is based on established criteria involving the risk level and immune status of the potentially exposed individual. This regimen can involve either immunisation following a designated vaccination schedule or vaccination combined with rabies human immunoglobulin administration. Further details can be found from a variety of resources [2-5].

High risk laboratory workers undergo close serological monitoring to verify that the rabies vaccination requirements of occupational health and safety guidelines are met. In the lower risk groups, such as bat handlers, serological monitoring has been infrequent and inconsistent.

Until 2002, rabies vaccination was supplied free of charge to licensed bat workers but not unlicensed bat handlers; the latter were required to pay for there own vaccines when and if they were administered. The Bat Conservation Trust carried out a rabies immunisation survey in November 2002 and found that the vaccination uptake rate in bat handlers of all types was low (circa 43 %, range 11-49 %) ($n = 193$). Of those who had been vaccinated only 25 % were within the 3-5 year recommended booster interval. In the non-licensed bat handlers ($n = 36$) 36 % were immunised, only 16 % had kept their reinforcing doses up to date, and cost had been reported as a significant factor in the lack of obtaining rabies vaccination [6]. Bat workers were not routinely blood tested to determine the level of circulating rabies virus neutralising antibody (VNA). Studies are currently underway to examine the rabies vaccinated bat worker cohort and immunisation now approaches 100 %. The majority of bat workers have participated in a recent study to assess their rabies VNA status. The project involved serological analysis followed by a reinforcing dose of rabies vaccine which for many was at an interval of 2 years after their primary immunisation course. It was shown that 11 % of vaccine recipients had below the recommended minimum level of neutralising antibody [7].

Serological testing is advised only for those who work with the live viruses, mainly laboratory staff. In this high risk occupational group VNA is assessed every 3-6 months and booster doses of vaccine given to maintain immune status. The WHO currently considers the minimal acceptable, measurable antibody titre to be 0.5 IU/ml [5-7]. At the VLA, and due to the hazardous nature of handling high titre lyssaviruses, local policy was implemented based on laboratory evidence. If handling classical rabies viruses (RABV), the requirement for laboratory staff is a minimum antibody titre of 1.0 IU/ml. For those handling non-RABV phylogroup I viruses (EBLVs, ABLV and DUVV) [8] a minimum titre of 5.0 IU/ml has been suggested in order that all staff have sufficient VNA to pass a virus specific (EBLV-1, EBLV-2 or ABLV) neutralisation assay (mFAVN) [9].

In this study we examined the RABV VNA longevity in 25 laboratory workers to determine the proportion that can be included in one of four categories; those requiring booster vaccinations in (i) > 5.0 years, (ii) 3-5 years (iii) 2-3 years and (iv) less than one year.

Data presented here has influenced the new policy recommendations outlined in the UK Department of Health guidelines [2] reducing reinforcing rabies vaccine dose intervals from 3-5 years to 2-3 years.

Materials and Methods

Serology samples

Sera from 25 laboratory staff, 15 males and 10 females, with an age range of 25-60 years who had been vaccinated with HDCV by the intramuscular route over a range of years (3-20) and sampling frequencies (3-12 months or years for a small number of individuals) were analysed to determine VNA longevity and booster requirements. The occupational environment of this group consists of rabies research staff working in laboratories or contingency personnel. All of the participants had received HDCV-PM based vaccine from (Aventis-Pasteur Ltd France) during the course of the study.

Serological testing

The anti-rabies VNA titres for each serum sample were established using the fluorescent antibody virus neutralisation (FAVN) assay employing the challenge virus standard (RABV-CVS) as previously described [10,11]. The results are expressed as international units per ml of serum determined in reference to the international WHO standard.

Results

Virus neutralising antibody level longevity was analysed for 25 laboratory staff, a summary of the vaccine booster intervals required to maintain an antibody level above 1.0 IU/ml in 13 representative individuals is shown in Figure 1. Complete longevity data (time course sampling) was not available for all participants. Of the

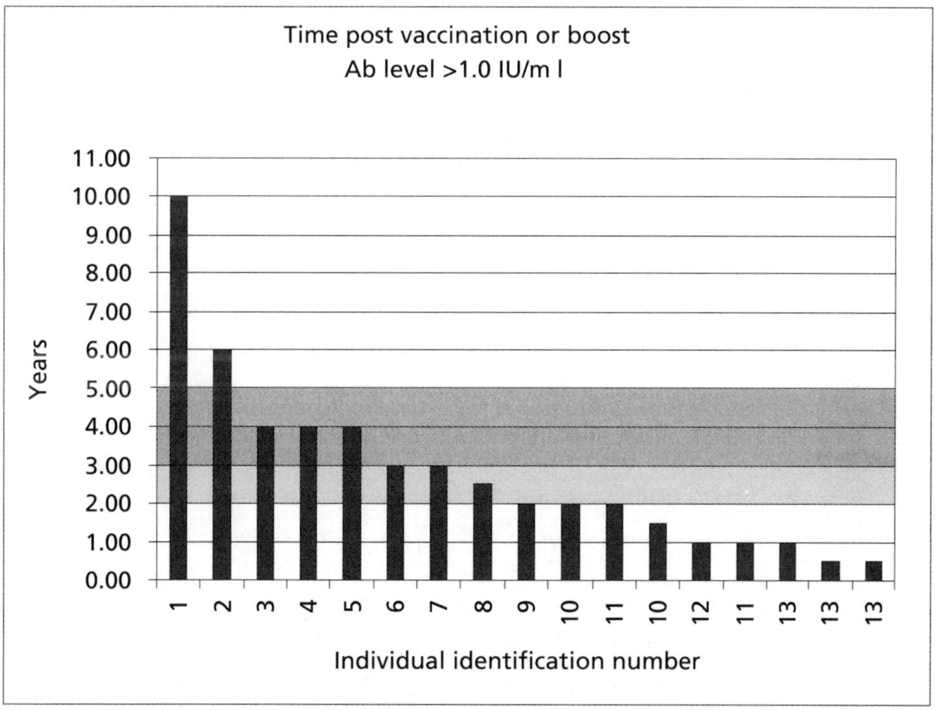

Fig. 1: The time required in years before each individual ($n = 13$) received a vaccine (HDCV) booster in order to maintain a VNA of > 1.0 IU/ml following serological monitoring at 3-6 month intervals.

broader group ($n = 25$); four required a booster vaccination at less than two years (0.92 ± 0.38 yrs), six during the 2-3 year interval, seven during the 3-5 year interval and eight had not required reinforcing dose in 5 years or more. Generally, 70 % ($n = 17/25$) required a booster in 2.5 years (range 6 months-4.5 years). Interestingly, of the 16 personnel for which primary post-vaccination blood samples were available, five (31 %) had a rapid titre decrease to below 1.0 IU/ml in less than one year following the primary vaccination course. Antibody titres (> 1.0 IU/ml) following the first reinforcing dose were sustained for 0.5-4 years in those where complete longevity data was available (test bleeds at 3, 6 or 12 month intervals). Examples of longevity profiles are shown in Figure 2 A-C. These longevity profiles illustrate the rapid decline in VNA following primary vaccination (Fig. 2A and 2C). A "poor" responder is shown in Figure 2A where booster doses were required every 5-8 months. The individual represented by Figure 2C has had two reinforcing doses in 7.5 years whilst the person represented by Figure 2B did not require a booster for over 5 years. Any differences occurring as a result of age or sex could not be determined due to the small sample size.

Inter-test variation was observed in individual VNA longevity profiles as a result of the biological nature of the FAVN assay and other factors relating to the individual's immune status at the time of sampling, such as hormonal fluctuations and pregnancy. In no cases were peaks observed which could have indicated exposure to virus during laboratory manipulation. In two cases individuals had received PEP (vaccine only) as a precautionary measure following separate virus spillage events. No cases of penetrating injuries involving virus occurred.

Discussion

After the primary course of classical rabies virus vaccination the literature suggests that a reinforcing dose at one year is important for the recipients ability to maintain a VNA titre of ≥ 0.5 IU/ml [12-14], the minimum measurable and recommended

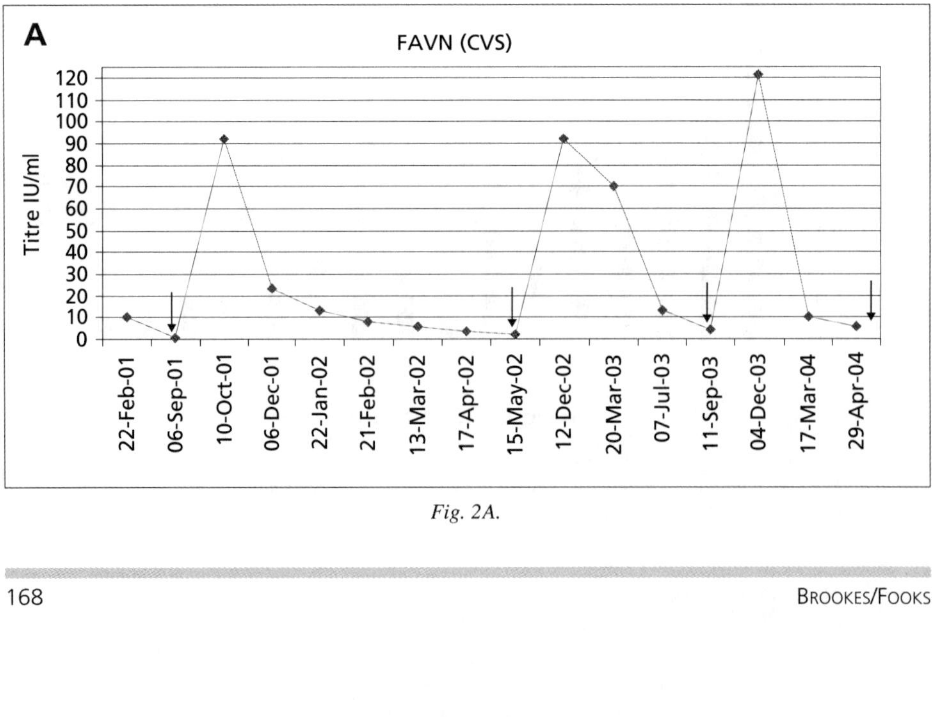

Fig. 2A.

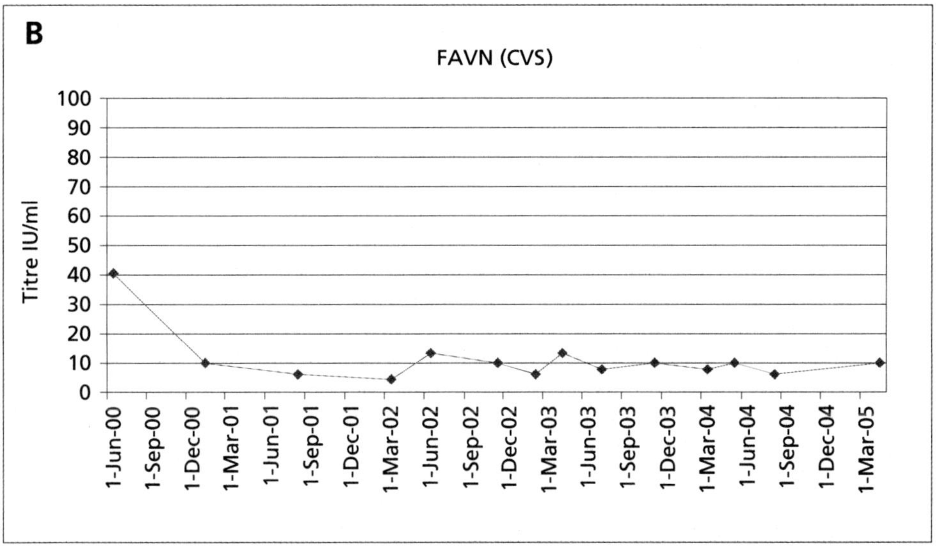

Fig. 2B.

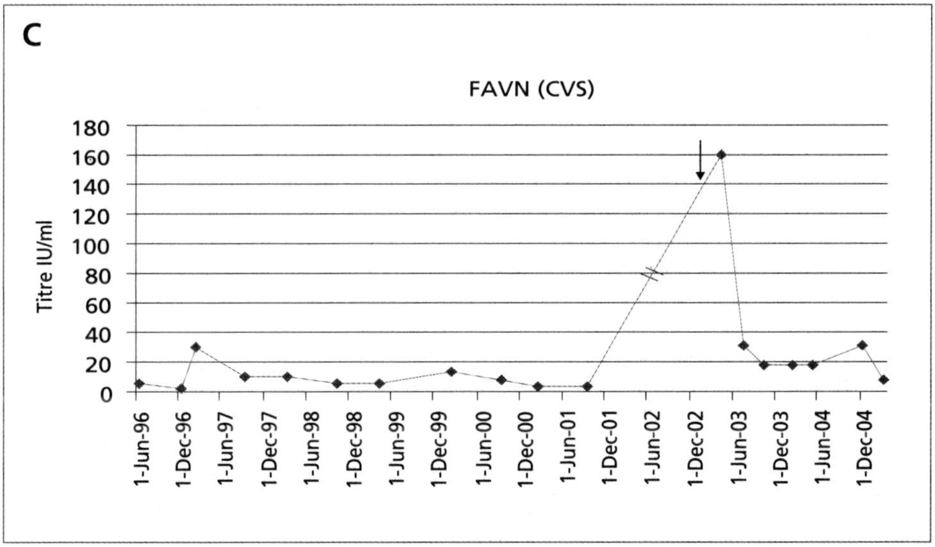

Fig. 2C.

Fig. 2 (A-C): Three individuals VNA titre (IU/ml) longevity plots of three individuals, each data point representing a serological result at either 3 or 6 month intervals. A – illustrates a poor responder, requiring repeated reinforcing doses in less than 1 year in order to maintain a minimum titre. B & C represent more common VNA longevity plots with time intervals between booster vaccinations at 3-5 years or more. Plots A & C clearly illustrate the requirement for the first booster, following the primary course, in less than 1 year. All three profiles include the first blood test following the primary vaccination series and booster immunisations are indicated with arrows. In plot C there was a break in VNA monitoring and vaccination related to a period of pregnancy and maternity leave (indicated by a double line pause).

titre [3-5]. However, the absence (or low titre) of neutralising antibody does not exclude the possibility of protection [15] as the antibody levels cannot be quantitatively correlated with protection in animals, including man. These VNA longevity data support the suggestion of a booster dose at one year post-immunisation in order to improve long term VNA levels.

Our studies apply only to the intra-muscular immunisation regime(s); the alternative intra-dermal rabies vaccination regimes have not been considered in these analyses [reviewed in 13].

We observed that approximately one-third of individuals demonstrated a rapid titre decrease during this early stage (one year post-primary vaccination) and 16 % demonstrated repeated rapid VNA titre declines during a 6-12 month period. Following the initial response to immunisation, booster recommendations vary form 3-5 years to 2-3 years, however most vaccine recipients, other than laboratory related staff are not routinely monitored for VNA levels. Our data indicates that 25 % of laboratory staff require boosters in the 2-3 year and 28 % in the 3-5 year time frames to maintain a titre of 1.0 IU/ml or more. A further 32 % did not require a reinforcing dose for over five years, some ($n = 4$) up to 10-20 years. These "high" responders have also been described by others, where an initial titre of > 30 IU/ml following the primary course and a booster at one year, VNA was maintained at a "protective" titre for at least 10 years [14,16,17]. A similar strategy (two primary doses plus a booster at one year) analysed samples from vaccine recipients at five years and found that 80 % had maintained a titre between 0.5-10 IU/ml and a single reinforcing vaccine dose at five years resulted in an anamnestic response of > 10 IU/ml [12]. Two to three year follow-up surveys have also been reported [7,18,19]. Previous studies have shown that if the first reinforcing dose at approximately one year is not administered after the primary course and the antibody titre tested at two years indicated that 11 % of the vaccine recipients were below the recommended 0.5 IU/ml and a further 12.5 % between 0.5-1.0 IU/ml [7]. The majority of the previous studies are different to that described here in that they analysed a single time point after vaccination and not a time course. Other groups examined serum VNA at 6-12 month intervals and pooled data for individuals [7,13,14,18,19]. Using these approaches anomalies may be obscured and poor responders not detected.

It has been suggested that the "poor" responders have a booster dose every three years [14]. This strategy, however, could potentially mean that a third of our cohort could be vulnerable if cryptic exposure occurred as PEP would not be administered. A booster dose even at two years would mean that 16 % would be in the non-protected group. An anamnestic response to challenge may be adequate and provide protection but this cannot be directly assessed. Taking into consideration data form this study and others [7], there may be approximately 14 % (11-16 %) of the population that do not respond well to HDCV vaccination and require a booster at less than two years irrespective of their having received a booster at one year post-primary immunisation or not. Repeated poor responses may be linked to recipient genetic factors such as haplotype [20].

Recommendations

High risk group (laboratory staff)

It is recommended that poor responders (requiring booster vaccination in < 2 years) be VNA tested every three months, intermediate responders (requiring booster vaccination in 2-5 years) be VNA tested every six months and good responders or those with infrequent exposure (requiring booster vaccination in 3-5 years) be VNA tested every 6-12 months. The minimum current WHO recommended and measurable titre is $\geq$0.5 IU/ml. For VLA laboratory staff the minimum is 1.0 IU/ml with the exception of those with regular potential exposure and poor cross-neutralising ability to non-RABV lyssaviruses where 5.0 IU/ml is suggested [9].

Lower risk group – (Bat workers)

Antibody testing of bat workers is not routinely undertaken (apart from an ongoing research project between the VLA and HPA [7]). With over 200 active bat workers in the UK, the occurrence of EBLV-2 (~ 3.5 % of UK Daubenton's bats) and a human death as a result of this virus in 2002, it became important to ensure that a high proportion of individuals in this occupational risk group were also vaccinated. Prior to 2002 the vaccination rate was less than 50 %, by 2005 this had increased substantially to > 90 % with improved maintenance of booster vaccinations (2-5 years) [6,7].

To put the risk of exposure in bat handlers into context, previous passive bat surveillance data from the UK has shown that between 0.5-3.0 % of bats had been involved in human contact (biting/scratching) incidents, approximately 12 persons per annum (2001-2004) [VLA, unpublished data]. However, not all dead or moribund bats are submitted to the VLA, it is estimated that only 10-25 % are submitted [21] and the contact cases are probably also under-reported. The frequency of reporting bat contact cases is increasing each year; as of July, 2005, the VLA had investigated 14 cases where a bat carcass was available and the BCT had reported 30 cases where a member of the public had been bitten by a bat within the last year (unpublished data). These data not only apply to bat handlers but also the general public; an audit of PEP following such incidents has recently been reported [22].

Regular rabies VNA testing could be undertaken in order to reduce the number of reinforcing doses of vaccine that an individual might require during their (working/travelling) lifetime. Instead of immunising with booster vaccine(s) at 2-3 or 3-5 year intervals, the primary course could involve three doses plus a reinforcing dose at one year followed by VNA testing at 6-12 month intervals for the majority of vaccine recipients. Booster rabies vaccine doses then only need be administered when the VNA titre had declined to between 0.5 and 5.0 IU/ml depending on the occupational setting. This scenario would help to reduce the number of potential adverse (systemic) reactions to the current vaccines; for HDCV this is approximately 6 % and < 2 % for PCECV [23,24]. The VNA longevity following immunisation with other vaccines has been less well studied [23-26].

The occupational risk for individuals other than laboratory workers is low, however the hazard is high and EBLV-2 is now considered endemic in the UK and constitutes a public health risk. Similar situations exist in mainland Europe and Eurasia where other non-classical rabies viruses are present in bat populations, in addition to RABV in terrestrial mammals in some countries. The detection of cryptic rabies in the USA that has later been diagnosed as bat RABV is becoming the main source of human exposure [27] and therefore could also be a factor in non-classical lyssavirus infection of humans and animals in Europe. Ongoing surveillance, molecular typing of isolates and vaccination monitoring is important in the management of rabies disease worldwide.

Acknowledgements

The authors would like to thank the rabies diagnostics-serology team for their assistance with routine FAVNs and serology data handling. We also appreciate the input of The Rabies Research Group, the Bat Conservation Trust for bat worker vaccination data, the UK Health Protection Agency and Department of Health collaborators and Department for Environment, Food and Rural Affairs (Defra) for funding this study (SE0418).

References

1 Fooks AR, Brookes SM, Johnson N, McElhinney LM, Hutson AM: European bat lyssaviruses: an emerging zoonosis. Epidemiol Infect 2003; 131 (3): 1029-1039.

2 Anonymous: Department of Health, UK 'Immunisation Against Infectious Disease 1996 – "The Green Book" 1996. Chapter 27 http://www.dh.gov.uk/assetRoot/04/11/09/70/04110970.pdf.

3 World Health Organization: WHO recommendations on rabies post-exposure treatment and the correct technique of intradermal immunization against rabies. WHO/EMC/ZOO.96.6, 1997. Available at: http://www.who.int/emcdocuments/rabies/docs/whoemczoo966.pdf

4 World Health Organization: Current WHO guide for rabies pre and post-exposure treatment in humans, 2000. Available at: www.who.int/emc/diseases/zoo/RabiesPET.pdf

5 World Health Organization. Rabies Bulletin Europe: http://www.who-rabies-bulletin.org/netscapestart.html

6 Bat Conservation Trust, London. Unpublished data, 2004.

7 Morris J, Crowcroft NS, Fooks AR, Brookes SM, Andrews N: Rabies antibody levels in bat handlers in the United Kingdom: A cross-sectional serological survey. Vaccine, in press.

8 Badrane H, Bahloul C, Perrin P, Tordo N: Evidence of two Lyssavirus phylogroups with distinct pathogenicity and immunogenicity. J Virol 2001; 75 (7): 3268-3276.

9 Brookes SM, Parsons G, Johnson N, McElhinney LM, Fooks AR: Rabies human diploid cell vaccine elicits cross-neutralising and cross-protecting immune responses against European and Australian bat lyssaviruses. Vaccine 2005; 23 (32): 4101-4109.

10 Cliquet F, Aubert M, Sagne L: Development of a fluorescent antibody virus neutralisation test (FAVN test) for the quantitation of rabies-neutralising antibody. J Immunol Methods 1998; 212 (1): 79-87.

11 Office International des Epizooties. Rabies. In "Manual of standards – Diagnostic tests and Vaccines". 4th edition, 2000.

12 Rodrigues FM, Mandke VB, Roumiantzeff M, Rao CV, Mehta JM, Pavri KM, Poonawalla C: Persistence of rabies antibody 5 years after pre-exposure prophylaxis with human diploid cell antirabies vaccine and antibody response to a single booster dose. Epidemiol Infect 1987; 99 (1): 91-95.

13 Briggs DJ, Schwenke JR: Longevity of rabies antibody titre in recipients of human diploid cell rabies vaccine. Vaccine 1992; 10 (2): 125-129.

14 Strady A, Lang J, Lienard M, Blondeau C, Jaussaud R, Plotkin SA: Antibody persistence following preexposure regimens of cell-culture rabies vaccines: 10-year follow-up and proposal for a new booster policy. J Infect Dis 1998; 177 (5): 1290-1295.

15 Aubert M: Can vaccination validated by the titration of rabies antibodies in serum of cats and dogs be an alternative to quarantine measures? Abstr Hyg Comm Dis 1993; 68: R1-R22.

16 Strady C, Jaussaud R, Beguinot I, Lienard M, Strady A: Predictive factors for the neutralizing antibody response following pre-exposure rabies immunization: validation of a new booster dose strategy. Vaccine. 2000; 18 (24): 2661-2667.

17 Strady C, Hung Nguyen V, Jaussaud R, Lang J, Lienard M, Strady A: Pre-exposure rabies vaccination: strategies and cost-minimization study. Vaccine 2001; 19 (11-12): 1416-1424.

18 Nicholson KG, Turner GS, Aoki FY: Immunization with a human diploid cell strain of rabies virus vaccine: two-year results. J Infect Dis 1978; 137 (6): 783-788.

19 Plotkin SA: Rabies vaccine prepared in human cell cultures: progress and perspectives. Rev Infect Dis. 1980; 2 (3): 433-448.

20 Kuwert EK, Barsenbach C, Werner I, Marcus N, Scheiermann N, Grosse-Wilde H, Krumbacher K: Early/High and Low/Late Responders among HDCS Vaccinees, in Kuwert EK, Wiktor TJ, Koprowski H (eds): Cell Culture Rabies Vaccines and their Protective effect in Man. Proceedings of WHO Consultations, Essen 1980. International Green Cross, 1981, pp 100-107.

21 Brown M: Bat Casualty Analysis 2003; Bat Care News 2004; 34: 12-18 and 2004; 36: 10-19.

22 Hossain J, Crowcroft NS, Lea G, Brown D, Mortimer PP: Audit of rabies post-exposure prophylaxis in England and Wales in 1990 and 2000. Commun Dis Public Health 2004; 7 (2): 105-111.

23 Bijok U, Barth R, Gruschkau H, Vodopija I, Smerdel S, Kukla H, Geursen R: Clinical trials in healthy volunteers with the new purified chick embryo cell rabies vaccine for man. J Commun Dis 1984; 16 (1): 61-69.

24 Dreesen DW, Fishbein DB, Kemp DT, Brown J: Two-year comparative trial on the immunogenicity and adverse effects of purified chick embryo cell rabies vaccine for pre-exposure immunization. Vaccine 1989; 7 (5): 397-400.

25 Scheiermann N, Baer J, Hilfenhaus J, Marcus I, Zoulek G: Reactogenicity and immunogenicity of the newly developed purified chick embryo cell (PCEC)-rabies vaccine in man. Zentralbl Bakteriol Mikrobiol Hyg [A] 1987; 265 (3-4): 439-450.

26 Sehgal S, Bhattacharya D, Bhardwaj M: Ten year longitudinal study of efficacy and safety of purified chick embryo cell vaccine for pre- and post-exposure prophylaxis of rabies in Indian population. J Commun Dis 1995; 27 (1): 36-43.

27 Messenger SL, Smith JS, Rupprecht CE: Emerging epidemiology of bat-associated cryptic cases of rabies in humans in the United States. Clin Infect Dis 2002; 35 (6): 738-747.

Dr. S.M. Brookes, Rabies and Wildlife Zoonoses Group, Veterinary Laboratories Agency (VLA), WHO Collaborating Centre for the Characterisation of Rabies and Rabies-Related Viruses, New Haw, Addlestone, Surrey, KT15 3NB, United Kingdom.
E-mail: s.brookes@vla.defra.gsi.gov.uk

Dodet B, Schudel A, Pastoret PP, Lombard M (eds): Rabies in Europe.
Dev Biol (Basel). Basel, Karger, 2006, vol 125, p 175.

Identification of a Human Monoclonal Antibody that Neutralizes a Broad Panel of Rabies Virus Isolates

D.M. Ambrosino[1], S.E. Schonhoff[1], M. Neizgoda[2], R.B. Mandell[1], W. Weldon[2], J. Blanton[2], C. Hanlon[2], G.J. Babcock[1], W.D. Thomas Jr.[1], C.E. Rupprecht[2]

[1] Massachusetts Biologic Laboratories, Jamaica Plain, MA, USA

[2] Division of Viral and Rickettsial Diseases, National Center for Infectious Diseases, Centers for Disease Control and Prevention, Atlanta, GA, USA

Abstract: Rabies is a significant zoonosis that results in millions of human exposures each year. Human monoclonal antibodies (HumAbs) that neutralize rabies virus may represent one viable strategy for post-exposure prophylaxis (PEP) in humans, and have many advantages over current human rabies or equine immune globulin (RIG). Transgenic mice carrying human immunoglobulin genes were used to isolate HumAbs that neutralized rabies virus. Mice (HumAb, Medarex) were immunized with commercial human rabies vaccine (RabAvert). Hybridomas were identified that produced IgGs recognizing the rabies virus glycoprotein. Several of these anti-rabies virus glycoprotein mAbs neutralized rabies virus infection in a Rapid Fluorescent Focus Inhibition Test (RFFIT) assay using the CVS-11 strain. All neutralizing HumAbs were further characterized by their ability to neutralize rabies virus variants from a broad panel of isolates of public health significance from North and South America, Europe, Africa and Asia. HumAb 17C7 was the most promising antibody identified, and neutralized all rabies virus isolates tested in a RFFIT assay. Moreover, HumAb 17C7 neutralized rabies virus variants at a much lower antibody concentration than RIG, suggesting that a single antibody may be as effective as RIG. HumAb 17C7 recognized a linear epitope in the ectodomain of the rabies virus glycoprotein between amino acids 20-422. In an experimental hamster model, HumAb 17C7 protected animals as effectively as commercial RIG, when tested alone or in combination with rabies vaccine. These results suggest that Humab17C7 could replace RIG as a safe, low cost, effective product for PEP of rabies.

Dodet B, Schudel A, Pastoret PP, Lombard M (eds): Rabies in Europe.
Dev Biol (Basel). Basel, Karger, 2006, vol 125, p 177.

Measurement of Rabies Neutralising Antibodies: Comparison of Titres Using Homologous vs Heterologous Challenge Virus Strain

S. Moore, D. Briggs, T. Ricke, R. Davis

Kansas State University College of Veterinary Medicine Manhattan, Kansas, USA

Abstract: The immune response to rabies vaccination includes cellular and humoral components. CD4 T lymphocytes primarily respond to the N antigen, and neutralizing antibodies to epitopes on the G protein. Both are needed for protection, but currently only assays measuring rabies virus neutralizing antibody are utilized for measuring immunity. CVS is recommended as the challenge virus for these assays. Monoclonal typing indicates that glycoproteins from different strains of CVS contain different epitopes. A previous study reported that different CVS challenge virus strains produced varying results when used to test serum from one source. When serum samples are tested using a CVS challenge virus strain, not only is the difference in antibody potency being evaluated, but the difference in antigenic determinants recognized by the antibodies is also being measured. The homology between virus strains used for rabies vaccine production and CVS reveals a closer relationship between the G proteins of PM strain than Flury strain. To determine the effect that differences in rabies vaccines have on the challenge virus used in assays measuring the immune response, serum samples from subjects vaccinated with rabies vaccines from two different parent strains were tested in parallel assays with the challenge virus strains CVS and Flury and their resulting titres compared. Though the difference in G protein homology between CVS and Flury strains has been reported to be only 5.8 %, the use of homologous challenge virus resulted in higher titres for samples from both sets of subjects compared to the titres obtained when heterologous strain was used.

Dodet B, Schudel A, Pastoret PP, Lombard M (eds): Rabies in Europe.
Dev Biol (Basel). Basel, Karger, 2006, vol 125, p 179.

SESSION V

Vaccinology and Immunology

Chairperson: *K. Gruzdev* (FGI, Russia)
Rapporteur: *P.P. Pastoret* (BBSRC, Belgium)

Dodet B, Schudel A, Pastoret PP, Lombard M (eds): Rabies in Europe.
Dev Biol (Basel). Basel, Karger, 2006, vol 125, pp 181-184.

Rabies Vaccinology and Immunology

A.I. Wandeler

CFIA Ottawa Laboratory Fallowfield, Nepean, Ontario, Canada

INTRODUCTION

Rabies was a sufficiently significant human health problem in the 18th and 19th centuries to attract the attention of the emerging medical sciences. A number of researchers engaged in the experimental study of the disease. This development was greatly advanced by Louis Pasteur's invention and application of post-exposure prophylaxis through immunization with partially inactivated virus. The impact of Pasteur's success was enormous. It influenced the development of virology and immunology, and most importantly of vaccinology. This brief introduction is not intended to give a comprehensive overview of the impressive achievements of modern rabies vaccinology and immunology. It is a very selective appraisal of some topics that may deserve further attention.

MEASURING THE IMMUNE RESPONSE

Rabies viruses are made up of the five structural proteins N, P, M, G, and L, and some host cell proteins. The mammalian immune system recognizes a number of antigenic sites on these proteins, a fact that is taken advantage of in the production of monoclonal antibodies. In vitro virus neutralization, in the absence of complement, is only mediated by antibodies to antigenic sites on the G protein. However, in vivo protection against challenge can also be provided by immunity to other viral proteins, e.g. the N protein.

Though the immune response to infection and vaccination includes cellular and humoral components, it is generally assessed by measuring neutralizing antibodies only. All methods have their advantages and drawbacks. Current tests are adequately described in OIE and WHO guidelines [1,2]. Neutralization tests provide reproducible results when applied to clean serum samples from humans or domestic animals. Unfortunately, it is frequently ignored that cytotoxicity in the assay system mimics neutralization. Nonspecific virus inactivation in neutralization tests has led WHO experts to postulate a 0.5 IU threshold to demonstrate seroconversion [3]. Relevant thresholds discriminating between specific and nonspecific virus inhibition should probably be much higher for most wildlife and domestic animal sera collected under field conditions. ELISAs bear a different set of complexities that largely depend on the assay system (indirect, competitive) chosen, on antigen and coating properties, and last, but not least, the quality of the sera tested. Better than just looking at thresholds would be to analyze Receiver Operating Characteristic (ROC) curves in terms of sensitivity and specificity of the test for each particular collection of data.

Pathogenesis and the Immune Response to Infection

There is usually no measurable immune response to rabies during incubation in humans, foxes and most domestic animals, except when animals are inoculated experimentally with relatively high doses (including massive amounts of dead antigen) or with a virus variant adapted to a different species. One can think of a number of explanations: our tests are not sensitive enough, there is indeed no or a very weak immune response because the virus is efficiently sequestered from immune detection, or because the inocula carry immunosuppressive properties. A measurable immune response is probably induced only when a large number of infected cells exhibit viral antigen on their surface and virions are released into the intercellular space. This does not happen before the virus starts to replicate in the CNS. Then, antibody and cellular immunity may become detectable. Chronically infected animals or those animals and humans surviving clinical disease exhibit high antibody titers not only in sera, but also in the cerebrospinal fluid. The scarcity of documented survival of clinical disease in experimentally and naturally infected animals contrasts with the frequent reports of neutralizing antibody in sera collected from wild animals in North America. There are several possible explanations: (i) survival of clinical disease in nature is more common than implied from observations of domestic animal and experimental wild animal rabies, this being more probable in some species such as bats and Caribbean mongoose; (ii) the antibodies are not the result of clinical rabies, but reflect the immune response to abortive peripheral infection and other (oral?) exposure to rabies antigen; (iii) the observed activities in neutralization tests, ELISAs, and hemagglutination inhibition assays are not specific or not even due to antibody.

The immune response to a neural infection strongly influences the development of clinical disease, generally enhancing structural and functional damage. These phenomena have also been described for rabies. In addition, pathways of cell damage and death are now better understood, though their exact involvement in neuronal dysfunction in rabies is slightly controversial. What we observe in laboratory rodents may well help to explain how properties of viral proteins are linked to pathogenicity in a host that is not particularly susceptible to rabies. Whether the immune response, apoptosis and related phenomena play a significant role in the highly susceptible principal hosts, such as foxes, is an unexplored question.

Pre- and Post-Exposure Immunization of Humans

The history of pre- and post-exposure vaccination against rabies is well documented [4-6]. Louis Pasteur initiated a new era of human rabies prevention when he used desiccated spinal cord of infected rabbits for immunization. The period in which animal brain vaccines dominated human postexposure prophylaxis lasted for almost a whole century. Pasteur's original regimen was modified numerous times. The modifications generally bear the names of their inventors, such as Fermi, Semple, Hempt, Fuenzalida, and others. Not all modifications were real improvements. Nevertheless, the change from partially inactivated to completely inactivated, and from adult animal brain to suckling mouse brain vaccines were significant developments. The most significant progress in the second half of the 20th century was the development of potent inactivated cell culture vaccines. They should by now completely replace all nervous tissue-derived products for use in humans.

Modern vaccines for human pre- and post-exposure prophylaxis all contain inactivated complete virus. All are highly effective. However, after severe exposures, active immunization must be supplemented with infiltration of the contaminated wound with virus neutralizing immunoglobulin preparations. These post-exposure prophylaxis regimens are largely empirical. They have become less cumbersome in recent decades through cautious and sensible modification of previously approved schedules [7]. Still, the necessity to administer immunoglobulin products simultaneously with a vaccine is somewhat awkward.

Vaccines for Animals

The development of animal vaccines has taken a different trajectory [8,9]. Animal brain-derived vaccines played, and still play, a variable role in dog rabies control. An important development was initiated in the 1940s with the attenuation of Flury strain virus through multiple passages in chicks, and then in chicken embryos. The Flury low-egg-passage (LEP) and Flury high-egg-passage (HEP) virus strains were soon joined by other live attenuated or modified live virus vaccines, of which ERA (Evelyn-Rockitnicki-Abelseth) was probably the most important. These attenuated vaccines were important for domestic animal rabies prevention and particularly for dog rabies control. Their application was largely discontinued when their residual pathogenicity became more evident. Today, potent and safe cell culture-derived vaccines dominate animal rabies prevention and control. A recombinant vaccine for cats is used to avoid some of the side-effects of killed vaccines in this species. Live attenuated vaccines are presently not recommended for parenteral vaccination.

Live vaccines made a come-back after George Baer's discovery that ERA immunizes when given per os [10], when systems for the oral immunization of wildlife were developed, and first field applications in Switzerland appeared to be successful [11]. The residual pathogenicity problem was partially resolved by developing rabies virus variants of lower pathogenicity [12] and recombinant vaccines [13,14]. For the oral immunization of wildlife and dogs it is necessary to apply live attenuated or recombinant vaccines. The vaccine virus must introduce rabies virus genes (mostly G) into host cells that are capable of expressing it. One step further would be the use of killed vaccines and non-infectious peptides for oral immunization. This will not be possible before new technologies are developed to allow for efficient transfer of ingested antigens through mucous membranes to immunocompetent cells. We are already capable of effective oral immunization with nonreplicating vectors that introduce a DNA equivalent of the rabies glycoprotein into host cells. There is no evident problem in devising genetically engineered vaccines, that are even safer and more effective, capable of selectively immunizing a narrower or wider range of target species.

CONCLUSIONS

Most of the presently available vaccines for parenteral immunization of animals and humans are excellent. Notwithstanding, research into designing even better vaccines is ongoing. Such research is partially driven by real and perceived deficiencies of present biologicals, but also by the ambitions and the inquisitiveness of the scientists involved. These new developments will not rapidly change the current situation, though the control of the disease in the principal reservoir species would indeed profit from the development of safer and more efficacious oral vaccines. However, there are also formidable obstacles to such developments. Concerns range from the sensible to the completely absurd. It is necessary that legislation addresses valid concerns and regulates the application of biotechnology. It is inevitable that legislation is occasionally a hindrance to further development. But the biggest deterrents are probably of an economical nature. Without relevant motivation commercial manufacturers that have spent considerable resources in the development and licensing of particular products are not likely to invest more capital or encourage competitive ventures. Of equal or even greater significance are the economic and cultural obstacles that prevent bite victims from receiving the proper post-exposure prophylaxis. A worldwide effort in public health education is needed.

REFERENCES

1 Meslin FX, Kaplan MM, Koprowski H (eds): Laboratory techniques in rabies (4th ed). Geneva, WHO, 476 pp.

2 Manual of standards for diagnostic tests and vaccines. Paris, OIE, 2000, 954 pp.

3 Sinnecker H, Atanasiu P, Bahmanyar M, Selimov M, Wandeler AI, Bögel K: Vaccine potency requirements for reduced immunization schedules and pre-exposure treatment, in Hennessen W, Regamey RH (eds): Joint WHO/IABS symposium on the standardization of rabies vaccines for human use produced in tissue culture. Dev Biol Stand. Basel, Karger, 1978, vol 40, pp 268-270.

4 Steele JH, Fernandez PJ: History of rabies and global aspects, in Baer GM (ed): The Natural History of Rabies. Boca Raton, CRC Press, 1991, pp 1-24.

5 Vodopija I, Clark HF: Human vaccination against rabies, in Baer GM (ed): The Natural History of Rabies. Boca Raton, CRC Press, 1991, pp 571-595.

6 Thraenhart O: Human rabies and its prevention, in King AA, Fooks AR, Aubert M, Wandeler AI (eds): Historical perspective of rabies in Europe and the Mediterranean Basin. Paris, OIE, 2005, pp 325-335.

7 WHO Expert Consultation on Rabies, First Report. Geneva, WHO, 2004, 121 pp.

8 Bunn TO: Canine and feline vaccines, past and present, in Baer GM (ed): The Natural History of Rabies. Boca Raton, CRC Press, 1991, pp 415-425.

9 Precausta P, Soulebot JP: Vaccines for domestic animals, in Baer GM (ed): The Natural History of Rabies. Boca Raton, CRC Press, 1991, pp 445-459.

10 Baer GM, Linhart SB, Dean DJ: Rabies vaccination of foxes. Annual Report of the Division of Laboratory Research. Albany, New York State Department of Health 1963: 145.

11 Wandeler AI: Oral immunization against rabies: afterthoughts and foresight. Schweiz Arch Tierheilk 2000; 142: 455-462.

12 Coulon P, Lafay F, Leblois H, Tuffereau C, Artois M, Blancou J, Benmansour A, Flamand A: The SAG: a new attenuated oral rabies vaccine, in Bögel K, Meslin FX, Kaplan M (eds): Wildlife Rabies Control. Proceedings of the International WHO Symposium on "Wildlife Rabies Control", Geneva, 2-5 July 1990. Chapel Place, Wells Medical, 1992, pp 105-111.

13 Kieny MP, lathe R, Drillien R, Spehner D, Skory S, Schmitt D, Wiktor T, Koprowski H, Lecocq JP: Expression of rabies virus glycoprotein from a recombinant vaccinia virus. Nature 1984; 312: 163-166.

14 Yarosh OK, Wandeler AI, Graham FL, Campbell JB, Prevec L: Human adenovirus type 5 vectors expressing rabies glycoprotein. Vaccine 1996; 14: 1257-1264.

Dr. A.I. Wandeler, CFIA Ottawa Laboratory Fallowfield, Nepean, Ontario, K0H 8P9, Canada.
E-mail: wandelera@inspection.gc.ca

Dodet B, Schudel A, Pastoret PP, Lombard M (eds): Rabies in Europe.
Dev Biol (Basel). Basel, Karger, 2006, vol 125, pp 185-193.

Ability of Rabies Vaccine Strains to Elicit Cross-Neutralising Antibodies

S.M. Brookes, D.M. Healy, A.R. Fooks

Rabies and Wildlife Zoonoses Group, Veterinary Laboratories Agency (VLA), WHO Collaborating Centre for the Characterisation of Rabies and Rabies-Related Viruses, Addlestone, Surrey, United Kingdom

Key words: Lyssaviruses, vaccines, cross-neutralisation.

Abstract: Two European Bat Lyssaviruses (EBLV-1 and EBLV-2) have been identified (*n* > *750* cases) in European bat species. In addition, EBLVs have been detected as "spillover" cases in three humans, one stone marten and four sheep. A further concern is the interaction of companion animals with infected bats and the possibility of subsequent lyssavirus infection. Cat-bat interactions represent ~32 % (*n* = *398*) of passive lyssavirus surveillance submissions at the Veterinary Laboratories Agency (VLA) (1987-2004). Cats therefore represent a potentially significant spillover host. This study evaluated the ability of rabies vaccine antibodies to neutralise EBLVs using modified fluorescent antibody virus neutralisation (FAVN) assays (EBLV-1, EBLV-2). We examined vaccinated human, dog and cat sera in two classes; (i) FAVN-CVS titres ≥ 0.5-5.0 IU/ml (*n* = *34*, *79* and *54*, respectively), and (ii) > 5.0 IU/ml (*n* = *22*, *21* and *32* respectively). Most sera (~80 %) with higher titres were able to neutralise both EBLV-1 and – 2 regardless of the vaccine received. Only a proportion of those with low titres were capable of neutralising either EBLV-1 (27-92 %) or EBLV-2 (38-92 %) or both EBLVs (27-79 %). The cat sera constitute the lower end of each range. More animals that had received LEP based vaccines were able to neutralise EBLVs than those that had received PV based vaccines. The continuing occurrence of non-classical lyssaviruses in Europe emphasizes the need for continual surveillance of bats and other species.

Introduction

Rabies vaccines are administered to companion animals (mainly dogs and cats) as part of the European Union pets travel scheme (PETS). We routinely test approximately 15,000 sera per annum for the level of classical rabies virus neutralising antibody (VNA). Any animal with ≥ 0.5 IU/ml of VNA is considered to have effectively sero-converted and passed the test [1]. Approximately 94-98 % of animals attain this threshold level following vaccination; the vaccinated population is composed mainly of dogs (about 88 %), with only around 12 % of samples tested from cats [2]. Protective antibody levels, however, are not defined, vaccinated animals occasionally do not reach the threshold pass level or antibody titres wane rapidly (within months) [3]. The absence (or low titre < 0.5 IU/ml) of neutralising antibody does not exclude the possibility of protection [4], as antibody levels cannot be quantitatively correlated with protection in animals. The majority of samples received are from animals vaccinated with Rabisin (Merial Animal Health, France) or Nobivac (Intervet, UK) rabies vaccines, while a small proportion receive Quantum (Schering-Plough Animal Health, UK) rabies vaccine or other licensed products [2].

In addition to classical rabies (RABV, genotype 1) in terrestrial mammals, other members of the genus *Lyssavirus* are capable of causing fatal rabies disease in mammals. These, with the exception of one, use bats as their reservoir hosts and include the European Bat Lyssaviruses (EBLV-1 and EBLV-2, genotypes 5 and 6), Duvenhage virus (DUW; genotype 4), Lagos bat virus (LBV; genotype 2), Australian bat lyssavirus (ABLV; genotype 7) and four as yet unclassified bat viruses form Eurasia [5]. In addition, RABV is found in bats from the Americas. The exception is Mokola virus (MOKV; genotype 3) for which the reservoir species is not known. All these Lyssavirus genotypes, with the exception of LBV, have been known to cross the species barrier and cause clinical disease and inevitable fatalities in humans [5]. The ability of these viruses to spillover into other mammals is limited but several cases have been reported, indicating that, while the risk is low, the hazard remains substantial in cases where the establishment of disease in another species could present a public health risk. Examples of bat rabies spillover into other mammals include; EBLV-1 in sheep (*n = 5*) [6,7], a stone marten [8] and evidence of infection in a cat; one with anti-EBLV-1 antibodies [9]. RABV of bat origin has been detected in skunks [10] and foxes [11] in North America. These two cases were important as they involved spillover with adaptation and subsequent spread in the spillover species. Spillover (without spread) of bat RABV is also a significant factor in the economic loss of livestock in Latin America as a result of vampire bats transmitting virus during blood meals [12]. Rabies due to a bat virus strain (RABV) has also been reported in a cat from Argentina [13].

In the United Kingdom there have been five cases of EBLV-2, four in bats and one in a human [2]. Surveillance of British bats (*Myotis daubentonii*) indicates that the prevalence of EBLV-2 in bats and previous exposure to virus in bats is approximately 3.5 % [14-16]. EBLV-1 has not been detected in the UK; however, preliminary seroprevalence data indicate that bats (*Eptesicus serotinus*) may have been previously exposed to this virus [14]. In mainland Europe there have been approximately 758 cases of EBLV-1 and 17 cases of EBLV-2 [14].

As part of continuing passive surveillance of lyssavirus in bats in the UK, for over 18 years, we have identified that at least 32 % (*n = 398*) of dead bats submitted to the VLA have had interactions with cats [17]. The Bat Care data (UK) suggest that the cat-bat interaction may be represented by 34 % (256/762) of injured bats, 55 % of which are fatally injured [18], which corresponds to the passive lyssavirus surveillance data.

The ability of currently available rabies vaccines to induce neutralising antibodies to other lyssaviruses and protect both humans and animals from infection has not been extensively investigated. While data suggest that human rabies vaccines will cross-neutralise and protect against viruses from phylogroup I (genotypes 1, 4, 5, 6, 7 plus Aravan, Khujand and Irkut viruses) but not phylogroup II (genotypes 2, 3 and West Caucasian bat virus) [reviewed by 19-21], very little data are available for animal vaccines [22]. It has also been suggested recently that a proportion (6 %) of individuals with antibody titres to RABV of < 5.0 IU/ml fail (< 0.5 IU/ml) to neutralise EBLVs in virus specific assays [23].

In this study we examined sera from rabies-vaccinated cats, dogs and humans for their ability to cross-neutralise EBLV-1 and/or EBLV-2. Pet sera were obtained as part of the PETS testing, following rabies vaccination with three authorised vaccines available in the UK; Nobivac, Rabisin or Quantum. These vaccines are based on two chemically inactivated virus strains; Nobivac and Rabisin contain Pasteur virus and Quantum contains Flury-LEP virus; all three are administered with adjuvant. Primary vaccination involves one dose in all three cases and blood tests are carried out at an interval prescribed by the vaccine manufacturers. Booster vaccinations are suggested at various intervals: Rabisin at one year for cats and two years for dogs; Nobivac every two years for both cats and dogs; and Quantum every three years for both cats and dogs. Human sera were obtained from laboratory staff following rabies vaccination with HDCV (Aventis Pasteur Ltd.) as part of the health surveillance programme. HDCV is based on the Pittman Moore (PM) virus strain and primary vaccination involves a three-dose course (days 0, 7, 28) followed by boosters at two to five years or as required by antibody level assessment.

Only sera that passed the RABV-fluorescent antibody virus neutralisation (FAVN) test were analysed. These were divided into two groups; above and below 5.0 IU/ml by RABV-FAVN. The sera were then tested for their ability to neutralise virus on modified FAVNs (mFAVN) specific for EBLV-1 or EBLV-2. Data indicate that the level of rabies vaccine induced antibodies required to cross-neutralise EBLVs is higher than that for adequate neutralisation of RABV-CVS.

Material and Methods

Virus

Initial RABV-FAVN data were obtained during PETS testing on the fixed laboratory strain; CVS. The bat virus isolates used in the mFAVNs were EBLV-1 (RV20 from Denmark, 1986), EBLV-2 (RV628, from the UK, 1996, Genbank U89478 and AY721613).

Serum samples

PETS serum (*n = 186*) consisted of samples from either dogs (*n = 100*) or cats (*n = 86*), recipients of vaccine PV-1 (*n = 25* dogs, *21* cats), PV-2 (*n = 16* dogs, *15* cats) or LEP (*n = 38* dogs, *18* cats) and titre levels (A) above 5.0 IU/ml (*n = 53, 21* dogs, *32* cats) on the routine fluorescent antibody test using classical RABV (FAVN-CVS) or (B) below 5.0 IU/ml (*n = 79* dogs, *54* cats).

In addition human sera (*n = 56*) were used for comparative purposes from one type of vaccine recipient (PM) and in titre groups A (*n = 22*) or B (*n = 34*). All the titres were determined in comparison to an OIE (positive dog serum) standard [23-25] and a naïve dog serum negative control (Harlan, UK). The human sera had also been previously tested on mFAVNs and compared to the WHO (positive human serum) standard [23].

Modified FAVN –

mFAVN were developed based on previous CVS protocols [24,25]. Details have been published elsewhere [15,23]. All sera were used in duplicate on each mFAVN assay.

Statistical analysis

EBLV specific mFAVN results were analysed using ANOVA, Minitab statistical software.

Results

Group A – antibody titre by CVS-FAVN > 5.0 IU/ml

Overall > 75 % (75-100 %) of sera produce positive results (> 0.5IU/ml) by EBLV-mFAVNs (Fig. 1). All pet sera above 15.0 IU/ml (*n* = *17*) on CVS passed on the mFAVNs. Sera between 5.0-15 IU/ml (*n* = *34*) came from 19 animals that had received LEP based vaccine and 15 that had received one of two PV based vaccines. Only 40 % of the animals that received PV based vaccine passed the EBLV-mFAVNs, in comparison with 79 % of the animals that received LEP based vaccine. All human sera in Group A passed both mFAVNs.

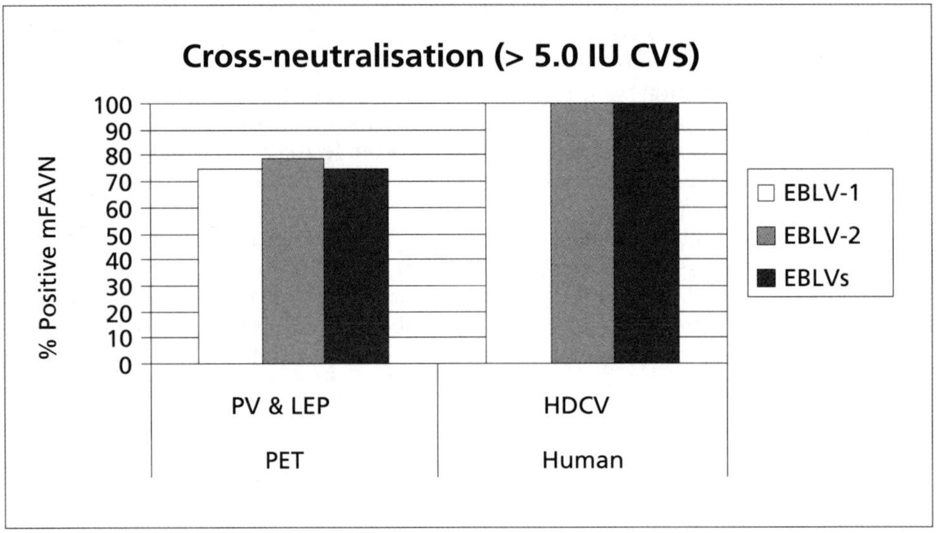

Fig. 1: High-titre RABV-induced antibody sera (< 5.0 IU/ml) ; a comparison of PET (dog and cat) sera and human sera using the OIE standard for pass/fail calculations. Data points are the percentage of sera that cross-neutralised EBLVs on specific mFAVNs (> 0.5IU/ml).

Group B – antibody titre by CVS-FAVN < 5.0 IU/ml

The ability of animal and human serum with lower VNA titres by CVS-FAVN varied considerably in their ability to neutralise EBLVs (Fig. 2). A general comparison of RABV-induced antibodies in the animal types, irrespective of the virus strain/vaccine used to induce the antibodies, and their ability to cross-neutralise EBLVs, is illustrated in Table 1. Sera from all recipients, dogs, cats and humans, cross-neutralised EBLV-1 more effectively than EBLV-2 ($p < 0.05$) (Table 1 and Fig. 2). Dog sera neutralised EBLVs more readily than cat sera ($p < 0.05$) (Table 1 and Fig. 2). Sera from more animals that had received LEP based vaccine neutralised EBLVs than that from those that had received PV based vaccines (Fig. 2). In dogs there was no significant difference between the two PV based vaccines ; however, in cats PV-1 was significantly better at neutralising EBLV-1 than EBLV-2 ($p < 0.05$) ; for PV-2 this situation was reversed ($p < 0.05$) (Fig. 2).

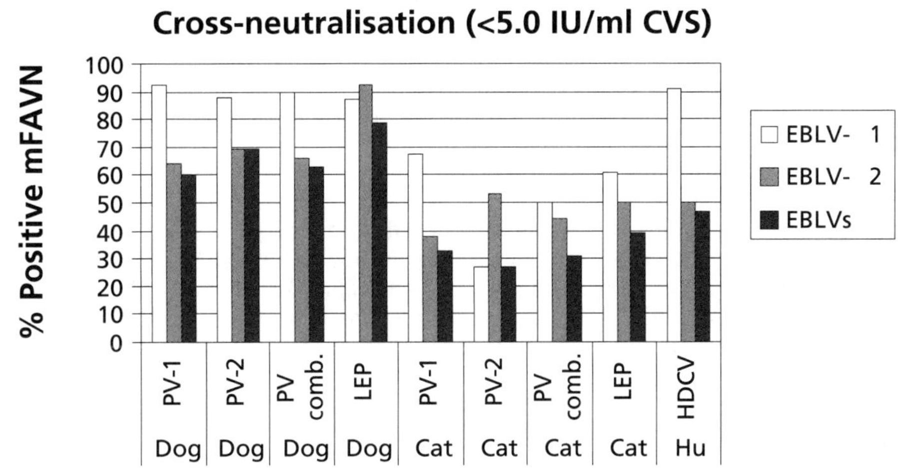

Fig. 2: Low-titre RABV-induced antibody sera (< 5.0 IU/ml); vaccine virus strain/animal type break down using the OIE standard for pass/fail calculations. Data points are the percentage of sera that cross-neutralised EBLVs on specific mFAVNs (> 0.5IU/ml).

Table 1: Low RABV-induced antibody titre serum (< 5.0 IU/ml); a comparison of animal types (pooled virus/vaccine type data) using the OIE standard for pass/fail calculations. Data points are the percentage (and range) of sera that cross-neutralised the EBLVs on specific mFAVNs (> 0.5IU/ml).

	Proportion of cross-neutralisation EBLVs		
Species	**EBLV-1**	**EBLV-2**	**Both EBLVs**
Dog	89.0 (87-92)	75.0 (64-92)	69.3 (60-79)
Cat	51.7 (27-67)	47.0 (38-53)	33.0 (27-39)
Pets (dog & cat)	70.3	61.0	51.2
Human	91.0	50.0	47.0
All	73.3	59.4	50.6

Discussion

The principal modality of protection in rabies infection is neutralising antibodies. All commercially available rabies vaccines are based on RABV virus strains belonging to phylogroup 1. The ability of human rabies vaccines to cross-protect against other lyssaviruses has been widely studied for the HDCV-PM vaccine [reviewed in 23]. Data suggest that immune responses elicited by HDCV-PM and other current rabies vaccines are capable of cross-protecting against some of the lyssavirus genotypes, principally those in phlyogroup I [19]. RABV based vaccines have not been shown to provide cross-protection for those lyssaviruses in genotypes 2 and 3, LBV and MOKV belonging to lyssaviruses phylogroup II [19] or the West Caucasian bat virus, respectively [21]. The latter is substantially divergent from other lyssaviruses and may be placed into a newly described phylogroup III (Kuzmin, unpublished data). In comparison there are limited data available on the ability of RABV-induced antibody to cross-neutralise or protect against other lyssaviruses [22,26].

Classically, the rapid fluorescent focus inhibition test (RFFIT) or FAVN assays are used to establish the levels of neutralising antibodies to RABV (CVS) generated following rabies vaccination of humans and animals. It has been suggested that in the case of exposure to EBLVs, the immune response should be monitored by a test specific for the virus in addition to classical CVS tests [23,27,28]. To address this issue and to monitor specific antibodies induced by vaccination this study used mFAVN assays for EBLV-1 and EBLV-2 [15,23].

Our previous studies using mFAVNs demonstrated that 96 % (*48* of *50*) of human sera from HDCV vaccine recipients were capable of neutralising (≥ 0.5 IU/ml) CVS, wRABV, EBLV-1, EBLV-2 and ABLV. For all recipients to cross-neutralise the viruses tested, it was necessary that they demonstrate a CVS VNA level of ≥ 4.5 IU/ml as determined against the WHO standard [23]. For this reason the PETS sera were also split into two groups; low titre < 5.0IU/ml and high titre > 5.0IU/ml as determined by CVS-FAVN; using the OIE standard, which is routine for animal sera. The EBLV-FAVN pass rate for the high titre sera, both pet (75-80 %) and human (100 %) (Fig. 1), was good, suggesting that the majority of vaccinated animals (80 % of those in the PETS travel scheme) and humans would be protected against EBLVs were exposure to occur. Antibody levels are a reasonable indicator for efficacy of protection [25], they do not necessarily equate to protection in challenge experiments. The correlation of antibody levels, immune response and protection against rabies is not well understood. Using the murine model, the commonly used rabies vaccine, HDCV, provided significant protection against peripheral challenge with EBLVs. Following the more severe form of challenge by the intra-cerebral route, HDCV provided significant protection against CVS and EBLV-2 but not EBLV-1 [23]. Veterinary-wildlife RABV vaccines (virus strains SAD, PV, PM, and LEP) have also been shown to provide acceptable levels of protection against EBLV-1 [22,26] and EBLV-2 [26].

Sera from animals with lower RABV antibody titres (about 20 % of PETS) were less able to neutralise EBLVs in vitro. This finding was more pronounced in cats than dogs and substantial differences were observed between the results for different vaccines and the virus strain used to prepare the vaccine (Table 1 and Fig. 2). Similar results have been reported for wildlife (foxes) following RABV vaccination [26].

From the duel analysis of human sera with mFAVNs, using either the WHO or OIE standards as titre calculation controls, substantial differences in results from low titre sera occurred; 96 % passed using the WHO control [23] compared to 47-91 % using the OIE control. The ability of the control standard sera to cross-neutralise the different EBLVs is apparent. Further analysis will be required to determine the impact of these factors on the data and subsequent recommendations.

CONCLUSIONS

Rabies vaccines induced antibodies that effectively neutralised EBLV-1 and EBLV-2 in vitro, with the exception of low titre sera from cats.

In almost all vaccine recipients (animal and human) the levels of neutralising antibody wane with time post-vaccination and some respond poorly to vaccination [3], either requiring repeated booster vaccinations or never attaining WHO recommended minimum titre [2,29,30].

Further studies may be required to set VNA thresholds for protection against non-RABV lyssaviruses following rabies vaccination of at-risk animal populations. If an individual animal has a VNA > 0.5 IU/ml it will most probably be protected (> 98% of vaccinated animals [2,3]). These data suggest that rabies vaccines are highly effective in protection against rabies and the related lyssavirus strains, at least for phylogroup I.

A relatively high proportion (60-70 %) proportion of cats, and pets combined (50 %), in the low titre group (20 % PETS travel scheme), that is, approximately 10-15 % of vaccinated animals, failed to neutralise the lyssaviruses tested. The reasons for this poor cross-neutralising response and its true prevalence in larger vaccinated populations is currently unclear and under investigation. It is, however, possible that a vaccine recipient's genetic background, e.g. major histocompatability complex (MHC) type [31], age, route of vaccination [3] and vaccine/virus strain may play a significant role in their ability to produce specific VNAs and potentially respond to lyssavirus challenge. These data also suggest that the LEP virus based vaccines may induce EBLV cross-neutralising antibodies in more recipients than do PV based vaccines. Further investigations are currently underway to examine this proposal.

In reference to the UK rabies/EBLV status, the presence of EBLV-2, but not EBLV-1, in Daubenton's bats (around 3.5 %) [5,15,32], and the proportion of vaccinated cat sera capable of neutralising EBLV-2 (47 % of low titre animals and 79 % of high titre sera, or, 73 % of pet sera, cross-neutralise, while 17 % do not), should be noted. The majority of cats in the UK are not vaccinated and approximately 33 % of detected moribund bats have been involved in cat contact incidents. The hazard is real; spillover of EBLV-2 in the UK has occurred from a Daubenton's bat to a human [5]; the level of risk, however, remains low as there is little evidence that cats can be infected by non-classical lyssaviruses [9,13] and the prevalence of EBLV-2 in the UK is low. The prevalence of EBLV-1 in mainland Europe < 1-20 % [14] and the more frequent spillover of this virus into non-bat hosts (human, sheep and stone marten [5-8]), is cause for concern. However, anti-RABV antibodies appear to neutralise and protect against EBLV-1 at a level of > 70 % and cross-protection data are similarly encouraging [review in 23]. The complete lack of cross-protection of RABV vaccines for lyssavirus phylogroup II and WCBV [21] and the potential for reduced protection (ABLV) and neutralisation (EBLVs) remains an area for further investigation. These findings imply that all those involved in lyssavirus surveillance in animal and human populations should remain vigilant as new lyssaviruses emerge and others are detected in new situations. Further research into the spillover of bat lyssaviruses into other mammalian hosts, the pathogenesis of disease and the protective ability of current vaccines, is required.

Acknowledgements

The authors would like to thank the rabies diagnostics-serology team for their assistance with routine FAVNs and serology data handling, the Rabies Research Group, the Bat Conservation Trust and Bat Care Workers groups for helpful discussion, and the Department for Environment, Food and Rural Affairs (Defra) for funding the work (SE0418).

References

1 Aubert M: Practical significance of rabies antibodies in cats and dogs. Rev Sci Tech 1992; 11: 735-760.

2 Fooks AR, McElhinney LM, Brookes SM, Johnson N, Keene V, Parsons G, Soldan A: Rabies antibody testing and the UK Pet Travel Scheme. Vet Rec 2002; 150 (14): 428-430.

3 Schweitzer K, Moore S, Bausch L, Davis R: Dogs and cats with repeat low rabies antibody levels studied. Kansas Vet Quart. 2003; 6 (1), 4-5. Accessed on 5/12/05 http://www.vet.ksu.edu/features/VetQuarterly/KVQSpr03.pdf.

4 Aubert MFA: Can vaccination validated by the titration of rabies antibodies in serum of cats and dogs be an alternative to quarantine measures? Abstr Hyg Comm Dis 1993; 68 (6): R1-R22.

5 Fooks AR, Brookes SM, Johnson N, McElhinney LM, Hutson AM: European bat lyssaviruses: an emerging zoonosis. Epidemiol Infect 2003; 131 (3): 1029-1039.

6 Ronsholt L, Sorenson KJ, Bruschke CJM, Wilenberg GJ, Van Oirschot JT, Johnstone P, Whitby JE, Bourhy H: Clinically silent rabies infection in (zoo) bats. Vet Rec 1998; 19: 519-520.

7 Ronsholt L: A new case of European Bat Lyssavirus (EBL) infection in Danish sheep. Rabies Bulletin Europe 2002; 2:15.

8 Muller T, Cox J, Peter W, Schafer R, Johnson N, McElhinney LM, Geue JL, Tjornehoj K, Fooks AR: Spill-over of European bat lyssavirus type 1 into a stone marten (*Martes foina*) in Germany. J Vet Med B Infect Dis Vet Public Health. 2004 Mar; 51 (2): 49-54.

9 Tjornehoj K, Ronsholt L, Fooks AR: Antibodies to EBLV-1 in a domestic cat in Denmark. Vet Rec 2004; 155 (18): 571-572.

10 Smith J: Molecular evidence for sustained transmission of a bat variant of rabies virus in skunks in Arizona. Abstract – 12th Annual Rabies in the Americas Conference, 2001, p 47.

11 Daoust PY, Wandeler AI, Casey GA: Cluster of rabies cases of probable bat origin among red foxes in Prince Edward Island, Canada. J Wildl Dis 1996; 32 (2): 403-406.

12 Mayen F: Haematophagous bats in Brazil, their role in rabies transmission, impact on public health, livestock industry and alternatives to an indiscriminat reduction of bat population. J Vet Med B Infect Dis Vet Public Health 2003; 50 (10): 469-472.

13 Amasino CF, Gury Dohmen F, de Gaetano J, Mena Segura C, Palazzolo A: A case of bat rabies in a cat in the province of Buenos Aires, Argentina. Rev Sci Tech 2003; 22 (3): 1021-1027.

14 Harris SL, Brookes SM, Jones G, Jolliffe TA, Aegerter JN, Smith GC, Moore NP, Mackie I, Swift SM, Racey PA, Fooks AR: Res Vet Sci 2005; 78 (Suppl. A): 30.

15 Brookes SM, Aegerter JN, Smith GC, Healy DM, Jolliffe TA, Swift SM, Mackie IJ, Pritchard JS, Racey PA, Moore NP, Fooks AR: European bat lyssavirus in Scottish bats. Emerg Infect Dis 2005; 11 (4): 572-578.

16 Fooks AR, Brookes SM, Healy D, Smith GC, Aegerter J, Harris SL, Jones G, Brash M, Racey P, Swift S, Mackie I, Pritchard S, Landeg F: Detection of antibodies to EBLV-2 in Daubenton's bats in the UK. Vet Rec 2004; 154 (8): 245-246.

17 Harris SL, Brookes SM, Jones G, Huston AM, Fooks AR: Passive surveillance for European bat lyssaviruses in UK bats 1987-2004. The Veterinary Record (in press).

18 Brown M: Bat Casualty Analysis 2003. Bat Care News 2004; 34: 12-18 – 36: 10-19.

19 Badrane H, Bahloul C, Perrin P, Tordo N: Evidence of two Lyssavirus phylogroups with distinct pathogenicity and immunogenicity. J Virol 2001; 75 (7): 3268-3276.

20 Fooks AR: The challenge of Emerging *Lyssaviruses*. Expert Rev Vaccines 2004; 3 (4): 89-92.

21 Hanlon CA, Kuzmin IV, Blanton JD, Weldon WC, Manangan JS, Rupprecht CE: Efficacy of rabies biologics against new lyssaviruses from Eurasia. Virus Res 2005; 111 (1): 44-54. Epub 2005 Apr 26.

22 Rooijakkers EJ, Nieuwenhuijs JH, Vermeulen AA, van Steenis G, Osterhaus AD: Potency of veterinary rabies vaccines in The Netherlands: a case for continued vigilance. Vet Q 1996; 18 (4): 146-150.

23 Brookes SM, Parsons G, Johnson N, McElhinney LM, Fooks AR: Rabies human diploid cell vaccine elicits cross-neutralising and cross-protecting immune responses against European and Australian bat lyssaviruses. Vaccine 2005; 23 (32): 4101-4109.

24 Cliquet F, Aubert M, Sagne L: Development of a fluorescent antibody virus neutralisation test (FAVN test) for the quantitation of rabies-neutralising antibody. J Immunol Methods 1998; 212 (1): 79-87.

25 Office International des Epizooties. Rabies, in Manual of standards – Diagnostic tests and Vaccines. 4th edition, 2000.

26 http://www.oie.int/eng/normes/mmanual/A_00042.htm.

27 Müller T, Burow J, Schameitat A, Selhorst T, Vos A: Cross-reactive antigenicity in orally vaccinated foxes and raccoon dogs against European bat lyssavirus type 1 and 2, in Dodet B, Schudel A, Pastoret PP, Lombard M (eds): Rabies in Europe. Dev Biol (Basel). Basel, Karger, 2006, vol 125, pp 195-204.

28 Herzog M, Fritzell C, Lafage M, Montano Hirose JA, Scott-Algara D, Lafon M: T and B cell human responses to European bat *Lyssavirus* after post-exposure rabies vaccination. Clin Exp Immunol 1991; 85 (2): 224-230.

29 Bunschoten H, Klapmuts RJ, Claassen IJ, Reyneveld SD, Osterhaus AD, Uytdehaag FG: Rabies virus-specific human T cell clones provide help for an in vitro antibody response against neutralising antibody-inducing determinants of the viral glycoprotein. J Gen Virol 1989; 70: 1513-1521.

30 Briggs DJ, Smith JS, Mueller FL, Schwenke J, Davis RD, Gordon CR, Schweitzer K, Orciari LA, Yager PA, Rupprecht CE: A comparison of two serological methods for detecting the immune response after rabies vaccination in dogs and cats being exported to rabies-free areas. Biologicals. 1998; 26 (4): 347-355.

31 Brookes SM and Fooks AR: Occupational lyssavirus risks and post-vaccination monitoring, in Dodet B, Schudel A, Pastoret PP, Lombard M (eds): Rabies in Europe. Dev Biol (Basel). Basel, Karger, 2006, vol 125, pp 165-173.

32 Kuwert et al: Early/High and Low/Late Responders among HDCS Vaccinees? in Kuwert EK, Wiktor TJ, Koprowski H (eds): Cell culture rabies vaccines & their protective effect in Man. Proceedings of WHO Consultations, Essen 1980. International Green Cross, 1981, pp 100-107.

33 Smith GC, Brookes SM, Harris SL, Aegerter JN, Jones G, Fooks AR: EBLV-2 prevalence in Great Britain as determined by surveillance testing, in Dodet B, Schudel A, Pastoret PP, Lombard M (eds): Rabies in Europe. Dev Biol (Basel). Basel, Karger, 2006, vol 125, pp 265-271.

Dr. S.M. Brookes, Rabies and Wildlife Zoonoses Group, Veterinary Laboratories Agency (VLA), WHO Collaborating Centre for the Characterisation of Rabies and Rabies-Related Viruses, New Haw, Addlestone, Surrey, KT15 3NB, United Kingdom.
E-mail: s.brookes@vla.defra.gsi.gov.uk

Dodet B, Schudel A, Pastoret PP, Lombard M (eds): Rabies in Europe.
Dev Biol (Basel). Basel, Karger, 2006, vol 125, pp 195-204.

Cross Reactive Antigenicity in Orally Vaccinated Foxes and Raccoon Dogs Against European Bat Lyssavirus Type 1 and 2

T. Müller[1], *T. Selhorst*[1] *J. Burow*[1], *A. Schameitat*[1], *A. Vos*[2]

[1] Friedrich-Loeffler-Institut, Federal Research Institute for Animal Health, WHO Collaborating Centre for Rabies Surveillance and Research, Wusterhausen, Germany

[2] Impstoffwerk Dessau Tornau GmbH (IDT), Rosslau, Germany

Abstract: For the first time, the effectiveness of oral rabies vaccines against European Bat Lyssaviruses Type 1 (EBLV-1) and Type 2 (EBLV-2) by means of cross-neutralization assays was investigated. Sera from orally vaccinated red foxes (*Vulpes vulpes*) and raccoon dogs (*Nyctereutes procyonoides*) with the Street Alabama Dufferin (SAD) B19 and SAD P5/88 live-modified vaccine viruses were used to study the cross reactive antigenicity against CVS-11 (genotype 1), EBLV-1 (genotype 5) and EBLV-2 (genotype 6). For comparison, similar crossneutralization assays with sera from EBLV-1 and EBLV-2 infected ferrets (*Mustela putorius furo*) and/or foxes were conducted. Sera from animals vaccinated with the two oral rabies vaccines were reactive against CVS-11 (homologous virus), EBLV-1 and EBLV-2 (heterologous virus). There was a positive relationship among the virus neutralising antibody titres (VNA); high VNA titres against CVS-11 also resulted in high VNA titres against each EBLV, whereas in general, the VNA-titres obtained with homologous virus were statistically higher than those with the heterologous virus except for SAD P5/88 vaccinated raccoon dogs. No significant difference was found between EBLV-1 and EBLV-2 VNA titres. A similar trend was observed when the results of the cross-neutralization data of the foxes and ferrets inoculated i.m. with EBLV-1 and/or EBLV-2 was analysed. Based on the similarity of the EBLV-VNA titres obtained in our study questions were raised on whether the genetic distance of genotype 5 & 6 within phylogroup 1 really does reflect their antigenetic characteristics or whether this is a feature of attenuated live vaccine viruses. This broad cross protection, however, demonstrated that the representatives of attenuated SAD strains of oral rabies vaccines currently used in Germany are most likely able to protect the reservoir species, red fox and raccoon dog, against EBLV-1 and EBLV-2 infection.

Introduction

The rabies situation in Germany has improved tremendously in recent decades; the incidence of rabies dropped from 10,484 to 34 rabies cases between 1983 and 2004 (Source: Rabies Bulletin Europe). The distribution of oral rabies vaccine baits has played a decisive role in the eradication of this infectious disease in Germany. At the moment, terrestrial wildlife rabies occurs only in a restricted area in a residual rabies focus in the border triangle of Hesse, Baden-Württemberg and Rhineland Palatinate, reflecting the topographical and geographical features of a fragmented landscape. The implementation of several corrective actions in 2005 has led to an improvement of vaccination protocols and a consistent vaccination strategy in the respective federal states, providing evidence that this residual focus will be eliminated in the near future.

Unfortunately, complete eradication of rabies seems to be impossible, due to the presence of bat rabies caused by the rabies viruses, European Bat Lyssavirus Type 1 (EBLV-1 – genotype 5) and Type 2 (EBLV-2 – genotype 6), in Germany and neighbouring countries [1]. Although in recent years several rabies cases of bat origin in terrestrial mammals, including humans [2], have been reported in Europe, routine rabies surveillance data suggest that such spill-over infections are rare. Furthermore, sustained transmission of bat rabies caused by EBLVs in terrestrial animals has never been documented. Moreover, experimental infection studies in animals with EBLVs indicate that such cross-species transmissions are most probably dead-end infections [3-5]. However, sustained spill-overs from bats to terrestrial animals cannot be completely ruled out, as has been shown in a recent rabies outbreak of bat origin in skunks (*Mephitis mephitis*) with genotype 1 (RABV) in Arizona, USA [6]. Actually, spill-over and subsequent host switching of lyssaviruses from bats to other mammals has repeatedly and successfully occurred in history [7]. To be prepared for such a situation, the question was raised of whether the currently used oral rabies vaccine in Germany would be able to effectively protect wildlife against an EBLV-infection. This issue became even more evident after the detection of a stone marten (*Martes foina*) infected with EBLV-1 in a rabies-free area in 2001, being the first and only reported spill-over of an EBLV into wildlife so far [8].

Vaccination failures with commercially available inactivated vaccines against rabies-related viruses have been documented in the past [9]. These failures may result from antigenic differences and lack of cross-reactivity between vaccines and different rabies viruses [10]. Virus strains of commercially available rabies vaccines, including oral rabies vaccines, all belong to genotype 1 (RABV). Also, the available recombinant rabies vaccines express the rabies glycoprotein G of RABV. Because the induction of virus neutralizing antibodies (VNA) is of primary importance in protection against rabies, antibody levels are a good indication of vaccine efficacy. Hence, the cross-neutralization assay was selected to investigate whether the oral rabies vaccine presently used in Germany would be able to protect the major rabies reservoir hosts, red fox (*Vulpes vulpes*) and raccoon dog (*Nyctereutes procyonoides*), against an EBLV-infection.

Material and Methods

Virus strains for vaccination and infection

Foxes and raccoon dogs were vaccinated orally against rabies with Street Alabama Dufferin (SAD) B19 and SAD P5/88. These vaccines strains are, as most commercial available live modified oral rabies vaccines, a derivative of the original SAD virus strain that was isolated from a dog in 1935 [11]. The EBLV-1 virus isolate, used to inoculate the foxes and ferrets, was obtained from a serotine bat (*Eptesicus serotinus*) from Germany in 2001. Additional ferrets were inoculated with an EBLV-2 isolate originating from a Dutch pond bat (*Myotis dasycneme*). The EBLV viruses were isolated from a 10 % brain suspension of the original brain material of the two bats by adaptation to and further passaging in murine neuroblastoma cells [4,5].

Antisera

The sera of the orally vaccinated foxes (N = 43) and raccoon dogs (N = 40) were taken from the sera bank at the Friedrich-Loeffler-Institut, Wusterhausen, Germany, from former efficacy studies [12-14]. Serum samples from ferrets (N = 21) and foxes (N = 8) inoculated i.m. with EBLVs were still available from previous experimental studies [4,5]. Thus, no additional animal experimentation was required for the specific purposes of this study.

Cross-neutralisation assays

Sera were evaluated for neutralising antibodies and relative cross-reactivity by modified versions of the Rapid Fluorescent Focus Inhibition Test (RFFIT) as described [15]. Test viruses used for the cross-neutralization assays were challenge virus standard-11 (CVS-11) and the same EBLV-1 and EBLV-2 isolates used to inoculate ferrets and foxes. CVS-11 is recommended for use in the detection of vaccine-induced rabies virus neutralising antibodies [16]. Each test virus was neutralized by its homologous antiserum and also by all the heterologous antisera. Pre-treatments for sera and use of standards were done as previously described [12]. For specificity reasons, the dilution showing a 100 % reduction of the test virus was used to calculate the respective homologous or heterologous VNA-titre of the antisera.

Statistical analysis

Geometric mean titres could not be calculated for all groups because sometimes the heterologous VNA-titre tested negative. Instead arithmetic mean titres were used, to allow for inclusion of VNA-negative animals as well. Differences between the individual homologous and heterologous VNA titres of a particular group and the level of cross-neutralization with EBLV-1, EBLV-2 and CVS-11 were analysed using the WILCOXON-test for paired data [17].

Results

Sera from animals vaccinated with SAD B19 and SAD P5/88 were reactive against CVS-11 (homologous titre), EBLV-1 and EBLV-2 (heterologous titre) (Table 1).

Table 1: Neutralisation titres of raccoon dogs and foxes orally vaccinated with SAD B19 and SAD P5/88.

Animal	Vaccine	CVS-11		EBLV-1		EBLV-2	
		Mean	Range	Mean	Range	Mean	Range
Foxes	SAD B19	100	10-640	37	10-160	47	0-320
Raccoon dogs	SAD B19	367	20-1280	186	10-640	163	20-640
Raccoon dogs	SAD P5/88	464	80-2560	224	80-640	387	80-1280

The comparative neutralisation pattern of sera from foxes and raccoon dogs orally vaccinated with live modified rabies vaccines showed individual variation when the homologous VNA titres were plotted against heterologous titres. While all serum samples of raccoon dogs vaccinated with either or both vaccines demonstrated neutralisation activity against EBLV-1 and -2, three out of the 43 SAD B19 vaccinated foxes did not show any neutralising activity against EBLV-2 (Figs. 1-3). All serum samples of foxes inoculated with EBLV-1 also showed neutralising activity against EBLV-2 and CVS-11. For the serum samples of ferrets infected with EBLV-1, 11 of 12 and nine of 12 showed reactivity to EBLV-2 and CVS-11, respectively, whereas one of nine sera of ferrets infected with EBLV-2 did not cross-reacted with CVS-11 (Table 2).

The statistical analysis of the data obtained with the orally vaccinated foxes and raccoon dogs showed a highly significant difference (WILCOXON test); the VNA-titres obtained with CVS-11 were higher than those with EBLV-1 and EBLV-2 except for SAD P5/88 vaccinated raccoon dogs (Table 3). No significant difference was found between EBLV-1 and EBLV-2. A similar trend was observed when the results of the cross-neutralization data of the foxes and ferrets inoculated i.m. with

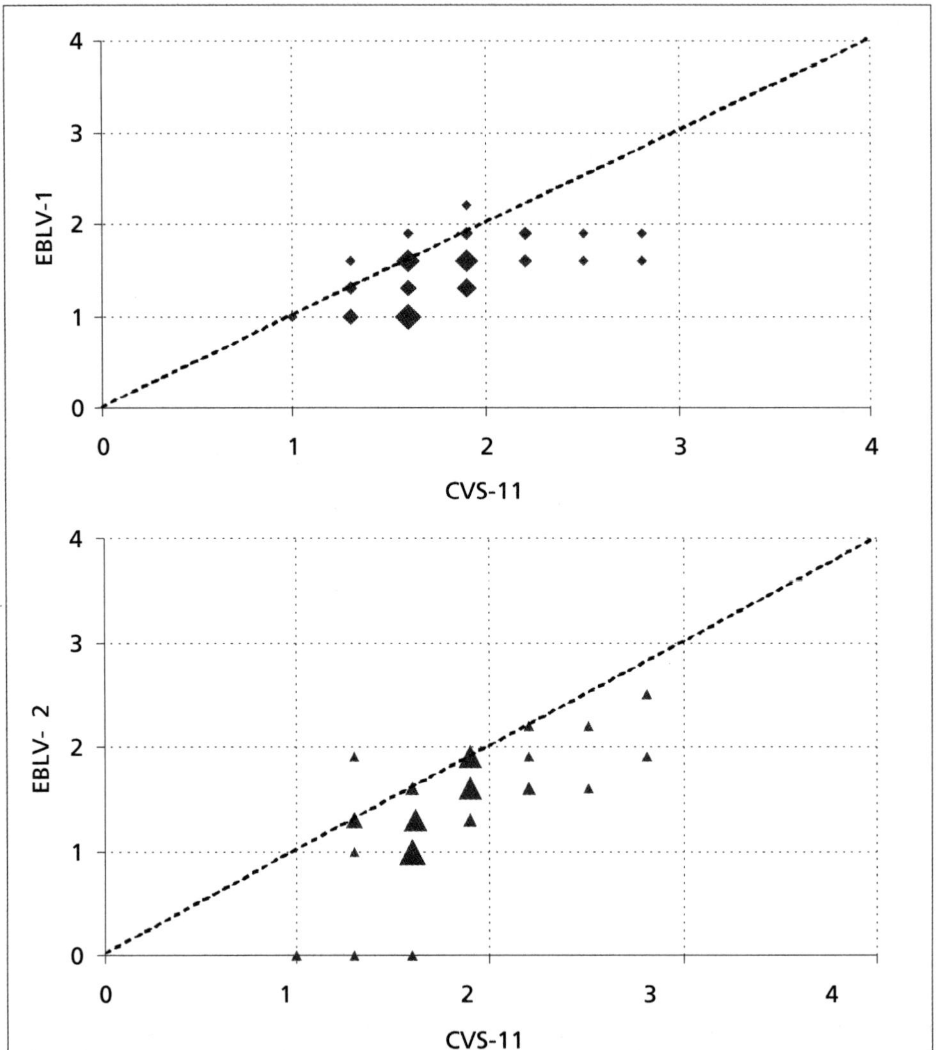

Fig. 1: Cross VNA titres in log10 (100 % reduction) of foxes orally vaccinated with SAD B19 against EBLV-1 and EBLV-2. The size of the symbols reflects the number of sera samples at a given data point. The equivalence equation (line) is also shown.

EBLV-1 and/or EBLV-2 were analysed (Table 3). However, as a result of the smaller sample sizes, the differences were less pronounced.

Furthermore, it was investigated whether there was a positive correlation between the cross-VNA titre of the sera samples pooled according to the inocula or animal species. The results of the statistical analysis are summarized in Table 4. For all (pooled) groups a significant positive correlation was found, except for orally vaccinated raccoon dogs.

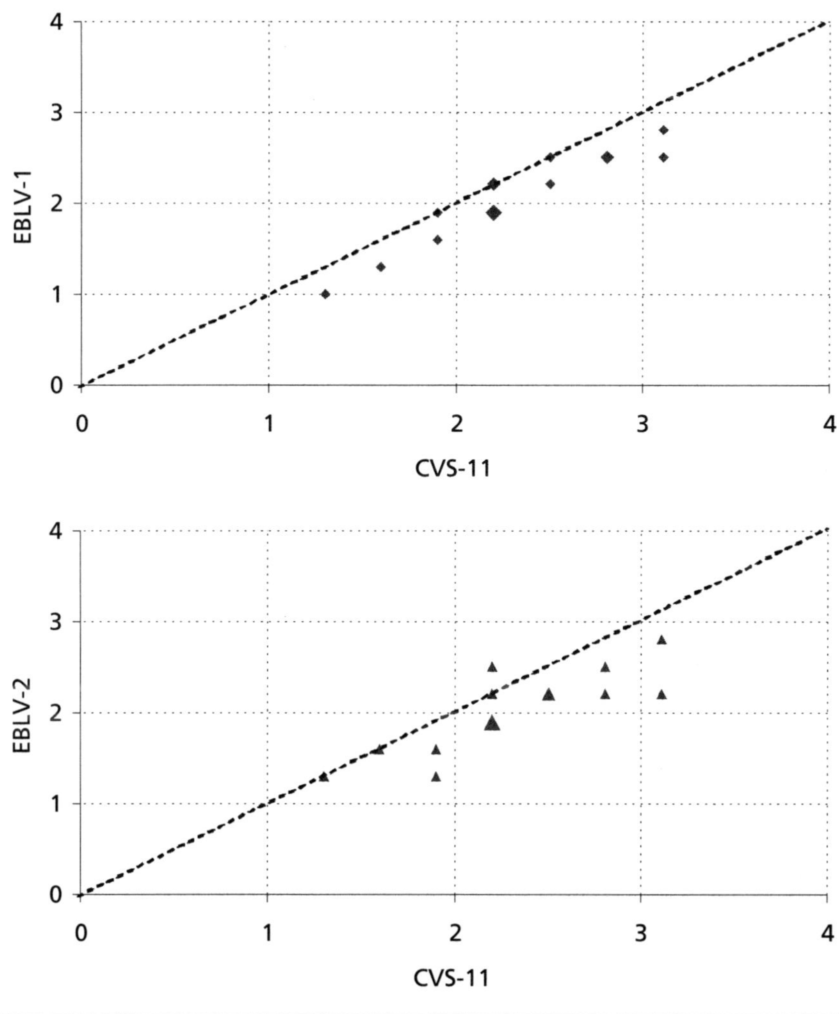

Fig. 2: Cross VNA titres in log10 (100 % reduction) of raccoon dogs orally vaccinated with SAD B19 against EBLV-1 and EBLV-2. The size of the symbols reflects the number of sera samples at a given data point. The equivalence equation (line) is also shown.

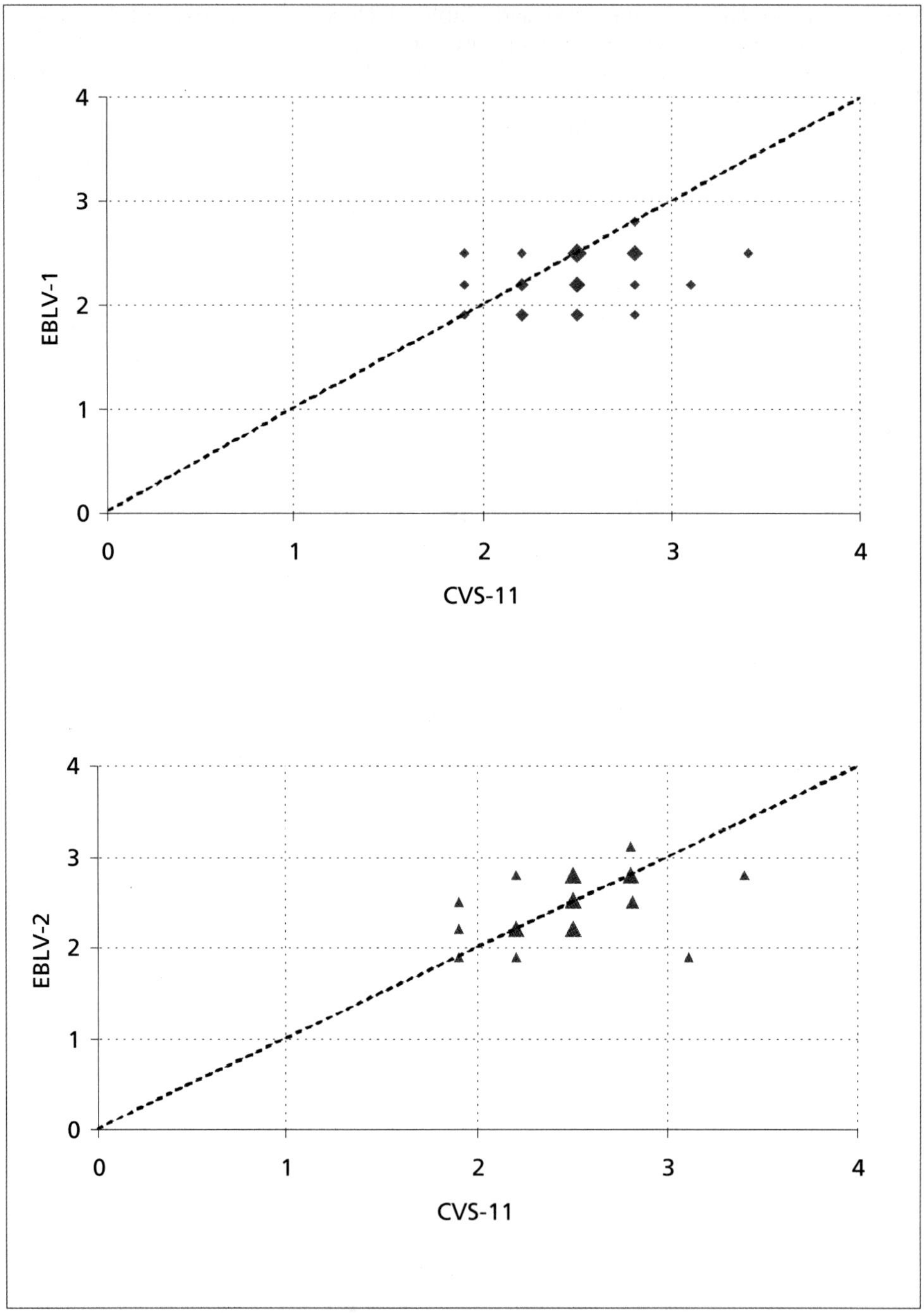

Fig. 3: Cross VNA titres in log10 (100 % reduction) of raccoon dogs orally vaccinated with SAD P5/88 against EBLV-1 and EBLV-2. The size of the symbols reflects the number of sera samples at a given data point. The equivalence equation (line) is also shown.

Table 2: Serological response (100 % reduction) of sera from foxes and ferrets inoculated i.m. with EBLV-1 and EBLV-2 to homologous and heterologous test virus strains (GMT – geometric mean titre).

	EBLV-1 infected foxes			**EBLV-1 infected ferrets**			**EBLV-2 infected ferrets**		
	VNA titres against			**VNA titres against**			**VNA titres against**		
Sample	**EBLV-1**	**EBLV-2**	**CVS-11**	**EBLV-1**	**EBLV-2**	**CVS-11**	**EBLV-2**	**EBLV-1**	**CVS-11**
1	100	40	20	20	40	< 5	10	20	10
2	100	40	10	40	80	< 5	20	80	< 5
3	100	80	40	80	160	10	20	80	20
4	800	320	320	40	< 5	10	40	80	10
5	40	40	10	80	40	10	40	160	20
6	640	640	160	40	40	20	40	10	10
7	20	40	10	20	40	10	40	20	10
8	640	640	160	40	40	< 5	160	320	80
9	–	–	–	40	80	20	160	40	10
10	–	–	–	40	40	10	–	–	–
11	–	–	–	40	80	40	–	–	–
12	–	–	–	40	80	80	–	–	–
GMT	**150**	**113**	**40**	**43**	**60**	**14**	**59**	**90**	**20**

Table 3: The result of the statistical analysis (WILCOXON test) of the sera investigated.

Inoculation virus	**Animal**	**CVS-11 vs. EBLV-1**	**CVS-11 vs. EBLV-2**	**EBLV-1 vs. EBLV-2**
SAD B19	Raccoon dog	***	***	n.s.
	Fox	***	***	n.s.
SAD P5/88	Raccoon dog	*	n.s.	**
EBLV-1	Fox	*	*	n.d.
	Ferrets	**	**	n.s.
EBLV-2	Ferrets	**	*	n.s.

Legend: n.d. – not determined, sample size too small for comparison, n.s. not significant.
* $P < 0.05$; ** $P < 0.01$; *** $P < 0.001$.

Discussion

In this study, the cross-neutralization assay was selected to test the efficacy of oral rabies vaccines against EBLVs. To demonstrate efficacy, a challenge experiment is normally required by the regulatory authorities. However, for our purposes such a model was not appropriate. During experimental studies it was shown that

Table 4: The result of the statistical analysis (WILCOXON test) of the sera investigated.

Inoculation virus	Animal	CVS-11 vs. EBLV-1	CVS-11 vs. EBLV-2	EBLV-1 vs. EBLV-2
SAD B19	Fox & raccoon dog	***	***	n.s.
SAD P5/88 & SAD B19	Raccoon dog	***	n.s.	n.s.
SAD P5/88 & SAD B19	Fox & raccoon dog	***	***	n.d.
EBLV-1	Fox & ferrets	***	***	n.s.

Legend: n.d. – not determined, sample size too small for comparison, n.s. not significant.

*** $P < 0.001$.

foxes and ferrets infected i.m. with EBLV-1 and/or EBLV-2 do not always succumb to rabies. An intracerebral infection would most probably be too severe and, more importantly, not stimulate the natural route of infection. For example, McElhinney et al. showed that mice vaccinated with a human vaccine (Human Diploid Cell Vaccine) were only partially protected against a challenge (intracerebral) with EBLV-1 [18]. When using a less severe route by administering EBLV-1 in the footpad, all animals were fully protected. Furthermore, a mouse model would have little relevance due to interspecific differences in susceptibility to EBLVs [5].

Several studies have already investigated the protective effect of inactivated rabies vaccines for human and veterinary use against EBLVs [3, 18-21], unfortunately, with sometimes conflicting results. In some of these experimental studies, the inactivated rabies vaccines tested were shown to fully protect the animals against EBLV-1; however, they elicited only partial protection against EBLV-2. Meanwhile, other studies showed the opposite; animals were fully protected against EBLV-2 but not against EBLV-1. Although differences in protection have been observed, it is generally believed that the commercially available rabies vaccines for human and veterinary use are effective against an EBLV infection. Recently, reduced protection with pre-exposure vaccination and with conventional rabies post-exposure prophylaxis was described against four new bat viruses, isolated from insectivorous bats in Asia, genetically different from EBLVs [22].

The fact that rabies vaccines are less efficient against EBLVs than against RABV is a result of antigenic differences between the genotypes 1, 5 and 6. The more homologous the vaccine strain is to the challenge virus, the higher the protective efficiency of the rabies vaccine. The genetic distance between RABV and EBLV-2 is smaller than between RABV and EBLV-1, thus commercial rabies vaccines are expected to generally induce better protection against EBLV-2 than against EBLV-1 [23]. However, the results of our cross-neutralization assays neither confirm nor contradict this, since no significant differences between EBLV-1 and -2 VNA titres in any of the SAD-vaccinated or EBLV-infected animals could be found. Only the SAD P5/88 vaccinated raccoon dogs showed significantly higher VNA-titres to EBLV-2 than to EBLV-1. In general, the cross-neutralisation patterns of the SAD-vaccinated animals yielded a positive relationship among the heterologous VNA-titres, e.g. high VNA against the homologous virus CVS-11 also resulted in high VNA titres against EBLV-1 and -2 and vice versa. This is in accordance with observations in human vaccinees [22,24]. Maybe the relative similarity of the EBVL-VNA titres obtained in our study better reflect the antigenetic characteristics of both types of EBLVs (genotypes 5, 6) within phylogroup 1, rather than their genetic distance to RABV (genotype 1) and to each other.

In contrast to the other cross-neutralization and protection studies performed, in which inactivated rabies vaccines were used, for the first time modified-live, attenuated, rabies vaccine viruses were tested which induced a "stronger" immune response than inactivated vaccine strains for human and veterinary use. On the other hand, sera were only tested against one isolate each as a representative of EBLV-1 and -2, hence a different neutralisation pattern using other EBLV-isolates cannot be completely ruled out.

In the event of sustained spillover as observed in skunks [6], it is necessary that the infected animals are capable of transmitting the virus. In contrast to ferrets and foxes experimentally infected with EBLV-1 and -2, the virus associated with the spillover in skunks could be isolated from their saliva after experimental infection with the virus associated with the spillover in this animal species [4,5,25]. Most oral rabies vaccines available in Europe are closely related to the vaccine virus used in these studies. Thus, it can be concluded that in the event of a sustained EBLV spillover from bats to terrestrial wildlife, oral vaccination campaigns as currently carried out will protect the major European rabies reservoir hosts, the red fox and raccoon dog, against infection against EBLV-1 and -2.

Conflict of Interest

AV is a scientific adviser for a company that produces the investigated oral vaccine viruses.

References

1 Bourhy H, Kissi B, Lafon M, Sacramento D, Tordo N: Antigenic and molecular characterization of bat rabies virus in Europe. J Clin Microbiol 1992; 30 (9): 2419-2426.

2 Fooks AR, Brookes SM, Johnson N, McElhinney LM, Hutson AM: European bat lyssaviruses: an emerging zoonosis. Epidemiol Infect 2003; 131 (3): 1029-1039.

3 Fekadu M, Shaddock JH, Sanderlin DW, Smith JS: Efficacy of rabies vaccines against Duvenhage virus isolated from European house bats (Eptesicus serotinus), classic rabies and rabies-related viruses. Vaccine 1988; 6 (6): 533-539.

4 Vos A, Müller T, Cox J, Neubert L, Fooks AR: Susceptibility of ferrets (Mustela putorius furo) to experimentally induced rabies with European Bat Lyssaviruses (EBLV). J Vet Med B Infect Dis Vet Public Health 2004a; 51 (2): 55-60.

5 Vos A, Müller T, Neubert L, Zurbriggen A, Botteron C, Pöhle D, Schoon H, Haas L, Jackson A: Rabies in red foxes (Vulpes vulpes) experimentally infected with European Bat Lyssavirus Type 1 (EBLV-1). J Vet Med B Infect Dis Vet Public Health 2004b; 51 (7): 327-332.

6 Smith JS, Messenger S, Davids A, Yager P, Rupprecht C: Bat rabies: spillover infection and reservoir establishment, in 12th International Meeting on Advances in Rabies Research and Control in the Americas. Peterborough, Canada, Nov. 12-16, 2001 pp 46.

7 Badrane H, Tordo N: Host switching in Lyssavirus History from the Chiroptera to the carnivores orders. J Virol 2001a; 75: 8096-8104

8 Müller T, Cox J, Peter W, Schafer R, Johnson N, McElhinney LM, Geue JL, Tjornehoj K, Fooks AR: Spill-over of European bat lyssavirus type 1 into a stone marten (Martes foina) in Germany. J Vet Med B Infect Dis Vet Public Health 2004; 51 (2): 49-54.

9 Foggin CM: Mokola virus infection in cats and a dog in Zimbabwe. Vet Rec 1983; 113: 115.

10 Lodmell DL, Smith JS, Esposito JJ, Ewalt LC: Cross-protection of mice against a global spectrum of rabies virus variants. J Virol 1995; 69: 4957-4962.

11 Blancou J, FX Meslin: Modified live-virus rabies vaccines for oral immunization of carnivores, in Meslin FX, Kaplan M, Koprowski H (eds): Laboratory Techniques in Rabies, 4th Ed. WHO, Geneva, 1996, pp 324-337.

12 Müller TF, Schuster P, Vos AC, Selhorst T, Wenzel UD, Neubert AM: Effect of maternal immunity on the immune response to oral vaccination against rabies in young foxes. Am J Vet Res 2001; 62 (7): 1154-1158.

13 Neubert A, Schuster P, Müller T, Vos A, Pommerening E: Immunogenicity and efficacy of the oral rabies vaccine SAD B19 in foxes. J Vet Med B Infect Dis Vet Public Health 2001; 48 (3): 179-183.

14 Schuster P, Muller T, Vos A, Selhorst T, Neubert L, Pommerening E: Comparative immunogenicity and efficacy studies with oral rabies virus vaccine SAD P5/88 in raccoon dogs and red foxes. Acta Vet Hung 2001; 49 (3): 285-290.

15 Cox JH, Schneider LG: Prophylactic immunization of humans against rabies by intradermal inoculation of human diploid cell culture vaccine. J Clin Microbiol 1976; 3 (2): 96-101.

16 Smith JS, Yager PA, Baer GM: A rapid reproducible test for determining rabies neutralizing antibody. Bull World Health Organ 1973; 48: 535-541.

17 Zöfel P: Statistik in der Praxis, 2. Auflage. Gustav Fisher Verlag Stuttgart, 1988.

18 McElhinney LM, Johnson N, Brookes SM, Mansfield K, Fooks AR: Serum neutralisation of lyssaviruses following vaccination with HDCV or a prototype peptide vaccine. 14th International Meeting on Research Advances and Rabies Control in the Americas, Philadelphia, USA, October 19-24, 2003, pp 62.

19 Schneider LG: Antigenic variants of rabies virus. Comp. Immun Microbiol Infect Dis 1982; 5: 101-107.

20 Lafon M, Bourhy H, Sureau P: Immunity against the European bat rabies (Duvenhage) virus induced by rabies vaccines: an experimental study in mice. Vaccine 1988; 6: 362-368.

21 Tordo N, Jacob Y, Jallet C, Desmezieres E, Perrin P: Potential of DNA-based immunization in Lyssavirus and transdisease vaccinology, in Third World Congress on vaccines and immunization. Opatija, Croatia, June 4-9, 2002, pp 61.

22 Hanlon CA, Kuzmin IV, Blanton JD, Weldon WC, Manangan JS, Rupprecht CE: Efficacy of rabies biologics against new lyssaviruses from Eurasia. Virus Res 2005; 111 (1): 44-54.

23 Badrane H, Bahloul C, Perrin P, Tordo N: Evidence of two Lyssavirus phylogroups with distinct pathogenicity and immunogenicity. J Virol 2001b; 75: 3268-3276.

24 Herzog M, Fritzell C, Lafage M, Montano Hirose JA, Scott-Algara D, Lafon M: T and B cell human responses to European bat lyssavirus after post-exposure rabies vaccination. Clin Exp Immunol 1991; 85: 224-230.

25 Niezgoda M, Hanlon CA, Hughes GJ, Orciari LA, Leslie M, Cheshier R, Rupprecht CE: Host switching of bat rabies viruses: Field and experimental observations of infected skunks. 14th International Meeting on Research Advances and Rabies Control in the Americas, Philadelphia, USA, October 19-24, 2003, pp 65.

Dr. T. Müller, Institute for Epidemiology, WHO Collaborating Centre for Rabies Surveillance and Research, OIE Reference Laboratory for Rabies, Friedrich-Loeffler-Institute – Federal Research Institute for Animal Health, Seestrasse 55, DE-16868 Wusterhausen, Germany.
E-mail: thomas.mueller@fli.bund.de

Dodet B, Schudel A, Pastoret PP, Lombard M (eds): Rabies in Europe.
Dev Biol (Basel). Basel, Karger, 2006, vol 125, pp 205-215.

Pre-Exposure Rabies Booster Vaccinations: a Literature Review

J. Morris, N.S. Crowcroft

Centre for Infections, Health Protection Agency, London, United Kingdom

Abstract: In Europe, more attention is turning towards human infection with European bat lyssaviruses (EBLVs). Following the death of a bat conservationist from EBLV in Scotland, in 2002, the Department of Health in the United Kingdom (UK) recommended that all bat workers receive prophylactic rabies vaccination. This systematic literature review aims to review the evidence base for current UK policy on rabies booster vaccination. Ten papers met the inclusion criteria and were reviewed. Most of the papers were prospective cohort studies with follow-up ending after the first booster vaccination. One year after a three dose intramuscular primary rabies vaccination course, 87.9-100 % of participants had a rabies antibody level ≥ 0.5 IU/ml, before the first booster. It may, therefore, be prudent for the UK to reduce its current recommended interval, primary course to first booster, from two years to one year. More research, with longer follow-up, is required to enable recommendations on subsequent boosters to be made.

INTRODUCTION

In Europe, human rabies infection has become less common since the establishment and monitoring of terrestrial rabies control programmes. Human infections with other lyssaviruses, particularly European bat lyssavirus 1 and 2 (EBLV1 and 2), have become more prominent over recent years. There have been four spill-over EBLV infections into humans over the past twenty years [1]. The most recent, in November of 2002, was a bat conservationist in Scotland who died from EBLV2 infection. None of these four cases had a history of prophylactic rabies vaccination [1].

Strict adherence to World Health Organization (WHO) rabies prophylaxis guidelines virtually guarantees protection against rabies infection [2]. Although it is impossible to test rabies vaccine efficacy in humans by routine methods, in the United States of America there have been no reports of human rabies infection with 50,000 doses of rabies vaccine administered to persons at increased risks of rabies [3]. This also suggests the WHO recognised rabies antibody level of 0.5 IU/ml ensures a reasonable safety margin.

Passive surveillance of bats in the UK has identified four Daubenton's bats (*Myotis daubentonii*) positive for EBLV2 antigen [4]. All four bats were behaving abnormally before their death. A recent study, undertaken by the Veterinary Laboratories Agency (VLA), has found that around 4.2 % of Daubenton's bat in the UK have rabies antibodies [5]. These bats may have had a rabies infection and recovered. Daubenton's bats are a less common bat species in the UK and, because of their natural behaviour, are unlikely to come into contact with humans. Only one other bat species has been found to be EBLV antibody positive in the UK, a serotine bat (*Eptesicus serotinus*) tested positive in 2005 [4].

Following the death of the bat conservationist in Scotland, the UK department of Health recommended that all bat workers have pre-exposure rabies vaccination. Current recommendations for pre-exposure vaccination is a primary three-dose intramuscular course (on days 0, 7 and 28) followed by the first rabies booster at two years and subsequent boosters every two to three years thereafter, if there is a continuing risk of rabies exposure. The human diploid cell rabies vaccine (HDCV) and purified chick embryo cell rabies vaccine (PCEC) are licensed for pre-exposure and post-exposure prophylaxis in the UK. The aim of this literature review is to identify the most appropriate interval for rabies booster vaccinations (first and subsequent boosters) and identify gaps in current knowledge requiring further research. The findings will evaluate the evidence base for current policy in the UK and assist with future recommendations.

Methods

To ensure that the literature review was systematic, a specific research question was defined: *"For pre-exposure immunisation of persons at continued rabies exposure risk, what is the optimal interval for rabies booster vaccinations?"* The databases Embase, Medline and the Cochrane Library were searched, from their year of inception until June 2005, using the search terms (and MESH terms) "rabies" and "booster". The search was limited to human subjects. Reference lists of all articles retrieved were also searched for relevant papers.

Given the wide variation in pre-exposure rabies vaccination courses worldwide over the last three decades, only articles with a similar vaccination course to the UK were included. Papers were excluded from this review if (i) the primary rabies vaccination course was given intradermally/subcutaneously or (ii) the course followed a different schedule from the UK. Each paper for inclusion was assessed according to SIGN (Scottish Intercollegiate Guidelines Network) guidelines [6] and a level of evidence score attributed.

Results

In total, 149 articles were identified and 59 were retrieved. Ten articles are included in this review. Forty-nine articles were excluded from review, 19 of which were not relevant to the research question and 30 of which evaluated rabies vaccinations solely administered intradermally/subcutaneously or given at different schedules from that in the UK. The design details of the studies included are shown in Table 1. Table 2 shows the main results of these studies. One article, discussed in the text, was identified from reference lists but did not fulfil the inclusion criteria and was not included in the tables.

In summary, the studies included in this review have a wide range in the number of participants, from 78 to 2,490 persons, and also a wide range in the length of follow-up, from no follow-up after the serology test to 10 years follow-up. Most of the studies included are prospective cohort studies, comparing different human rabies vaccines along with different schedules and routes of vaccination. In these studies, most initial rabies booster vaccinations were given at one year following the primary

Table 1 : Design details of papers included in the rabies booster vaccination literature review.

Authors (year, country)	Aim	Type of study	Inclusion & exclusion criteria	Methods	Length of follow up
Simani S (2004, Iran) [10]	Evaluate effectiveness of pre-exposure rabies vaccination	Prospective serological survey	Rabies vaccinated high-risk staff working in treatment centres	Single serological test at one point in time. Four study groups – complete/incomplete primary course +/- booster	Not followed up after blood test
Strady A (1998, France) [7]	Determine persistence of rabies antibodies following pre-exposure rabies immunisation with booster immunisation at 1 year	Prospective, comparative trial	Subjects were volunteers at risk due to their profession (livestock breeders, forestry workers, veterinary workers). All from Northern part of France. Had no contraindications to vaccination	Four study groups – each received either HDCV or PVRV by 2 or 3 dose IM primary course with booster at 1 year. Serological testing on days 0, 42, 379 then every year	10 years
Sabchareon A (1999, Thailand) [12]	Evaluate the safety and immunogenicity of CPRV in comparison to HDCV	Randomised double-blinded controlled trial	Healthy children aged 5-13 years attending 3 schools in Bangkok. No recent immunoglobulin therapy, blood or blood products, immunosuppressive treatment or required other vaccines between days 0 and 42 or days 365 and 379	Two study groups – each received either CPRV or HDCV by 3 dose IM primary course with booster at 1 year. Serological testing on days 0, 28, 42, 180, 365, 372 and 379	379 days
Lang J (1998, France) [14]	Demonstrate that CPRV did not produce an inferior immunological response in comparison to PVRV	Randomised double-blinded controlled trial	Healthy first-year veterinary students, aged at least 18 years. No fever on day of vaccination or immune deficiency, immunoglobulin therapy, blood or blood products, immunosuppressive treatment within past 6 months or severe, chronic disease	Two study groups – each received either CPRV or PVRV by 3 dose IM primary course with booster at 1 year. Serological testing on days 0, 28, 42, 180, 365 and 379	379 days
Sabchareon A (1998, Thailand) [13]	Evaluate the safety and immunogenicity of intradermal PVRV in comparison to intramuscular PVRV	Randomised, comparative trial.	Healthy children aged 5-12 years attending 2 schools in Bangkok. No recent immunoglobulin therapy, chloroquine or malaria prophylaxis or recent immunisations	Two study groups – each received either PVRV ID or PVRV IM by 3 dose primary course with booster at 1 year. Serological testing on days 0, 56, 180 and 365 Testing also days 7, 180, 365 and 730 after the booster vaccination.	3 years
Klietmann W (1988, Germany) [8]	Evaluate the safety and immunogenicity of PVRV using various immunisation schedules	Prospective, comparative trial	Students or employees of the Veterinary Faculty of the University of Giessen, aged between 22 to 48 years	Four study groups – 3 groups received primary course of PVRV IM, 1 group received booster PVRV IM (previously immunised with HDCV as primary course) Serological testing on treatment days and 14 days later, with an additional test on day 70 in group IA)	104 days

HDCV human diploid cell vaccine ; PVRV purified Vero cell rabies vaccine ; CPRV chromatographically purified rabies vaccine ; PCEC purified chick embryo cell vaccine.

Table 1 (continued): Design details of papers included in the rabies booster vaccination literature review.

Authors (year, country)	Aim	Type of study	Inclusion & exclusion criteria	Methods	Length of follow up
Picot N (2001, France) [15]	Evaluate the safety and immunogenicity of one and two dose CPRV boosters	Prospective, comparative trial	Healthy adults – veterinary students, staff and travellers	Two study groups – both groups had received primary HDCV or PVRV course at least one year previously. Had 1 or 2 booster doses of CPRV at 1 year. Serological testing days 0 and 14 (1 booster dose) or days 0, 3 and 10 (2 booster doses)	14 days
Bernard KW (1987, USA) [16]	Evaluate the safety and efficacy of intradermal HDCV in comparison to intramuscular HDCV	Prospective, randomised, comparative trial	Adult volunteers	Five study groups – receiving HDCV on days 0, 7 and 28. Dose (0.1/0.25/1.0ml) and route (ID/SC/IM) differs between each group. Half of each group had ID HDCV booster at one year, the other half an ID HDCV booster at two years. Serological testing on days 0, 49, 90, 365 and 730 and 14 days after booster	730 days
Dreesen DW (1989, USA) [9]	Study the antigenicity and side effects of PCEC in comparison to HDCV	Prospective, randomised, comparative trial	Adult volunteers	Four groups – PCEC/HDCV IM (1.0ml)/ID (0.1ml) on days 0, 7 and 28. Two years later given PCEC IM booster (day 756) Serological testing on days 0, 28, 50, 92, 365, 756 and 763	763 days
Briggs DJ (1996, USA) [17]	Determine the safety and immnuogenicity of Lyssavac-HDCV	Prospective, comparative trial	Veterinary students. Exclusion criteria: history of atrophy, asthma, allergy or immunosuppressive disease; viral disease; autoimmune disease; pregnancy; prior rabies vaccination; contraindication to vaccine/immunoglobulin.	Two study groups – Lyssavac-HDCV IM as pre-exposure course and booster dose at 1 year or post-exposure course with immunoglobulin, no booster. Serological testing prior to study and on days 7, 14, 42, 90 (pre-exposure only), 360 and days 367 and 381 for those who had the pre-exposure course	381 days

HDCV human diploid cell vaccine; PVRV purified Vero cell rabies vaccine; CPRV chromatographically purified rabies vaccine; PCEC purified chick embryo cell vaccine.

Table 2 : Main results of papers included in the rabies booster vaccination literature review.

Authors (year, country)	Sample size and attrition	Main outcome measure	Main results	Notes	Level of evidence
Simani S (2004, Iran) [10]	2490 subjects tested	Seroconversion – rabies antibody level ≥ 0.5IU/ml (using ELISA)	73 % of those with complete course and booster had rabies antibody level of ≥ 0.5IU/ml	Unclear when booster was given Maximum interval from last vaccination to serological test 21 years. Would benefit from further statistical analysis	3
Strady A (1998, France) [7]	312 subjects at day 0 divided into the 4 groups. 8.3 % lost to follow up at 1 year, 33.3 % at 5 years and 46.5 % at 10 years	Seroconversion – rabies antibody level ≥ 0.5IU/ml (using rapid fluorescent focus inhibition test [RFFIT])	Of the 32 vaccinated with 3 dose HDCV 100 % had rabies antibody level of ≥ 0.5IU/ml, of the 69 vaccinated with 3 dose PVRV 87.9 % had rabies antibody level of ≥ 0.5IU/ml (100 % 14 days after booster). The seroconversion rate decreased more rapidly for the 2 injection than 3 injectiongroups ($p < 0.001$) and for those vaccinated with PVRV than those vaccinated with HDCV ($p < 0.006$). No significant difference for the 3 dose groups vaccinated with PVRV or HDCV	Predictive analysis : a titre of 30IU/ml on day 379 (75 % of vaccinated subjects) corresponded to a positive predictive value of 100 % and negative predictive value of 18 % of remaining seroconverted at 10 years	2 ++
Sabchareon A (1999, Thailand) [12]	400 subjects, 90 (22.5 %) did not complete the study	Seroconversion – rabies antibody level ≥ 0.5IU/ml (using rapid fluorescent focus inhibition test [RFFIT])	88.1 % CPRV subjects had rabies antibody level ≥ 0.5IU/ml on day 365, 100 % on day 379. 96.8 % HDCV subjects had rabies antibody level ≥ 0.5IU/ml on day 365, 100 % on day 379	All children lost to follow up accounted for. Short follow up after first booster. Only children included	1-
Lang J (1998, France) [14]	330 subjects, 15 (4.5 %) did not complete the study	Seroconversion – rabies antibody level ≥ 0.5IU/ml (using rapid fluorescent focus inhibition test [RFFIT])	97.5 % CPRV subjects had rabies antibody level ≥ 0.5IU/ml on day 365, 100 % on day 379. 98.8 % HDCV subjects had rabies antibody level ≥ 0.5IU/ml on day 365, 100 % on day 379	Subjects immunised with CPRV had significantly more local reactions and significantly fewer systemic reactions than the subjects immunised with PVRV. Short follow up after first booster	1-
Sabchareon A (1998, Thailand) [13]	190 subjects. 18.0 % lost to follow up at 1 year, 26.3 % at 2 years and 38.0 % at 3 years	Seroconversion – rabies antibody level ≥ 0.5IU/ml (using rapid fluorescent focus inhibition test [RFFIT]).	90.7 % PVRV IM subjects had rabies antibody level ≥ 0.5IU/ml on day 365, 100 % on day 379, 100 % two years after booster	Only children included	2 +

HDCV human diploid cell vaccine ; PVRV purified Vero cell rabies vaccine ; CPRV chromatographically purified rabies vaccine ; PCEC purified chick embryo cell vaccine.

Table 2 (continued): Main results of papers included in the rabies booster vaccination literature review.

Authors (year, country)	Sample size and attrition	Main outcome measure	Main results	Notes	Level of evidence
Klietmann W (1988, Germany) [8]	82 subjects, all completed study.	Seroconversion – rabies antibody level ≥ 0.5IU/ml (using rapid fluorescent focus inhibition test [RFFIT])	Of the 10 subjects in group III, 9 had a rabies antibody level ≥ 0.5IU/ml at most 38 months after the primary rabies vaccination course All of these subjects had a rabies antibody level ≥ 0.5IU/ml 14 days after the booster vaccination	Small study size. Date of previous vaccination for 2 subjects in group III not given. Short length of follow up	2 -
Picot N (2001, France) [15]	517 subjects, 1.7 % did not complete the study	Seroconversion – rabies antibody level ≥ 0.5IU/ml (using rapid fluorescent focus inhibition test [RFFIT])	100 % subjects had seroconverted by day 14/10, depending on study	Short report. No pre-booster rabies antibody levels given. No further serological follow up after booster dose	2 +
Bernard KW (1987, USA) [16]	124 subjects, 9.7 % did not complete the study	Seroconversion – rabies antibody level ≥ 0.5IU/ml (using rapid fluorescent focus inhibition test [RFFIT])	18 subjects had a primary IM course. All subjects had rabies antibody level ≥ 0.5IU/ml on day 365 (lowest 1.1IU/ml) and the 8 due a booster at 2 years had rabies antibody level ≥ 0.5IU/ml on day 730 (lowest 0.5IU/ml).	Small numbers in each group	2 -
Dreesen DW (1989, USA) [9]	78 subjects, 11.5 % did not complete the study	Seroconversion – rabies antibody titre ≥ 1:11 (using rapid fluorescent focus inhibition test [RFFIT])	100 % subjects receiving an IM primary course had a rabies antibody titre ≥ 1:11 at 2 years (prior to first booster). There was an anamnestic response following the booster dose with a titre range 270-9500 7 days following	Small numbers in each group	2 -
Briggs DJ (1996, USA) [17]	318 subjects, 6.9 % did not complete the study	Seroconversion – rabies antibody titre ≥ 1:5 (using rapid fluorescent focus inhibition test [RFFIT])	100 % of the three dose regime subjects (n = 146) had a rabies antibody titre > 1:5 at 1 year (prior to first booster). They demonstrated a significant anamnestic response to the booster dose		2 +

HDCV human diploid cell vaccine; PVRV purified Vero cell rabies vaccine; CPRV chromatographically purified rabies vaccine; PCEC purified chick embryo cell vaccine.

rabies vaccination course with serological testing for rabies antibody levels fourteen days later. The WHO recognised level of 0.5 IU/ml was taken as the appropriate level for demonstrating rabies immunity. Where pre-booster antibody levels are stated, at one-year post primary intramuscular vaccination course, the proportion of the study population that has an antibody level ≥ 0.5 IU/ml varies from 87.9 % to 100 %. Where possible, this information is represented in Figure 1. Fourteen days after the booster vaccination, 100 % of these study subjects have rabies antibody levels of ≥ 0.5 IU/ml. Generally, the geometric mean of these boosted antibody titres is much higher due to a marked anamnestic response, indicating good immunological memory. The proportion of the study population followed-up for at least one year and has a rabies antibody level ≥ 0.5 IU/ml after the first booster vaccination is represented in Figure 2.

Out of all the studies, Strady [7] followed their participants for the longest period of time. If the participant had a rabies antibody titre of 30 IU/ml or more 14 days after the first booster (given on day 365), their antibody level would remain ≥ 0.5 IU/ml for the next 10 years. This study concluded that most study subjects would remain ≥ 0.5 IU/ml at 10 years post first booster vaccination. An algorithm is provided to assist identification of individuals that will require boosters at an earlier date.

Klietmann [8] followed 10 adults who had received a primary course of rabies before their involvement with the study. The interval between primary course and first booster varied from five months to three years (mostly three years). Nine of the adults had rabies antibody levels of ≥ 0.5 IU/ml before their first booster. All had rabies antibody levels of ≥ 0.5 IU/ml and had a greater than four-fold increase of antibody levels two weeks after the booster vaccination.

Dreesen [9] undertook a small study with 78 adults. Thirty-nine participants received a primary three-dose rabies vaccination course intramuscularly. Two years following the primary course, 100 % of these participants had rabies antibody levels of ≥ 0.5 IU/ml before their first booster.

One prospective serological survey has been included in this review. Simani [10] checked the rabies antibody level of 2,490 adults. These participants were divided into four study groups: those with a complete primary course and those without a complete primary course; these were divided further into those with and without a rabies booster vaccination. Most of the participants (n = 1,865) had received a complete primary vaccination course without booster vaccinations. Of these, 614 individuals (36 %) had antibody levels below 0.5 IU/ml. The time from the last rabies vaccination to serological testing was variable; for the whole group this ranged from several days to 21 years. This interval is not given specifically for those with a complete primary course and no booster vaccinations. The paper states that the antibody titre level decreased with time. However, there was no differentiation in the results between the groups; all four groups were included in this analysis.

The study by Ajjan [11], which was identified after reviewing the reference lists of the papers retrieved, followed 144 participants for 21 months following their primary rabies vaccination course, but no rabies booster vaccination was given. The participants received either HDCV or purified Vero rabies vaccine (PVRV) intramuscularly as a primary course. At 21 months, 51 out of 54 (94 %) subjects who had received HDCV had an acceptable rabies antibody level of ≥ 0.5 IU/ml. Out of the subjects who received PVRV, 43 of the 44 tested (98 %) had an acceptable rabies antibody level. Forty-six participants (32 %) were lost to follow-up by this time.

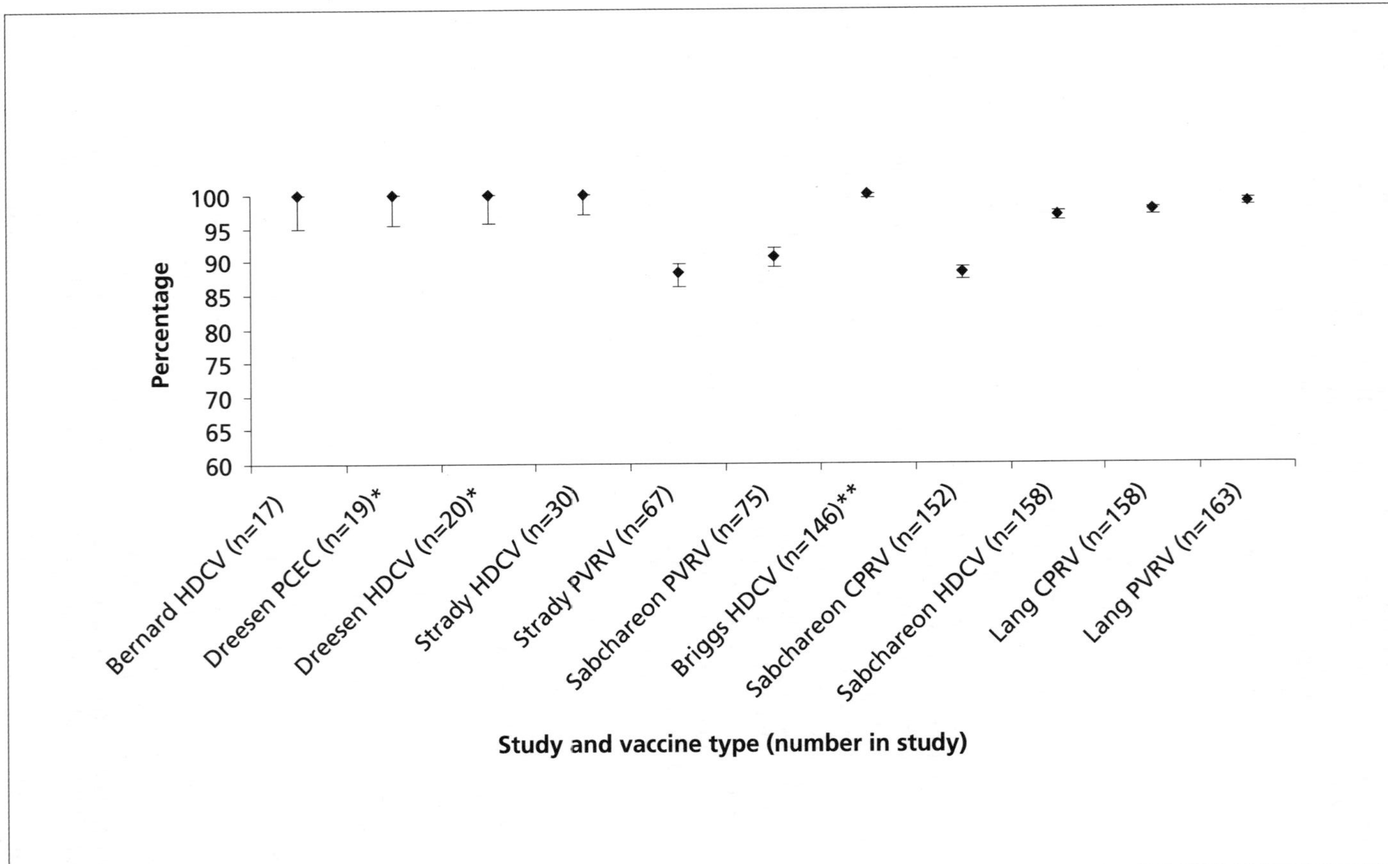

Fig. 1: Proportion of study subjects with a rabies antibody level ≥ 0.5 IU/ml taken 12 months after the primary rabies vaccination course.

* Seroconversion: rabies antibody titre ≥ 1:11; **Seroconversion: rabies antibody titre ≥ 1:5.

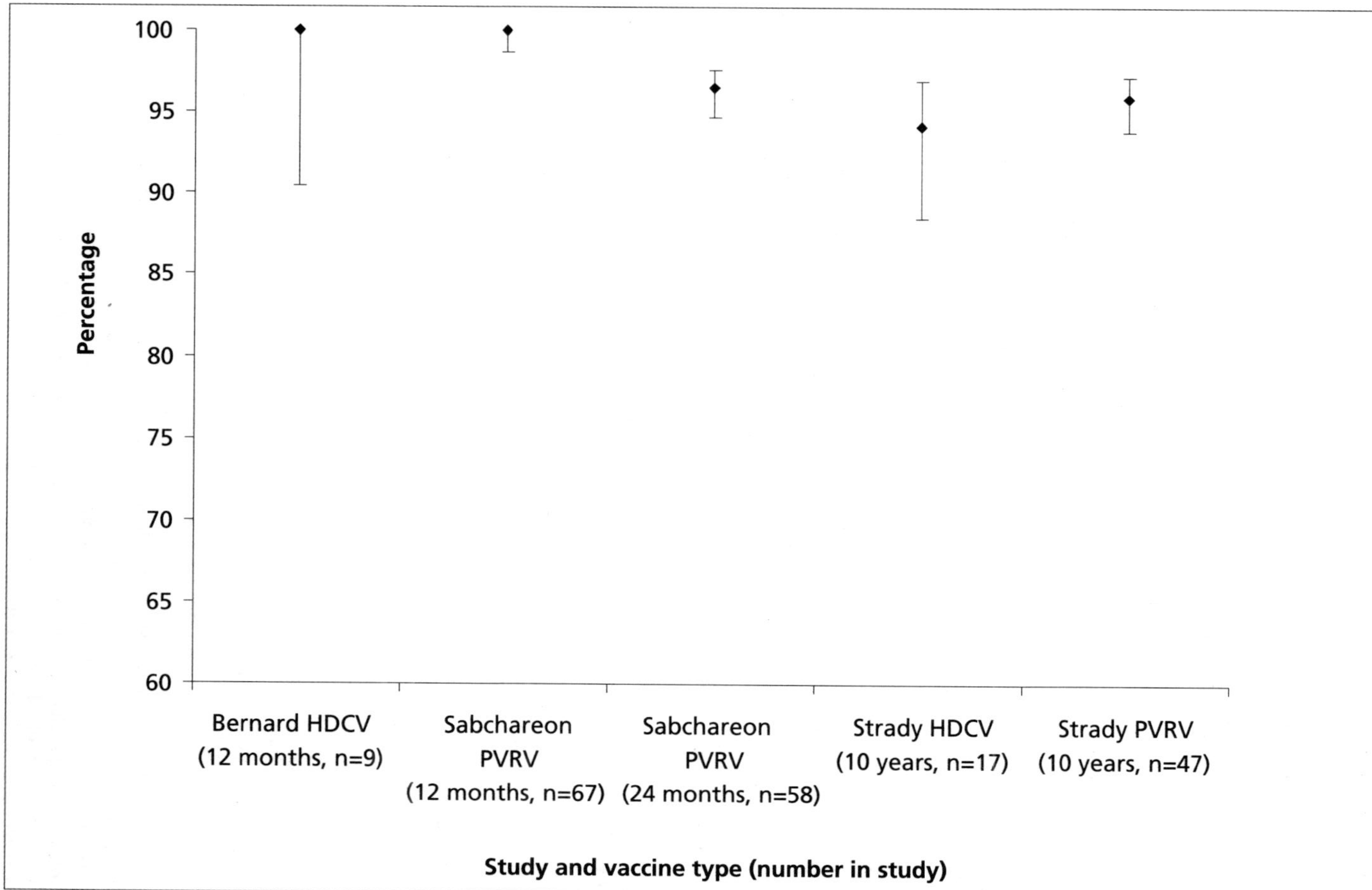

Fig. 2: Proportion of study subjects with a rabies antibody level ≥ 0.5 IU/ml taken 12 months after the rabies booster vaccination (given at 1 year).

Discussion

This systematic review has identified literature on the timing of rabies booster vaccinations in those persons requiring pre-exposure rabies prophylaxis. However, there are some limitations to the methods used for this review. This review included only published literature. "Grey" literature was not searched and this may lead to a publication bias. Hand searching of specific journals was not undertaken and therefore some relevant studies may have been missed.

This review also has a number of strengths. Due to the explicit methodology, as described previously, this review is both comprehensive and reproducible. Established guidelines, produced by the SIGN Network, were used to assess each article qualitatively and attribute a level of evidence score assisting with the comparability of the papers.

There are some problems associated with the studies included in this review. The small number of participants in many of the studies, particularly when further dividing the participants into groups, reduced the statistical power of the results. Also, two of the studies [12,13] looked only at healthy children, making these results difficult to extrapolate to adults. Few of the studies followed participants for longer than one year, most ending after the first booster vaccination. Given these limitations, recommendations for the timing of subsequent booster vaccinations, following the first booster, are difficult to make on the basis of existing knowledge. It would be cautious to recommend that the first rabies booster vaccination be given one year after the primary course in the UK, rather than the current two years. More research is needed, with longer follow-up periods, to determine the interval for subsequent boosters.

Acknowledgements

We would like to thank our colleagues at the Veterinary Laboratories Agency, Bat Conservation Trust and English Nature for their assistance with this literature review. We would also like to thank David Brown for reading the drafts of this paper.

References

1 Fooks AR, Brookes SM, Johnson N, McElhinney LM, Hutson AM: European bat lyssaviruses: an emerging zoonosis. Epidemiol Infect 2003; 131: 1029-1039.

2 WHO Expert Consulation on Rabies. First Report. Geneva, World Health Organization, 2004 (WHO technical report series, 931).

3 World Health Organization. Vaccines and Immunization. Available at <http://www.who.int/rabies/vaccines/en/>. Accessed 26th July 2005.

4 HPA. First serotine bat from southern England found to be positive for EBLV1 antibodies. Commun Dis Rep CDR Wkly [serial online] 2005 [cited 3 June 2005], 15 (22): news. Available at <http://www.hpa.org.uk/cdr/archives/archive05/News/news2205.htm#bats>.

5 Preliminary results of study into bat rabies (European bat lyssavirus) in England. Press release 215/05. London: DEFRA, 21 May 2005. Available at <http://www.defra.gov.uk/news/2005/050521a.htm>.

6 Scottish Intercollegiate Guidelines Network (SIGN). SIGN 50: A guideline developers' handbook. Available at http://www.sign.ac.uk/guidelines/fulltext/50/index.html>. Accessed 26th July 2005.

7 Strady A, Lang J, Lienard M, Blondeau C, Jaussaud R, Plotkin SA: Antibody persistence following preexposure regimens of cell-culture rabies vaccines: 10-year follow-up and proposal for a new booster policy. J Infect Dis 1998; 177: 1290-1295.

8 Klietmann W, Klietmann B, Cox J, Charbonnier C: Effectiveness and tolerance of pre- and postexposure treatment with purified inactivated rabies vaccine prepared on Vero cell line. Vaccine 1988; 6:39-43.

9 Dreesen DW, Fishbein DB, Kemp DT, Brown J: Two-year comparative trial on the immunogenicity and adverse effects of purified chick embryo cell rabies vaccine for pre-exposure immunisation. Vaccine 1989; 7: 397-400.

10 Simani S et al: Evaluation of the effectiveness of preexposure rabies vaccination in Iran. Arch Iranian Med 2004; 7 (4): 251-255.

11 Ajjan N, Pilet CH: Comparative study of the safety and protective value, in pre-exposure use, of rabies vaccine cultivated on human diploid cells (HDCV) and of the new vaccine grown on Vero cells. Vaccine 1989; 7: 125-128.

12 Sabchareon A et al: A new Vero cell rabies vaccine: results of a comparative trial with human diploid cell rabies vaccine in children. Clin Infect Dis 1999; 29: 141-149.

13 Sabchareon A et al: Persistence of antibodies in children after intradermal or intramuscular administration of preexposure primary and booster immunisations with purified Vero cell rabies vaccine. Pediatr Infect Dis J 1998; 17 (11): 1001-1007.

14 Lang J et al: Immunogenicity and safety in adults of a new chromatographically purified Vero-cell rabies vaccine (CPRV): a randomised, double-blind trial with purified Vero-cell rabies vaccine (PVRV). Biologicals 1998; 26: 299-308.

15 Picot N et al: Booster effect of a new chromato graphically purified Vero-cell rabies vaccine (CPRV): immunogenicity of a single or double injection. Trans R Soc Trop Med Hyg 2001; 95: 342-344.

16 Bernard KW et al: Preexposure immunisation with intradermal human diploid cell rabies vaccine. JAMA 1987; 257 (8): 1059-1063.

17 Briggs DJ et al: Safety and immunogenicity of Lyssavac Berna human diploid cell rabies vaccine in healthy adults. Vaccine 1996; 14 (14): 1361-1365.

Dr. N.S. Crowcroft, Centre for Infections Health Protection Agency, 61 Colindale Avenue, London, NW9 5HT, United Kingdom.
E-mail: natasha.crowcroft@hpa.org.uk

Dodet B, Schudel A, Pastoret PP, Lombard M (eds): Rabies in Europe.
Dev Biol (Basel). Basel, Karger, 2006, vol 125, pp 217-220.

Determination of Efficacy of Rabies Vaccine in the Saratov Region

A.V. Borisov, A.V. Savvin, V.V. Mikhalishin, K.N. Gruzdev, I.A. Domsky

Federal Centre for Animal Health (FGI ARRIAH), Vladimir, Russia

Abstract: The most complicated situation concerning rabies is seen in the Saratov region. The basic reservoir of rabies in this region is wild carnivores. A study was conduted in three districts of the Saratov region to define the efficiency of measures taken with the " Sinrab " rabies vaccine containing " RV-97 " used for oral immunisation of wild animals. As a result of the experiment it was established that specific prevention of rabies in wildlife in enzootic territories resulted in a decrease of rabies cases.

INTRODUCTION

In Russia, as well as in many countries of the world, rabies is considered to be one of the most dangerous zoonotic diseases. In recent years irregularity of rabies distribution in regions of the Russian Federation has become extremely obvious, with a high prevalence of rabies determined in some regions [2].

In the dynamics of rabies, there have been notable periods when the number of cases have increased – 1989-1990, 1994-1995, 1998-1999, and 2001. Rabies control measures among its facultative and obligatory hosts has not in fact yielded the expected results. Since 1998 such vaccines as "Lyssvulpen" and "Sinrab" have been used in 25-28 subjects of the Russian Federation for oral vaccination of foxes (about 941-1050 thousand doses every year) within the framework of the rabies prevention system.

The vaccines were used in different seasons at various intervals and using various doses in areas over 1 km^2. Under such conditions it was difficult to unambiguously evaluate the efficacy of the vaccines [1].

MATERIALS AND METHODS

The oral "Sinrab" vaccine containing strain "PB-97" produced by ARRIAH was used in the experiment. Considering the epizootic situation at 1.12.2002, three districts in the Saratov region consistantly effected by rabies, Kalininsk, Lysogorsk and Ekaterininsk, were chosen for the experiment. Bait with oral "Sinrab" rabies vaccine was distributed three times a year, taking into account the seasonal increase of rabies cases. The bait with vaccine (15 – 20 baits per 1 km^2) was distributed, according to the directions, by hand, around the habitats of carnivores; later the consumption of bait containing the vaccine was checked. The total vaccination area was 595 km^2.

The experiment was based on a complex epizootic approach including descriptive and historical methods, epizootic statistics, epizootic investigation, virology analyses and experimental investigations [5].

Results

As shown in Figure 1, the situation for rabies in the Saratov region is very complex. It is established that 33.2 % of cases involve wild animal reservoirs, 24.2 %, dogs and 25.9 %, farm animals.

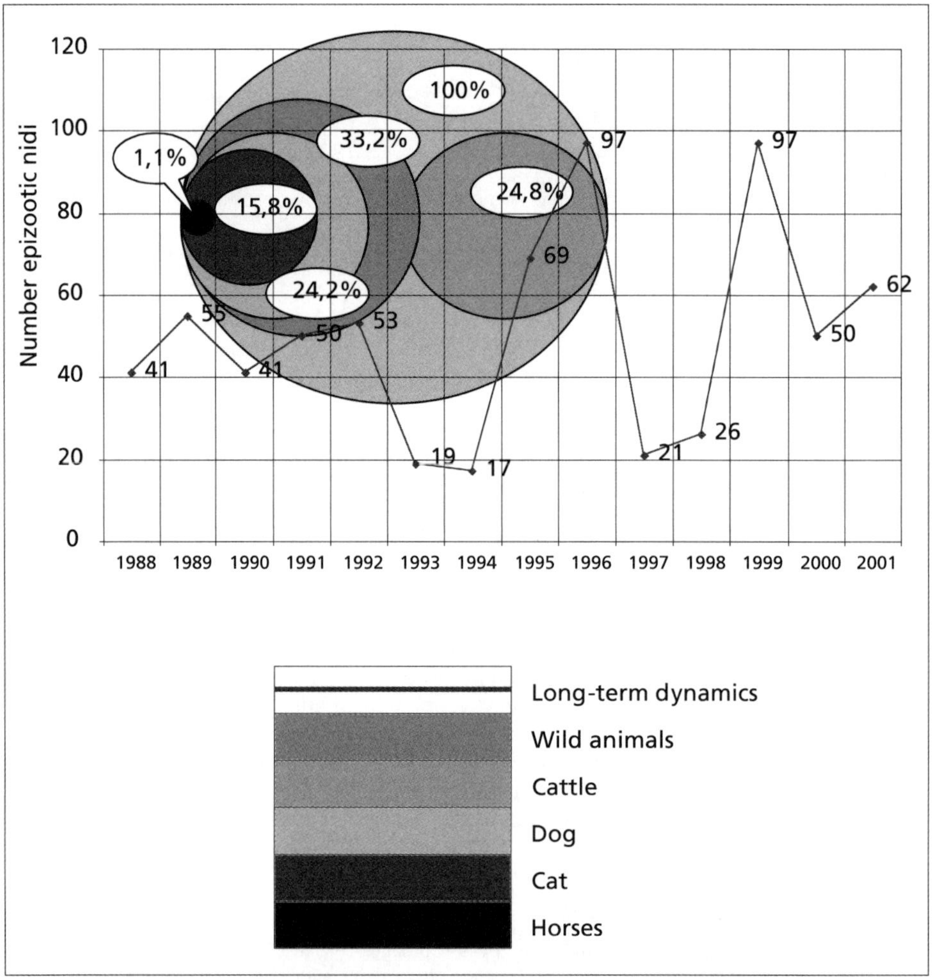

Fig. 1: Retrospective analysis of rabies infection in the territory of the Saratov region (dynamics, parasite-host relationship) from 1988 to 2001.

Oral vaccination of wild carnivores in the Saratov region started in 1998. The vaccines were used in different seasons with various frequencies and with various doses used over 1 km. Instead of 15-20 doses, three to eight baits per 1 km^2 were distributed. Due to the random use of vaccine, the number of rabies cases in wildlife did not decrease: in 1998 fifteen rabies nidi were reported in seven districts of the region; in 2002 seventy-three nidi were reported in 22 districts.

For more effective and rational rabies vaccination of wild carnivores, the seasonal pattern of rabies spread in wildlife in the Saratov region was studied.

Figure 2 shows rabies cases in wildlife reported during year-round with an increase of cases occurring in March-April and October-November-December every year.

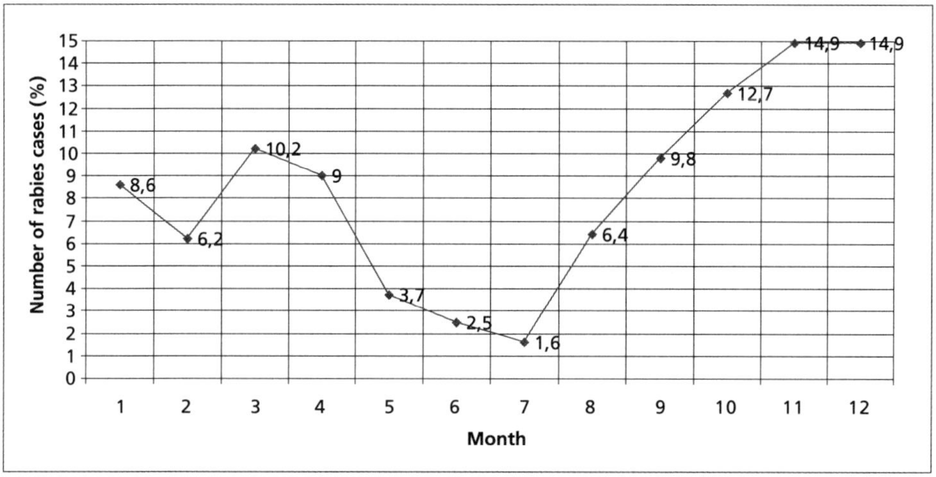

Fig. 2: Annual dynamics of rabies infection in the Saratov region between 1995 and 2002.

To determine the anti-epizootic efficacy of control measures using the "Sinrab" oral rabies vaccine, an experiment to ascertain the optimal immunization periods and frequency was carried out in the territory of the Saratov region.

In 2002, 28 cases of rabies were reported in 11 effected areas of the Kalininsk district. Rabies was detected in 23 foxes, three farm animals and two cats. In 2002 nine cases of rabies were reported in the Ekaterininsk district, including five cases in foxes. In 2002 seven rabies cases were reported in the Lysogorsk district: six in foxes and one in a dog.

The data in Table 1 prove that prevention measures using the "Sinrab" rabies vaccine in 2002-2003 in the Kalininsk district helped to reduce the number of autochthonous rabies nidi in wildlife (foxes) 4.6-fold (from 23 to five cases), the total number of cases decreasing three-fold, from 28 to nine. Moreover, in 2003, four out of nine rabies epizootic nidi were reported in other effected areas where immunization was not carried out.

In the Lysogorsk district the number of autochthonous nidi decreased by half (from six to three), the total number of cases decreased by 42.9 %. In the Ekaterininsk district the number of nidi in wildlife dropped by 40 % and the total number of cases dropped by 11.2 %.

The number of rabies cases in domestic animals remained more or less the same.

Table 1: Development of rabies infection in three districts of the Saratov region after immunization of wild carnivores using anti-rabies "Sinrab" vaccine.

District	**Number of rabies cases before immunization**					**Number of rabies cases after immunization**				
	Fox	Dog	Cat	Farm. animals	Total	Fox	Dog	Cat	Farm. animals	Total
Kalininsk	23	–	2	3	28	5	1	2	1	9
Lysogorsk	6	1	–	–	7	3	1	–	–	4
Ekaterininsk	5	1	1	2	9	3	1	–	4	8

Discussion

For the last 30-40 years particular attention has been paid, worldwide, to specific measures for the prevention of wildlife rabies, with specific oral rabies vaccines being developed and methods for their use evaluated [4].

In the Saratov region, rabies virus affects mainly wild animals (33.2 % of cases), that is 1.24 times more often than all species of farm animals, 1.4 times more often than in dogs and 2.1 times more often than in cats. The increase of cases always starts in autochthonous nidi, then the infection spreads to anthropurgic nidi in dogs and cattle. The drop of infection in wildlife always results in a drop of infection in domestic animals.

The data presented demonstrate that, while rabies cases in wildlife are reported year-round, a considerable increase of cases occurs in March-April and October-November-December, coinciding with the life activity of the fox population.

As a result of this experiment it was established that the specific prevention of rabies in wildlife in enzootic territories resulted in a decrease of rabies epizootic nidi even without a considerable reduction in the density of the fox population. Before using of the vaccine it was necessary to study the seasonal pattern of the disease.

References

1 Avilov VM, Gusyev AA, Savvin AV: Epizootic status and efficacy of rabies control measures on the territory of Russia in 1981-2000. Vet Pathol 2002; 72-77.

2 Makarov VV, Dzhupina SI, Vedernikov VA, et al: Rabies in different animal species under contemporary conditions – epidemiology and clinical picture. Vet Pathol 2002; 65-71.

3 Makarov VV: Rabies: nosoarea and outline of control. Vet Pathol 2002; 12-20.

4 Matouch O: Control of rabies in foxes by oral vaccination in Czech Republic. Veterinarstvi 1995; 45 (4): 178-179.

5 Urban VP, Kalishin NM: Methods of epidemiological investigation. L, 1991; 26.

Dr. A.V. Borisov, Federal Centre for Animal Health (FGI ARRIAH), Yur`evets, RU-600901Vladimir, Russia.
E-mail: borisof.al@mail.ru

Dodet B, Schudel A, Pastoret PP, Lombard M (eds): Rabies in Europe.
Dev Biol (Basel). Basel, Karger, 2006, vol 125, pp 221-231.

Rabies DNA Vaccination by the Intranasal Route in Dogs

E. Tesoro Cruz[1,3], R. Hernández González[1], R. Alonso Morales[2], A. Aguilar-Setién[3]

1 Departamento de Investigación Experimental y Bioterio del Instituto Nacional de Ciencias Medicas y Nutrición " Salvador Zubirán ", Mexico

2 Laboratorio de Genética Molecular de Facultad de Medicina Veterinaria y Zootécnia, UNAM, Mexico

3 Unidad de Investigación Médica en Inmunología, Unidad Médica de alta especialidad, Hospital de Pediatría, Centro Médico Nacional Siglo XXI, IMSS, Mexico

Abstract: A DNA vaccine, using a pCI-neo plasmid encoding the glycoprotein gene of a Mexican isolate of rabies virus, was developed to induce long-lasting protective immunity against rabies virus in dogs. The aim of this work was to evaluate the intranasal (IN) vaccination route in mice and dogs. Mice and dogs were immunized via the intramuscular (IM) and IN routes. Mice received 50 μg of DNA vaccine, a booster on day 30, using the same doses and routes, and on day 90 they were challenged. Dogs received 100 μg of DNA vaccine, with a booster on day 180, and immune responses were studied on day 210. Virus-neutralizing antibodies were detected in blood sera (up to 0.5 IU) in animals immunized via the IN route and when the animals were submitted to a booster, the levels of neutralizing antibodies increased. Animals vaccinated via the IM route presented higher neutralizing antibody titres than those vaccinated IN. Control groups lacked anti-rabies antibodies. On day 90, mice were challenged. From these, a 100 % of the IM vaccinated mice, and an 80 % of the IN vaccinated mice survived the challenge. No animals from the control group survived. Dogs revealed significant virus-neutralizing antibody titres (up to 0.5 IU) on day 30 and, after booster, on day 210 neutralizing antibody titre was higher than 1.8 IU. The main advantage of using DNA vaccines over traditional live ones is that there is no contamination with viruses that could be disseminated in the environment and reproduced in susceptible animals. This study demonstrated that pGQH was succesful when administrated via the IN route. IN vaccination seems attractive due to its easy application and mucosal protection. This form of vaccination could also be advantageous in domestic animal vaccination campaigns, for it is less stressful than the parenteral route (no painful shots).

Introduction

Rabies is a fatal viral encephalitis which affects humans and wild and domestic homeothermic animals [1]. Domestic animal rabies (especially dogs) has been controlled in industrialized countries using traditional parenteral vaccination [2], but wild animal rabies has been more difficult to control due to host inaccessibility. It has, thus, remained an important problem for public health [3]. Countries that have successfully controlled domestic animal rabies still face the threat of viral foci in wild animal species such as red foxes (*Vulpes vulpes*) in Europe, and raccoons (*Procyon lotor*) and bats in North America [4-6]. Strategies for the control of sylvatic rabies have concentrated on the development of oral vaccines in wild rabies reservoir species. Oral vaccination in foxes led to the virtual elimination of sylvatic rabies in most Western European Countries [7]. Bats are frequent hosts to lyssavirus, and insectivorous bats play an important role in the epidemiology of rabies and rabies-like lyssaviruses [8,9].

Dissemination of rabies virus between infected and non-infected bats can occur through other routes than the classical bite, such as aerosol [10], mutual grooming, or food sharing of regurgitated ingested blood [11].

Recently, the IN route of DNA administration has drawn attention towards developing genetic vaccines and other gene therapy fields. The IN route, by providing substantial absorption for DNA, may be promising as a non-invasive delivery route of DNA vaccines and for genic therapy. Moreover, the significant distribution and expression in the different lymph nodes indicate that the IN administration of DNA may be legitimate for inducing systemic responses [12].

Mucosal immunization (MI) is, therefore, an important way of vaccination for these species and could be important in preventing viral dissemination.

MI effector immune mechanisms include secretory antibodies, mainly immunoglobulin A (IgA) isotype, cytotoxic T cells, as well as cytokines, chemokines, and their receptors.

MI stimulates both mucosal and systemic immune responses; meanwhile, systemic immunization only induces systemic responses without activating the mucosal immune system. The epithelial surfaces of the nasal lymphoid tissue (NALT) contain specialized antigen sampling cells that transport antigens from the mucosal surfaces into the underlying lymphoid tissues [13]. After entering into the NALT, antigens are rapidly internalized and processed by sub-epithelial dendritic cells and macrophages, and are presented to B and T cells located in the NALT [13,14]. In a previous report, we demonstrated the possibility of vaccinating vampire bats by aerosol, using recombinant vaccinia-rabies virus [15]. Furthermore, it has been proven that DNA vaccines are efficient when administered via the IN route [12].

DNA immunizations have some advantages over traditional vaccines: they are innocuous, because at no time is the rabies virus handled, and they induce both cell-mediated and humoral immune responses. Different inoculation routes for DNA vaccines have been explored, but efficacy varies with the animal model and the inoculation route used.

DNA vaccines could be a possible solution for the problems associated with controlling canine rabies. For instance, in national anti-rabies campaigns, vaccines are sometimes inadequate and fail to maintain detectable neutralizing antibody levels. This, together with the difficulty in locating dogs for booster vaccinations, suggests that an inexpensive rabies vaccine, which elicits long-term immunity after a single-dose vaccination, could improve the control of canine rabies in developing countries. In addition, Osorio et al. determined that cats and Beagle dogs vaccinated with a DNA vaccine produce neutralizing antibodies [16]. Other studies also demonstrated that a single DNA vaccination elicits life-long protection in mice against the rabies virus [17]. Beagle dogs receiving first and booster IM immunizations with a rabies DNA vaccine were protected against challenge with a wild-type dog rabies virus [18]. These data suggest that a rabies DNA vaccine is an excellent choice to help in the control of canine rabies in developing countries. The purpose of this work is to evaluate the efficacy of an anti-rabies DNA vaccine administered intranasally to mice and dogs.

Materials and Methods

Plasmid construction

The DNA vaccine against rabies consists of a mammalian expression pCl-neo vector into which the glycoprotein-encoding gene of a Mexican rabies isolate (obtained from a child who died of vampire bat-transmitted rabies) [19] was inserted as previously described by Perrin and Bahloul [18,20]. This vaccine has a potent eukaryotic promoter from the cytomegalovirus, and when administered via the parenteral route led to high titres of antibodies and protection against rabies in mice and dogs [18,20].

Viruses and cells

BHK-21 cells were grown in Eagle's minimal essential medium (MEM) containing 10 % foetal bovine serum (FBS). Rabies PV/BHK-21 were maintained by serial passages in BHK-21 cells, as previously described [21]. Challenge Virus Standard (CVS) strain was maintained by serial passage in BALB/c suckling mice.

Mice and administration of plasmid DNA

Forty BALB/c, female, 8-10 week-old, 25 g mice were used in this study. Twenty received 50 μg of DNA vaccine diluted in 25 ul of phosphate-buffered saline (PBS) (experimental group) through the IN route, by instillation, and twenty received 25 μl of PBS alone (control group) IN. The experimental group received a booster consisting of the same DNA vaccine previously applied, using the same dose and route of inoculation, 30 days after the first vaccination.

Four randomly selected mice from each group were used to study rabies virus glycoprotein expression in tissues three days after the first vaccination, and another six mice, also randomly selected from each group, to detect specific IL-2 and IFN-γ, after the first vaccination (days 0, 7 and 15). Seroconversion studies and challenge tests were performed on the remaining mice. Serum was obtained from retro-orbital plexus blood at days 0, 15, 30, 45, 60, and 90.

Approximately 120 μl of blood were collected from each mouse. On the same dates, nasal and oral fluids were obtained by introducing 40 μl of PBS with a thin pipette and gently withdrawing it. Nasal and oral fluids were stored at - 20 °C and centrifuged before assay.

Rabies glycoprotein expression in tissues

Four mice were sacrificed by cervical dislocation, 72 hours after the first vaccination in order to search for rabies virus glycoprotein expression in mucosal tissue, brain, and immune cells from lymphoid tissue (regional submaxilar lymph nodes, mesenteric lymph nodes, and spleen). Glycoprotein expression was found in the different tissues studied, in 5 μc slices, using an FITC-hyperimmune (fluorescein isothiocyanate) anti-glycoprotein serum, obtained from an immunized rabbit.

Dogs and administration of plasmid DNA

Nine female Beagle dogs (one year old, weight 8-10 kg and free of anti-rabies antibodies) were used. The dogs, randomly assigned to three experimental groups of three dogs per group, were exercised daily, fed commercial dog food, and given free access to water. The dogs had previously received Parvigen® Virbac (canine parvovirus) and Canigen® MH2L Virbac (canine distemper, hepatitis, adenovirus 2, and canine leptospirosis) vaccines, but they had not been vaccinated against rabies. All dogs were healthy and were housed in individual cages (0.9 x 1.20 x 1.0 m), with an enriched environment, located in an animal facility at the Instituto Nacional de Ciencias Médicas y Nutrición "Salvador Zubirán" (INCMNSZ). The Animal Resources Laboratory and the animal care and programmes used at the INCMNSZ are fully accredited by the Office of Laboratory Animal Welfare (OLAW) of the USA. Public Health Services under the animal welfare assurance: # A5600-1. Group 1 received by intramuscular injection 100 μg/DNA in 0.5 ml PBS in the quadriceps muscle. Group 2 received 100 μg/DNA in 0.5 ml phosphate buffer solution (PBS) by IN instillation. Group 3 received

1ml PBS alone, IM, and was used as a control group. The dogs were bled before vaccination and 15, 30, 60, 90, 120, 150, 180 and 210 days after the initial vaccination. Animals from groups 1 and 2 received a booster on day 180 (same doses and routes). Blood samples from all dogs were taken from the safena vein, and sera were stored at - 20 °C and centrifuged before assay.

Rabies virus neutralizing antibodies

Virus neutralizing antibody titres (VNAb) were determined using the rapid fluorescent focus inhibition test (RFFIT) and results were expressed in International Units (IU)/ml of rabies virus neutralizing antibody (protective titre >0.5 IU/ml), as described by Smith [21].

Rabies hyperimmune dog serum and a human rabies immunoglobulin solution were used as positive controls in all assays. Three-fold serial dilutions of both the serum samples and the positive and negative controls, were prepared in the microplates, each serum dilution being added to four adjacent wells. Fifty µl of a dilution of challenge rabies virus (CVS) strain containing from 15 to 30 fluorescent foci were also added to each well. After 60 min of incubation at 37° C in a humidified incubator with 5 % CO_2, a 50 µl volume of the cell suspension containing 4 x 105 cells/ml was added to each well and the plates were incubated for 48h at 37° C. After fixation for 30 min at room temperature in 80 % acetone, the microplates were stained by adding FITC anti-rabies monoclonal antibody (Laboratorios BAER, S.A. de C.V. México) to each well. Staining was carried out in an incubator at 37°C for 30 min.

ELISA and Western blot

Simultaneously, enzyme-linked immunosorbent assay (ELISA) and Western blot (Wb) tests were applied to all fluid samples. These were made using partially purified rabies glycoprotein. The PV strain of rabies virus was grown in BHK-21 cells. Cell-culture supernatants containing high titres of rabies virus were clarified by low-speed centrifugation at 500 g for 10 min to remove cellular debris. After clarification, the virus was partially purified by ultracentrifugation at 70,000 g, at 4° C for 2 hrs.

ELISA

The obtained button was resuspended in PBS, quantified, and 1 µg of protein was added per well, in 96-well plastic plates, as decribed by Atanasiu and Perrin [22,23].

The wells of the sensitised plates were rinsed five times with a washing buffer (consisting of NaCl, 0.9 % and Tween 20, 0.1 %) and shaken until dry. Sera samples (100 µl prediluted 1 : 100) were added to the wells. Each was tested at a single dilution in duplicate. After 1 h incubation at 37° C, serum samples were removed and the plates washed five times.

HRPO-conjugated anti-mouse IgG (100 µl prediluted to 1 : 4000) was added to each well and left for 1 h at 37° C. After five additional washing steps, 100 µl peroxidase substrate (consisting of 0.05 % o-phenylenediamine and 0.05 % hydrogen peroxide) were added to the wells.

For ELISA reading a Dynatech MR5000 spectrophotometer was used. The reaction was stopped by adding 50 µl of 4N H2SO4 to each well.

ELISA tests were performed to know whether IgA or IgG was produced in oral fluid and sera, respectively.

Also tracheal lavages were performed in six mice that were sacrificed at the beginning of the experiment to study some interleukines, two before vaccination, two on day 7, and two on day 15 after the first vaccination. The obtained tracheal lavages were used to know the IgA content by ELISA.

To perform the ELISA tests, rabbit anti-mouse IgG and anti-IgA peroxidase conjugates (Sigma, St. Louis, MO) were used.

Western blot (Wb)

Wb was performed to all samples [24].

The obtained button was resuspended in 200 µl of lysis-buffer solution (0.05 M Tris-HCl, 0.15 M NaCl, 0.1 % SDS, 1 % Triton-X and 1 % deoxycolic acid) and 200 µl of sample buffer solution (3.2 ml Tris-HCl 0.5 M pH 6.8, 4 ml 10 % SDS, 2ml glycerol, bromophenol blue and 0.8 ml of bidistilled water).

Next, 300 µl (2.5 µg protein/µl) (Bradford reactive) of the viral suspension were placed per polyacrylimide gel (SDS, PAGE 3 %) with 5 µl of the molecular weight marker (Bio-Rad, Cat. 161-0318; Hercules, CA) and proteins were run at 120 V for 1 h.

Antigens were transferred to a nitrocellulose membrane (*sandwich-like*), of which the middle part contained the gel, while on both sides there were nitrocellulose membranes. The *sandwich* obtained was wrapped in cling film plastic and aluminium foil. The package was placed under 12 kg of weight approximately and left for three days at room temperature.

Following the transferral of the viral proteins, the nitrocellulose membranes were blocked with bovine albumin (3 % in PBS at 37° C for 1 h with constant agitation) and cut into 3 mm wide strips. Each strip was incubated with 25 µl of sample serum diluted in 1 ml of buffer solution (PBS with 0.2 % Tween 20 plus 1 % bovine albumin), for 1 h at 37° C and constantly stirred. Next, peroxidase-marked mouse anti-IgG (Sigma, St. Louis, MO) was added to each nitrocellulose strip (1: 2000) (at 37° C for 1 h with constant agitation). Diaminobenzidene (0.05 %) in PBS and 0.05 % hydrogen peroxide (H_2O_2) were used as revealers.

Detection of IL-2 and INF – γ

Six vaccinated and six non-vaccinated mice from each group were sacrificed by cervical dislocation: two before vaccination, two on day 7, and two on day 15 after the first vaccination.

Spleens were removed from immunized and non-immunized mice. Splenocytes (1 ml aliquots containing 6 x 10^6 cells per well for IL-2 and INF-γ) were stimulated with 0.5 µg rabies antigen or 5 µg of ConA in 24-well plates (Nuclon-Delta, Nunc) and cultivated as described [25] in RPMI-1640 medium (Gibco) supplemented with 10 % foetal bovine serum (FBS), 1mM sodium pyruvate, non-essential amino acids, 5 x 10 -5 M 2-mercapto-ethanol and 10 mM Hepes buffer (Flow Laboratories). Cells were incubated at 37° C in a humidified atmosphere. IL-2 and INF-γ concentrations were determined in spleen cell culture supernatants by ELISA commercial kits (Duoset ELISA R & D SYSTEMS) according to manufacturer's recommendations.

Challenge

The remaining 10 animals from the vaccinated group received a booster 30 days after the first vaccination, and on day 90 they were challenged by intra-cerebral inoculation with 50-100 LD 50 % rabies challenge virus standard (CVS). Inoculated animals were observed daily and when the first unmistakable sign of rabies was detected, they were sacrificed by cervical dislocation. Rabies was confirmed by direct immunofluorescent test in brain smears.

Results

Rabies glycoprotein expression in tissues

Four mice were sacrificed three days after the first vaccination and nasal tissues, brain smears (frontal lobules), and immune cells from regional sub-maxillar lymph nodes, mesenteric lymph nodes, and spleen were harvested. Rabies virus glycoprotein was detected in 0.001 % immune cells from regional sub-maxillar lymph nodes, mesenteric lymph nodes and spleen. In nasal tissue only a few fluorescent cells (1-2 fluorescent cells in each microscope field) were observed. On the other hand, in frontal lobe smears, 15 fluorescent cells in each microscope field were observed (Fig. 1).

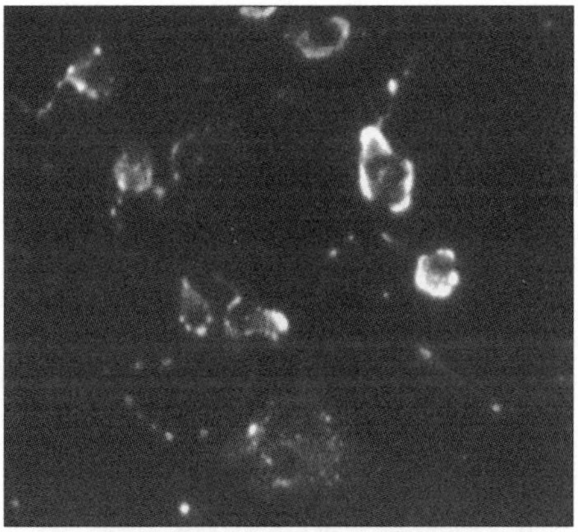

Fig. 1: Detection of rabies virus glycoprotein expression in brain smears (frontal lobes) from vaccinated mice via the IN route.

Rabies virus neutralizing antibodies in mice

Rabies antibodies were detected in blood sera but only in the vaccinated group; 15 days post-vaccination the titre was 0.35 UI, DS 0.10, and on day 30 0.65 UI, DS 0.12. Antibody titres increased on day 45 (1.2 UI, DS 0.16) due to booster applications, on day 60 (1.55 UI, DS 0.24) and on day 90 (1.85 UI, DS 0.39). The control group lacked anti-rabies antibodies (Fig. 2).

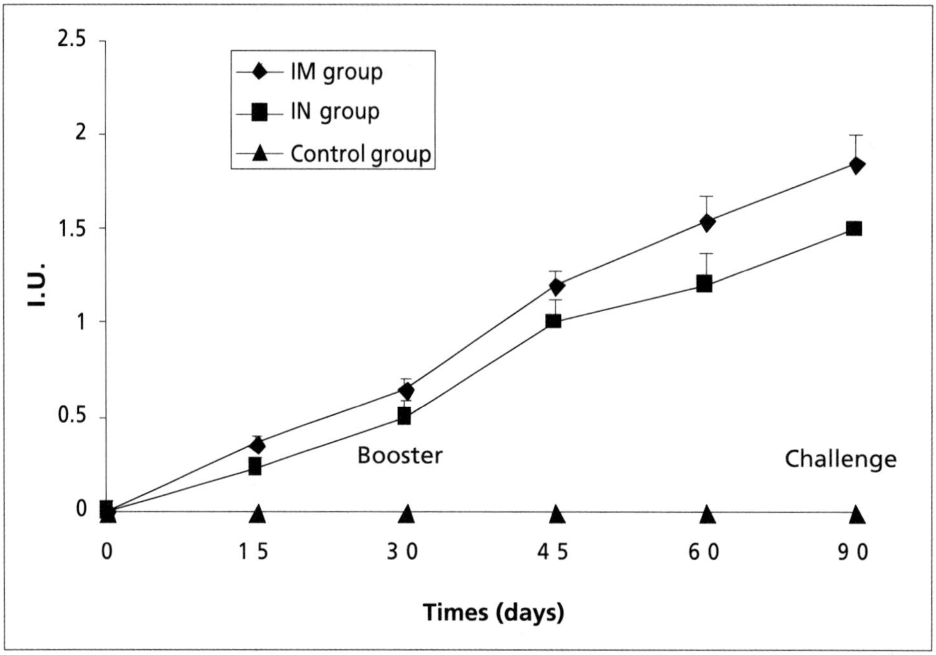

Fig. 2: Seroconversion expressed in IU from mice vaccinated with genetic vaccine against rabies via IM and IN routes.

ELISA and Western blot

Mice immunized IN with a Mexican rabies DNA vaccine were found to contain low titres of specific IgA in nasal and oral fluids, but high titres were detected in tracheal lavages. High titres of specific IgG isotype were detected in sera until day 30.

Specific IgA and IgG antibodies were not detected in nasal and oral fluids nor in the serum samples from non-immunized mice (Fig. 3).

Western blot tests were performed in order to recognize specific seroconversion; only sera from vaccinated animals revealed an intense glycoprotein band (67 Kd) 45 days after intranasal immunization.

Detection of IL-2 and INF-γ

Cytokines IL-2 and INF-γ play an interesting key role in the induction of protective immune responses against rabies virus. IFN-γ and IL-2 kinetics were determined in supernatants of spleen cell cultures using ELISA commercial kits. These cytokines were produced by spleen lymphocytes in vaccinated animals. Before vaccination they were not detected, but after vaccination both were present in low levels in the first samples, then in increased levels in the following samples (2.6 ng/ml IFN-γ. and 3.1 ng/ml IL-2) (Fig. 4).

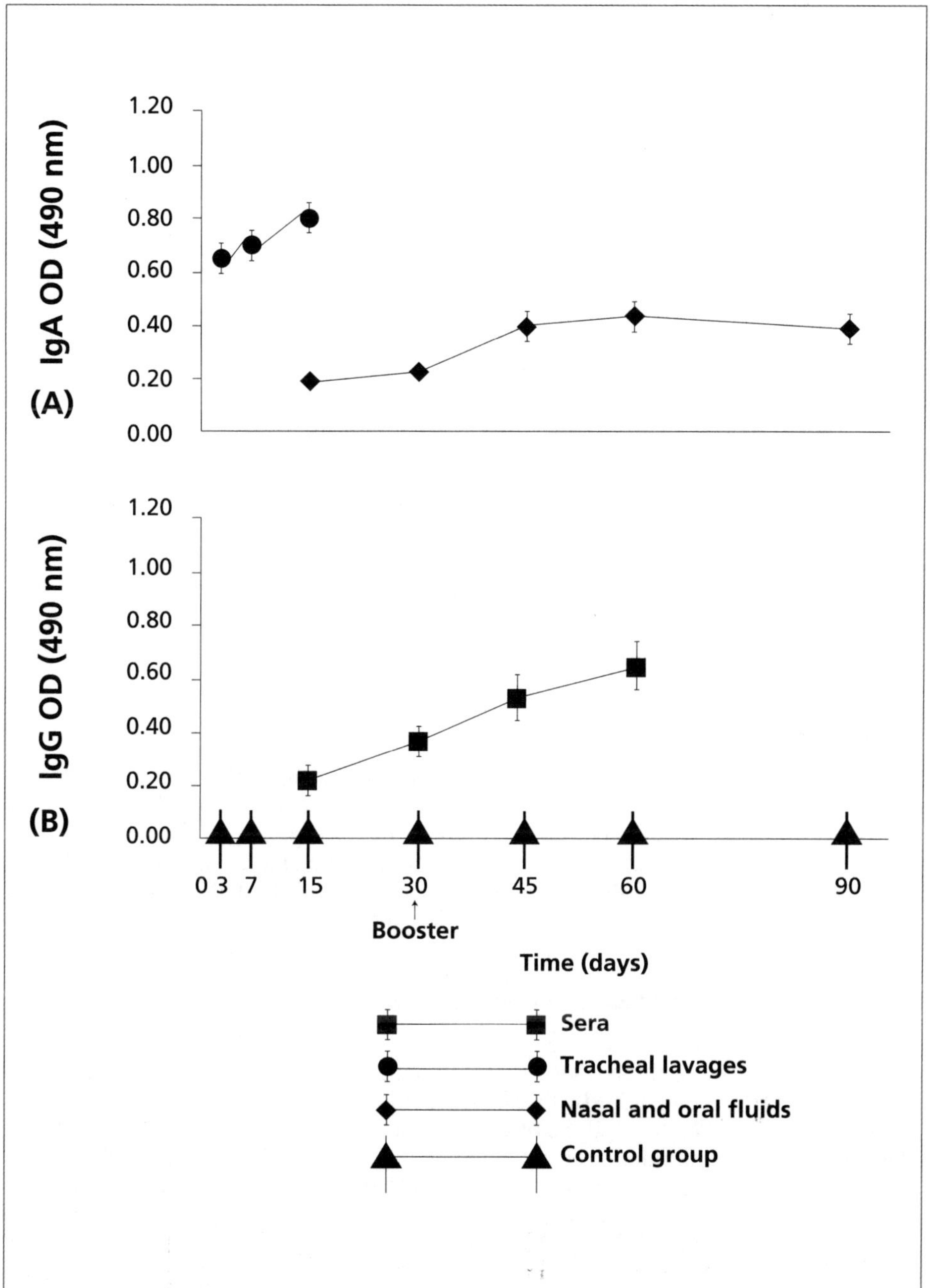

Fig. 3: (A) IgA production in nasal and oral fluids and tracheal lavages, from mice IN vaccinated with DNA vaccine against rabies. (B) IgG production in sera, from mice IN vaccinated with DNA vaccine against rabies.

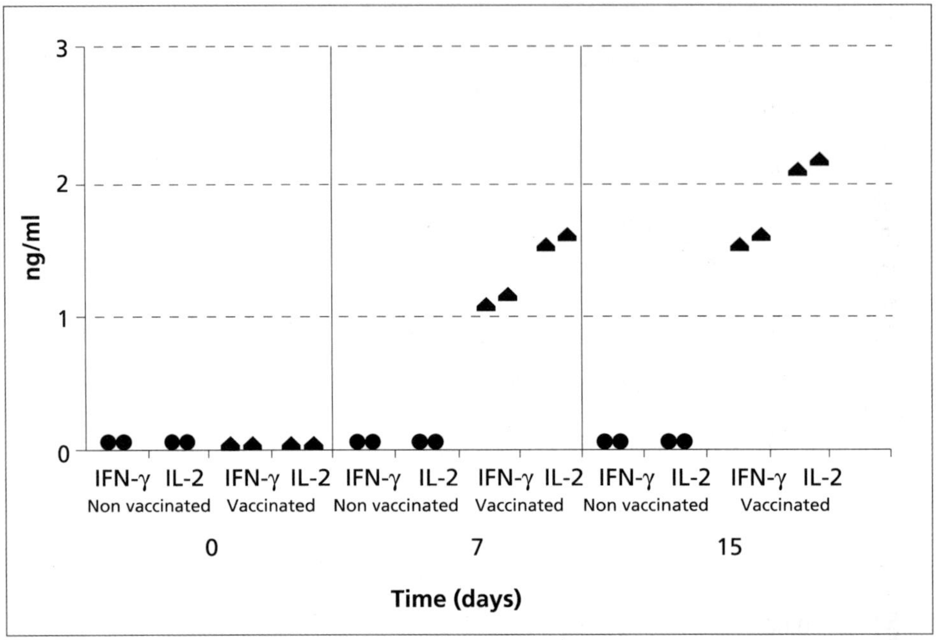

Fig. 4: IL-2 and INF-γ, detection in mice vaccinated with DNA vaccine against rabies through the IN route.

Challenge

Sixty days after booster, 10 mice from each group were challenged using 50-100 LD 50 % rabies challenge virus standard. Seventeen days after the challenge, none of the intramuscularly vaccinated mice presented rabies signs with a survival rate of 100 %. From the IN vaccinated group, 11 days after the challenge, 2 of the 10 mice presented rabies signs and died, the other 80 % survived the lethal challenge. Both groups were observed for 21 days. All control non-vaccinated animals died with signs of rabies and were positive to direct immunofluorescent test using brain smears.

Rabies virus neutralizing antibodies in dogs

Rabies antibodies were detected on day 15 in only one of the three dogs IM vaccinated; on day 30 the three dogs presented neutralizing antibodies higher than 0.5 IU. After neutralizing antibody titres increased, on day 180 (up to 1.3 IU) dogs received a booster. On day 210 the titre of neutralizing antibodies was 2.6 IU. On the other hand, rabies antibodies were detected on day 30 (up to 0.5 IU) in the three dogs IN vaccinated. After boosting, the titres of neutralizing antibodies increased on day 210 (up to 1.8 IU). Dogs from the control group lacked anti-rabies antibodies (Fig. 5).

Discussion

There are some advantages in the administration of a rabies vaccine via the IN route: (i) simple administration (no need for injections); (ii) small doses are

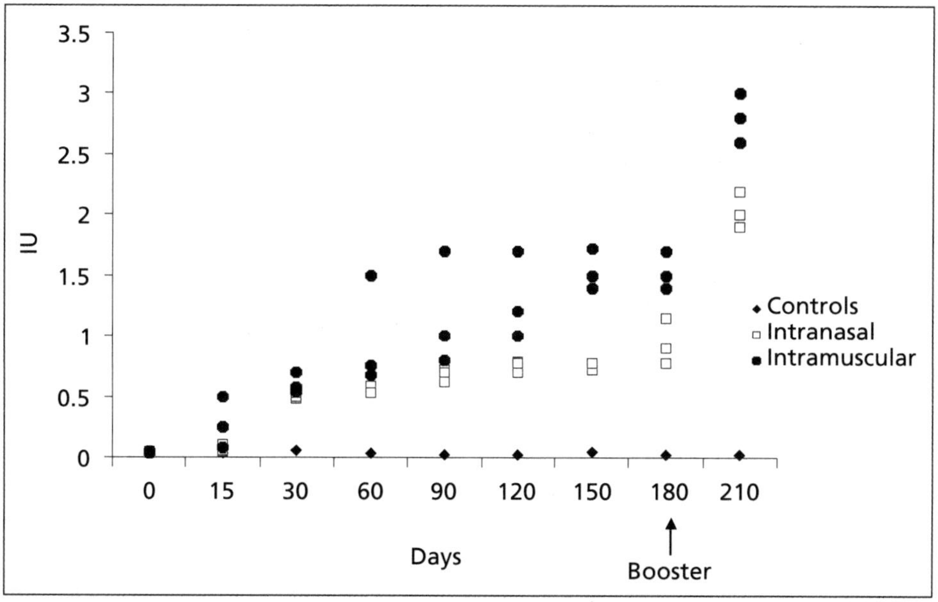

Fig. 5: Seroconversion, expressed in IU, from dogs vaccinated with genetic vaccine against rabies via IM and IN routes.

required; (iii) both mucosal and systemic immune responses are obtained; (iv) immune responses occur at a pathogen-entry site; (v) responses at other mucosal sites (common system) are evident; (vi) there are some functional advantages of secretory IgA over conventional IgA and IgG; and (vii) long term memory is obtained [12,26].

In this work, we demonstrated that a DNA vaccine encoding rabies glycoprotein G can elicit antigen-specific immune responses when administered via the IN route in mice and dogs.

The IN administered DNA plasmid is absorbed by the systemic circulation and is distributed to different body tissues, including the brain (12). IN antigen administration, together with cholera toxin or heat-labile *E. coli* enterotoxin as adjuvant, leads to the localization of both antigen and toxin, in the olfactory nerve and the olfactory bulb for an extended period [27,28].

The glycoprotein was expressed in brain tissue when the DNA vaccine was applied via the IN route. The rabies virus is neurotropic and causes damages to the nervous system; therefore, locating the antigens or DNA in the brain could be advantageous in protecting these specific tissues.

The IN vaccination route was successfully used in human beings against influenza virus, however the risk of Bell´s Palsy was reported when this type of vaccine was applied in combination with *E. coli* toxin [29].

The mechanism by which a large DNA plasmid molecule is absorbed remains unknown. DNA plasmid might interact with the epithelial membrane and transiently effect tight junctions. Alternatively, a transport system which facilitates the absorption of DNA plasmid across the nasal mucosa may be operating.

All mice intramuscularly vaccinated survived the challenge; on the other hand, eight of the ten mice intranasally vaccinated survived the challenge. Challenge was performed via the intracerebral (I.C.) route as recommended by WHO [30], while immunization was locally applied. Challenge studies using the oral, IN, and/or aerosol routes must be performed in the future.

IN vaccination seems attractive for bats due to its easy application and mucosal protection. This form of vaccination could also be advantageous for domestic animals, such as dogs and cats, for it is less stressful than the parenteral route (no painful shots).

The main advantage of using DNA vaccines over traditional live ones is that there is no contamination with viruses that could be disseminated in the environment and reproduced in susceptible animals. DNA is not transfected into the cells and is degraded by the environment.

Acknowledgements

This work was supported by a grant of the CONACYT of Mexico (Z-006).

References

1 Soulebot JP, Brun A, Chappuis G, Guillermin F, Tixier G: Rabies virus pathogenicity and challenge. Influence of the method of preparation the route of inoculation, and the species. Comparison of the characteristics of the modified fixed and wild strains. Comp Immunol Microbiol Infect Dis 1982; 5: 71-78.

2 Acha PN, Arambulo PV: Rabies in the tropics – history and current status, in Kuwert E, Merieux C, Koprowski H, Bogel K (eds): Rabies in the Tropics. New York, Springer-Verlag, 1985, pp 780-786.

3 Brochier B, Blancou J, Thomas I, Languet B, Artois M, Kieny M P, Lecocq JP, Costy F, Desmettre P, Chappuis G, Pastoret PP: Use of recombinant vaccinia-rabies glycoprotein virus for oral vaccination of wildlife against rabies. Innocuity to several non-target bait consuming species. J Widl Dis 1989; 25: 540-547.

4 Toma B, Andral I: Epidemiology of fox rabies. Adv Virus Res 1977; 21:1-15.

5 Rupprecht CE, Hamir AN, Jhonston DH, Koprowski H: Oral efficacy of a vaccinia – rabies glycoprotein recombinant virus vaccine in raccoons (*Procyon lotor lotor*). Rev Infect Dis1988; 10: S803-S808.

6 Pastoret PP, Boulanger D, Brochier B: Field trials of recombinant rabies vaccine. Parasitology 1995; 110: S37-S42.

7 Brochier B, Kieny MP, Costy F, Coppens P, Bauduin B, Lecocq JP, Languet B, Chappuis G, Desmettre P, Afiademanyo K, Libois R, Pastoret PP: Large-scale eradication of rabies using recombinant vaccinia-rabies vaccine. Nature 1991; 354: 520-522.

8 Badrane H, Tordo N: Host switching in Lyssavirus history from the Chiroptera to the Carnivora orders. J Virol 2001; 75: 8096-8104.

9 Morimoto K, Patel M, Corisdeo S, Hooper DC, Fang Fu Z, Rupprecht C, Koprowski H, Dietzschold B: Characterization of a unique variant of bat rabies virus responsible for newly emerging human cases in North America. Proc of the Ntl Acad Sci USA 1996; 93 (11): 5653-5658.

10 McColl KA, Tordo N, Aguilar-Setién A: Bat lyssavirus infections. Rev Sci Tech OIE 2000; 19 (1): 177-196.

11 Wilkinson GS: Reciprocal food sharing in the vampire bat. Nature 1984; 308: 181-186.

12 Yu-Kyoung O, Jong-Oil K, Tae Sun H, Jung Jae K, Jung Mogg K, Ji-Sun Y, Chong-Kook K: Nasal absortion and biodistribution of plasmid DNA: an alternative route of DNA vaccine delivery. Vaccine 2001; 19: 4519-4525.

13 Frey A, Neutra MR: Targeting of mucosal vaccines to Peyer´s patch M cells. Behring Ins Mitt 1997; 98: 376-389.

14 Walker RI: New strategies for using mucosal immunization to achieve more effective immunization. Vaccine 1994; 12: 387-400.

15 Aguilar-Setién A, León-Campos Y, Tesoro-Cruz E, Kretschmer R, Brochier B, Pastoret PP: Vaccination of vampire bats using a recombinant vaccinia-rabies virus. J Widl Dis 2002; 38: 539-544.

16 Osorio JE, Tomlinson CC, Frank RS, Haanes EJ, Rushlow K, Haynes JR, Stinchcomb DT: Immunization of dogs and cats with a DNA vaccine against rabies virus. Vaccine 1999; 17: 1109-1116.

17 Lodmell DL, Ewalt LC: Rabies vaccination: comparison of neutralizing antibody responses after priming and boosting with different combinations of DNA, inactivated virus, or recombinant vaccinia virus vaccines. Vaccine 2000; 18: 2394-2398.

18 Perrin P, Jacob Y, Aguilar-Setién A, Loza-Rubio E, Jallet C, Desmézières E, Aubert M, Cliquet F, Tordo N: Immunization of dogs with a DNA vaccine induces protection against rabies virus. Vaccine 2000; 18: 479-486.

19 Aguilar-Setién A, Aguila-Tecuatl H, Tesoro-Cruz E, Ramos-Ramírez L, Kretscmer R: Preservation of rabies virus RNA from brain tissue using glycerina. Transact Trans R Soc Trop Med Hyg 2003; 97: 547-549.

20 Bahloul Ch, Jacob Y, Tordo N, Perrin P: DNA-based immunization for exploring the enlargement of immunological cross-reactivity against the lyssaviruses. Vaccine 1998; 16: 417-425.

21 Gallegos Gallegos RM, Espinosa Larios EL, Ramos Ramirez L, Kretschmer SR, Aguilar-Setien A: Rabies veterinary virus vaccine produced in BHK-21 cells grown on microcarriers in a bioreactor. Arch Med Res 1995; 26: 59-63.

22 Smith JS, Yager PA, Baer GA: A rapid fluorescent focus inhibition test (RFFIT) for determining rabies neutralizing antibodies, in Meslin F-X, Kaplan MM, Koprowski H (eds): WHO Geneva, Laboratory Techniques in Rabies, 1996, pp 181-192.

23 Atanasiu P, Perrin P: Microméthode immunoenzymatique de titrage des anticorps antirabiques: utilisation de la glycoprotéine rabique et de la protéine conjuguées à la peroxydase. Ann Microbiol (Institut Pasteur) 1979; 7: 213-220.

24 Grassi M, Wandeler A, Peterhans E: Enzyme – linked immunosorbent assay for determination of antibodies to the envelope glycoprotein of rabies virus. J Clin Microbiol 1989; 27: 899-902.

25 Dietzschold B: Techniques for the purification of rabies virus, its subunits and recombinant products, in Meslin F-X, Kaplan MM, Koprowski H (eds): WHO Geneva, Laboratory Techniques in Rabies, 1996, pp 175-179.

26 Perrin P, Joffret ML, Leclerc C, Oth D, Sureau P, Thibodeau L: Interleukin -2 increases protection against experimental rabies. Immunobiology 1988; 177: 199-209. (27) Kyd JM, Foxwell AR, Cripps AW. Mucosal immunity in the lung and upper airway. Vaccine 2001; 19: 2527-2533.

27 Eriksson AM, Schon KM, Lycke NY: The Cholera toxin-derived CTA1-DD vaccine adjuvant administered intranasally does not cause inflammation or accumulate in the nervous tissues. J Immunol 2004; 173: 3310-3319.

28 Apostolaki M, Williams NA: Nasal delivery of antigen with the B subunit of Escherichia coli heat-labile enterotoxin augments antigen-specific T-Cell clonal expansion and differentiation. Infect Immun 2004; 72: 4072-4080.

29 Mutsch M, Zhou W, Rhodes P, Bopp M, Chen RT, Linder T, Spyr C, Steffen R: Use of the inactivated intranasal influenza vaccine and the risk of Bell's palsy in Switzerland. N Engl J Med 2004; 350 (9): 896-903.

30 Wilbur LA, Aubert MFA: The NIH test for potency in Meslin F-X, Kaplan MM, Koprowski H (eds): WHO Geneva, Laboratory Techniques in Rabies, 1996, pp 360-368.

Dr. E. Tesoro Cruz, Unidad de Investigación Médica en Inmunología, Hospital de Pediatria, CMN-Siglo XXI, IMSS, Av. Cuauhtemoc 330, Col. Doctores, México D.F. 06725.
E-mail: emiliano_tesoro@hotmail.com.mx

Dodet B, Schudel A, Pastoret PP, Lombard M (eds): Rabies in Europe.
Dev Biol (Basel). Basel, Karger, 2006, vol 125, pp 233-239.

Studies on an Inactivated Vaccine Against Rabies Virus in Domestic Animals

F. Monaco, P.M. Franchi, R. Lelli

Virology and Biotechnology Laboratory, Istituto Zooprofilattico Sperimentale dell'Abruzzo e del Molise " G. Caporale ", Teramo, Italy

Key words: Rabies inactivated vaccine, cattle, equine, ovine, neutralizing antibodies.

Abstract: An inactivated vaccine against rabies virus was prepared from the attenuated ATCC PV-12 viral rabbit Pasteur strain. The virus was grown on Baby Hamster Kidney (BHK_{21}) cells, and the supernatant was purified by filtration and inactivated with β-propriolactone. The inactivated product was checked according to the NHI and European Pharmacopoeia methods.
Part of the product was then lyophilised and the other part was adjuvanted with $Al(OH)_3$. Both parts were used to vaccinate and boost groups of horses, cattle and sheep at different intervals. Their immunogenicity was compared with a similar commercial product.
Blood samples were collected on a regular basis and the antibody titre was determined by the Fluorescence Antibody Virus Neutralisation (FAVN) test.
No significant differences were found between species after both inoculations even though the immune response increased in intensity and duration after the booster dose in all the animals tested and was stronger and lasted longer with the adjuvanted aliquot.

INTRODUCTION

Rabies is a severe and fatal disease of the central nervous system of warm-blooded animals, including man. In urban areas the disease is strictly associated with dogs which constitute a major public health problem as they are most often responsible for the transmission to humans. In contrast, in rural areas rabies occurs mainly in herbivores as a paralytic disease and is transmitted to livestock by different animals in different regions of the world. In North America foxes and skunks transmit the virus to cattle [1], while in Latin America bats are the main vector [1]. In Europe, the epidemiology indicates the fox as a major source of transmission [2].

Vaccination against rabies is of capital importance in protecting both animals and humans against the disease and for this reason much attention focuses on vaccine quality. It is generally accepted that killed vaccines provide satisfactory protection of animals [3,4] and their use is strongly recommended in countries where there is no evidence of viral circulation.

The aim of this study was to measure and compare the antibody response elicited by vaccinating cattle, horses and sheep with two different vaccine preparations of an inactivated vaccine, to define a preliminary vaccination protocol.

Materials and Methods

Virus growth and titration

A Pasteur strain seed virus, ATCC PV-12, attenuated by several passages on rabbit brain was adapted on BHK_{21} cells. The viral titre was determined by infecting BHK_{21} 96 well plate monolayers with serial dilutions of the viral suspension. For each dilution six replicates were made and after five days of incubation at 33° C, cells were fixed and stained with a rabies anti-nucleocapsid monoclonal antibody conjugated with FITC, since the virus did not show any cytopathic effect. Fluorescent wells were recorded and the $TCID_{50}$/ml calculated by the method of Reed and Munch [5].

Preparation of vaccine

The vaccine was produced using four hour-old BHK_{21} monolayers cultivated in rolling roux with Glasgow medium supplemented with 10 % foetal calf serum and antibiotics. Roux were incubated at 33°C and checked daily. Maximal yield of infective virus in the medium was obtained after five days of incubation and the virus harvested at this time was used for vaccine preparation.

The viral suspension was clarified by 0.8 µm filtration and inactivated with β-propriolactone. The product was checked for its sterility, safety, toxicity and innocuity. The potency was also determined, in mice, according to the NHI and European Pharmacopoeia methods [6]. Two different aliquots were produced: the first was lyophilised and the remaining part kept in fluid form and adjuvanted with $Al(OH)_3$.

Animals

Adult horses, bovines and sheep derived from local farms were screened for rabies using a sera neutralization test, and seronegative animals were selected. They were distributed into three different groups homogeneous for sex and age.

The vaccination procedure consisted of a subcutaneous injection of 1 ml of vaccine in the region of the neck. The first group, which included eight horses, 15 cattle and 20 sheep, was vaccinated with the lyophilised aliquot. A second inoculation was given to all animals 240 days post vaccination (dpv) except for five sheep which were inoculated 365 dpv.

A second group, of 11 sheep, was injected with the adjuvanted aliquot: four received the booster dose 110 dpv, while the other seven received it 365 dpv. A third group, of seven sheep, was vaccinated with a single injection of a commercial product.

Clinical examination was performed daily and local reaction at the injection sites recorded. Blood samples were collected from all animals on days 0, 14, 28, 60, 120, 180 and 240 after each injection. Sera were separated, and aliquots were prepared and stored at - 20° C until tested.

Serological tests

Antibody titre was determined from blood samples by the Flourescence Antibody Virus Neutralisation (FAVN) test [7] as described in the Manual of Diagnostic Tests and Vaccines for Terrestrial Animals, OIE, 2004 [8].

Analysis of variance was used to verify whether or not the antibody response following vaccination in the different species with either lyophilised or adjuvanted aliquots elicited different immuno-responses. The Tukey test was applied to confirm the difference between the antibody responses induced by the adjuvanted, the lyophilised and the commercial vaccines.

Results

The product was free of any bacteria, mycoplasma or fungi, the viral inactivation was complete and no toxic effect was observed; furthermore the vaccine did not show any secondary effect even when a double dose was injected. The antigen titre was 1.4 UI/ml.

Lyophilized vaccine

Species difference

All the animals developed a detectable immune response in the four weeks following the vaccination and none of the vaccinated animals showed any unfavourable local or systemic reaction to the vaccine.

During the second week following the first injection with the lyophilised aliquot, the antibody titre reached the protective threshold of 0.5 UI/ml in only four cattle (26 %), four sheep (20 %) and three horses (37.5 %). However, all animals tested unprotected two weeks later (Fig. 1).

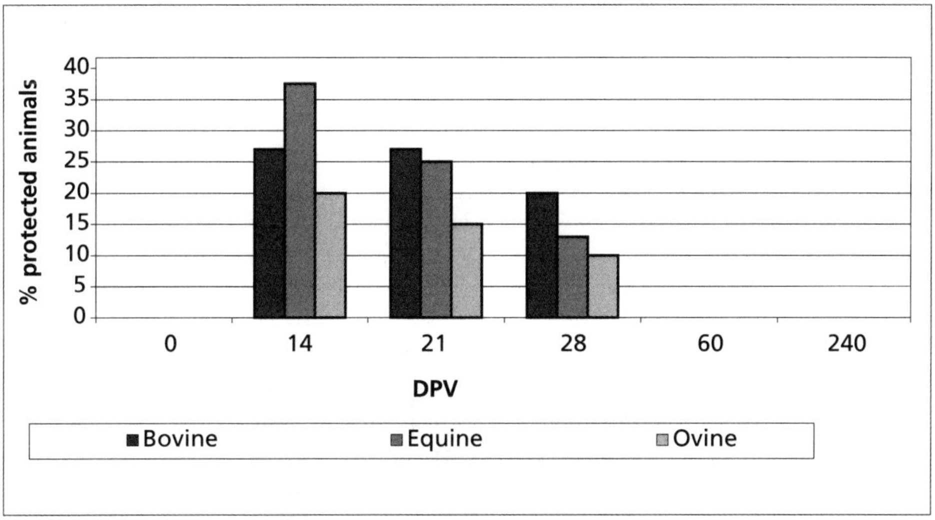

Fig. 1: Percentage of protected animals after first injection with lyophilised aliquot.

The second injection, given 240 dpv, enhanced the antibody titre in all species. All equines seroconverted with a peak in the mean antibody titre of 16.12 UI/ml 14 days after the booster. At 60 days post booster, all horses (100 %) were protected, three (37.5 %) of which showed effective protection until the end of the experiment (240 days post booster) (Fig. 2). The capacity of the vaccine to stimulate an immune response in ovines was promising, 11 animals exceeding 0.5 UI/ml after 14 days but only three (25 %) of them remaining positive until the end of the trial. Only two cattle (15 %) maintained a protective immuno-response 240 days post booster while thirteen (85 %) were protected for 14 days and seven (47 %) for 60 days post booster (Fig. 3).

According to statistical analysis the antibody response following vaccination with lyophilised vaccine showed no significant difference between species after both inoculations ($P < 0.005$). In the ovines, the booster dose resulted in a secondary response with high antibody levels in all animals but there was no significant difference in the reaction induced by re-vaccinating at either 240 days or 365 days after the initial injection (Fig. 4).

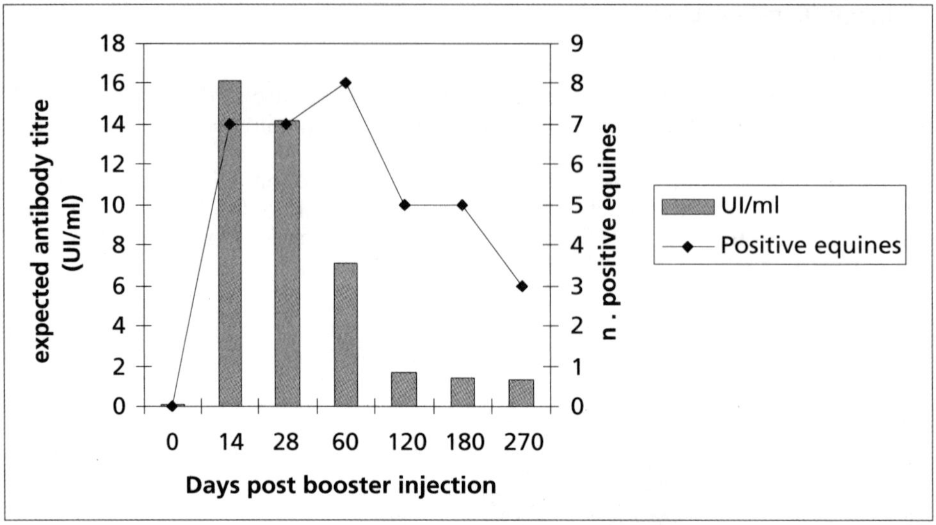

Fig. 2: Antibody response after booster injection in equines 240 days after first vaccine dose.

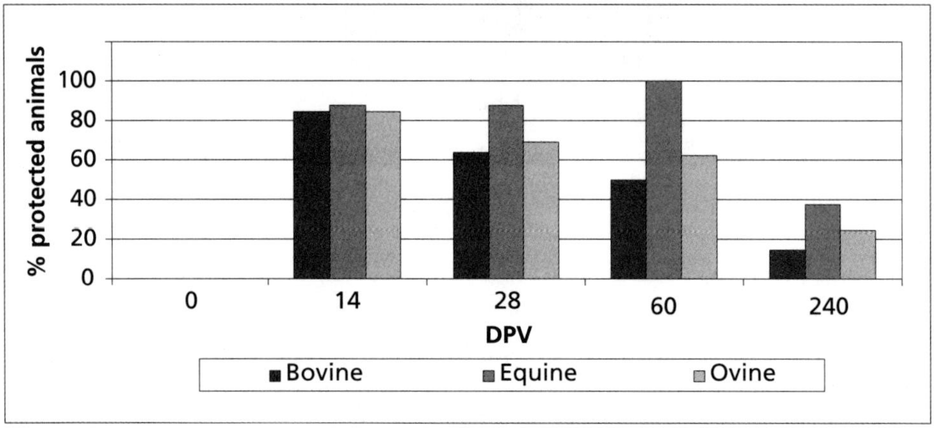

Fig. 3: Percentage of protected animals after second injection with lyophilised aliquot.

Adjuvanted vaccine

All the sheep inoculated once with the adjuvanted vaccine reached the protective threshold 14 dpv. Four animals in the group given the booster at 110 dpv showed an effective antibody titre at the time of the booster, while all five sheep injected at 365 dpv lacked protection at the time of the second vaccine injection.

Among the animals boosted after one year, three developed an effective immune response from 14 dpv up to six months. The sheep injected with a second dose of adjuvanted vaccine 110 days after the first inoculation improved the protective antibody response for the following 180 days. In both groups the secondary responses

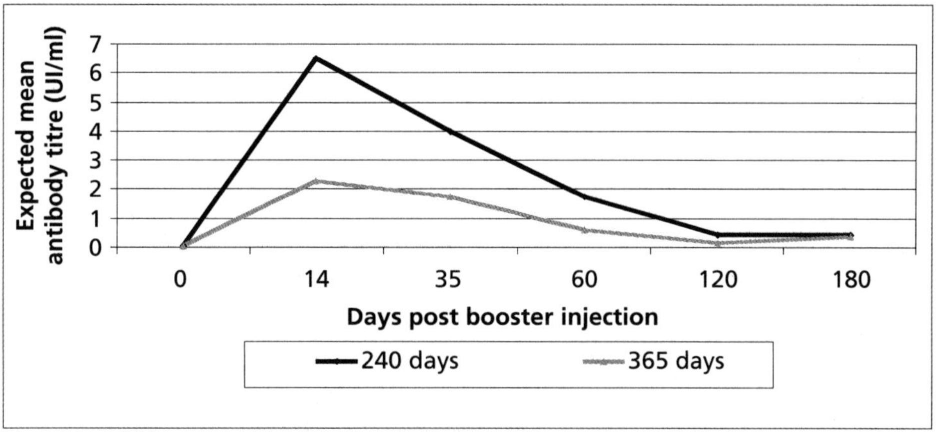

Fig. 4: Antibody response after booster injection in sheep 240 and 365 days post vaccination with lyophilised aliquot.

resulted in higher and long-lasting antibody levels but the differences observed in the antibody response due to the different intervals between vaccinations was not significant (Fig. 5).

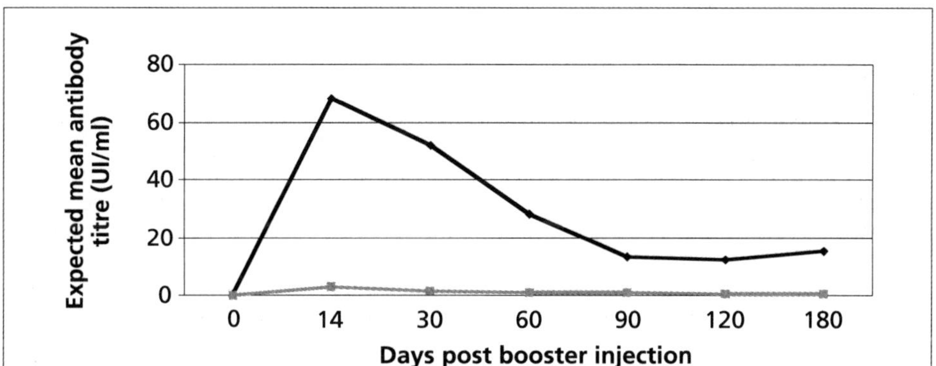

	0	14	30	60	90	120	180
110 days	0,44	68,2	51,69	28,135	13,3	12,44	15,485
365 days	0,195	2,73	1,42	1,06	1,043	0,51	0,617

Fig. 5: Antibody response after booster injection in sheep 110 and 365 days post vaccination with adjuvanted aliquot.

Commercial vaccine

Six of the seven sheep vaccinated with a commercial product developed an immune response, with antibodies detected 14 days post vaccination, when the maximum titre was reached. Data analysis showed a difference between the adjuvanted vaccine and the other two vaccines ($P < 0.001$) (Fig. 6).

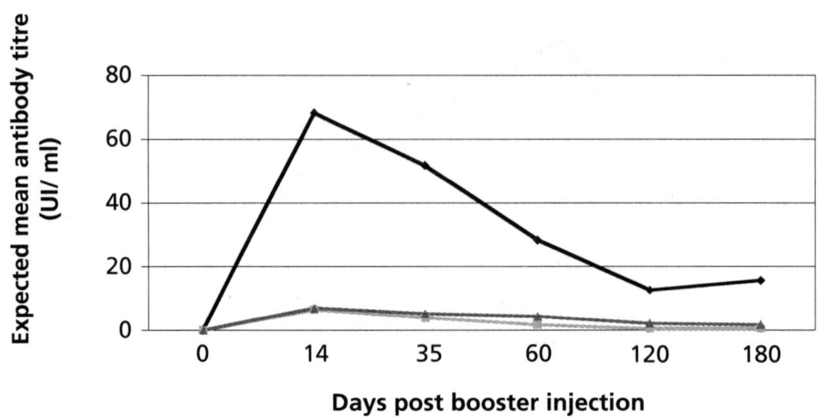

	0	14	35	60	120	180
adjuvanted	0.44	68.2	51.69	28.135	12.44	15.485
lyophilised	0.043	6.528	4.001	1.744	0.418	0.415
commercial	0.05	6.826	5.342	4.272	2.17	1.554

Fig. 6: Comparison of the antibody response after booster injection 110 days post vaccination with adjuvanted aliquot and after 240 dpv with lyophilised aliquot, and with a single injection of commercial vaccine.

Discussion

The present study showed that the inactivated vaccine prepared from a Pasteur strain of rabies virus was safe, innocuous and capable of eliciting an effective immune response in horses, cattle and sheep. Neither pyrexia nor other clinical signs or local reactions were observed, confirming that although adjuvants could be considered as one of the causes of the development of fibrosarcomas in cats [9] they are well tolerated by large animals [10,11].

The antibody response in the horses, cattle and sheep was similar in terms of percentage of protected animals and duration of antibody response after both inoculations.

No differences were observed in sheep despite the different vaccination protocols used; however, a second inoculation increased the intensity and duration of the protective immune response.

The results of this study confirmed that inactivated rabies vaccine can achieve high VNA titres and protective rates in livestock [1,12-14]. Furthermore, the immunogenicity of the inactivated product was increased using an adjuvant which elicited a significantly stronger protective immune response in terms of duration and mean antibody titre compared to the non-adjuvanted lyophilised aliquot.

Unexpectedly, the commercial product was not as immunogenic as the adjuvanted aliquot in terms of intensity of the antibody response; the reason is probably due to the fact that the booster antibody response of the adjuvanted aliquot was compared with the response induced by a single dose of the commercial vaccine without any booster. Furthermore, in this study, data recorded for six months following vaccination was analysed, however, over a longer period, the difference between the antibody titre induced by both vaccines would probably decrease and the two curves overlap.

Although none of the animals were challenged, the level of neutralizing antibodies was accepted as evidence of immunity [15]. Further studies are necessary to test other vaccination protocols and adjuvants, and to prove the efficacy of the vaccine with a challenge trial.

References

1 Larghi OP, Nebel AE: Duration of immunity afforded to cattle by a binary-ethylenimine inactivated rabies vaccine. Zentralbl Veterinarmed B 1985; 32: 609-615.

2 Pepin M, Blancou J, Aubert MFA: Rage expérimentale des bovines: sensibilité, symptômes, réactions immunitaires humorales, lésions et excrétion du virus. Ann Rech Vet 1984; 15: 325-333.

3 Mantovani A, Caporale V, Ciuchini F, Di Trani L, Irsara A, Prosperi S: A summary of antibody titration experiments in some animal species treated with ERA vaccine. Comp Immunol Microbiol Infect Dis 1982; 5 (1-3): 139-141.

4 Di Tran L, Irsara A, Ciuchini F, Pestalozza S, Orfei Z: Antibody levels following ERA Rabies Vaccine in cattle. Comp Immunol Microbiol Infect Dis 1982; 5: 199-203.

5 Reed LJ, Muench H: A simple method of estimating fifty percent endpoints. Am J Hyg 1938; 27: 493-497.

6 European Pharmacopoeia 5th ed, 2005.

7 Cliquet F, Aubert M, Sagne L: Development of antibody virus neutralization test (FAVN) for the quantitation of rabies virus neutralising antibodies. J Immunol Methods 1998; 212: 79-89.

8 Manual of Diagnostic Tests and Vaccines for Terrestrial Animals, OIE. 5th ed, 2004, chapter 2.2.5.

9 Couto CG, Griffey SM, Duarte PC, Madewell BR: Feline vaccine-associated fibrosarcoma: morfologic distinctions. Vet Pathol 2002; 39: 33-41.

10 De Angelis Cortes J, Rweyemamu MM, Ito FH, Umerara O, Medeiros Neto RR, De Lucca Neto D, Baltazar MC, Vasconcellos SA: Immune response in cattle induced by inactivated rabies vaccine adjuvanted with aluminium hydroxide either alone or in combination with avridine. Rev Sci Tech 1993; 12 (3): 941-955.

11 Prosperi S, Irsara A, Battelli G, Sanguinetti V: Vaccination of cattle with live and inactivated rabies vaccine: a study of antibody response. Vet Res Commun 1984; 8 (3): 181-185.

12 Ribeiro Neto A, Nilsson MR, Cortes JA, Mizumo M, Miguel O: Comparative study of cattle antirabies vaccines. II. Protection conferred by Alurabifa, ERA and Formidogel vaccine. Zentralbl Veterinarmed B 1973; 20: 378-404.

13 Marx MB, Sikes RK: Immunizing horses against rabies. J Am Vet Med Assoc 1966; 149: 1159-1161.

14 Rodriguez Da Silva AD, Caporale GM, Goncalves CA, Targueta MC, Comin F, Zanetti CR, Kotai I: Antibody response in cattle after vaccination with inactivated and attenuated rabies vaccines. Rev Inst Med Trop Sao Paulo 2000; 42 (2): 95-98.

15 Baer GM: Serum neutralizing antibody after rabies post-exposure prophylaxis, in Baer GM (ed): The Natural History of Rabies. New York, Academic Press, 1975, vol 2, p 387.

Dr. F. Monaco, Virology and Biotechnology Laboratory, Istituto Zooprofilattico Sperimentale dell'Abruzzo e del Molise "G. Caporale", Via Campo Boario, IT-64100 Teramo, Italy.
E-mail: f.monaco@izs.it

Dodet B, Schudel A, Pastoret PP, Lombard M (eds): Rabies in Europe.
Dev Biol (Basel). Basel, Karger, 2006, vol 125, p 241.

Three Rs Approaches in the Quality Control of Inactivated Rabies Vaccines: The Report and Recommendations of an ECVAM Workshop

K. Cussler[1], *L. Bruckner*[2], *M. Halder*[3]

1 Advisory Group on Alternatives to Animal Testing in Immunobiologicals, Utrecht, The Netherlands

2 Institute of Virology and Immunoprophylaxis, Mittelhäusern, Switzerland

3 European Centre for the Validation of Alternative Methods, Institute for Health & Consumer Protection, European Commission Joint Research Centre, Ispra, Italy

Abstract: Rabies vaccines are prepared from infectious materials; their production is a biological process and therefore inherently variable. All the processes have to be strictly controlled to ensure safe, reliable, efficacious and consistent vaccine production. Consequently, each batch of vaccine is checked by a panel of quality control tests. Among them are safety, inactivation, pyrogenicity, and potency, tests which are legally stipulated and require the use of animals. In practice, a very large number of animals is necessary, in particular for potency testing with at least 120 mice needed for each batch of vaccine. There is an urgent need for replacement of the NIH test and its variants applied to batch potency testing, stability tests and in process testing. Furthermore many possibilities for reducing animal testing and the refinement of procedures are mentioned in the scientific literature.

The ECVAM workshop on Three Rs Approaches in the Quality Control of Inactivated Rabies Vaccines was held in Langen, Germany, on 19-21 April 2002 to collect information about the state-of-the-art of non-animal test development and validation, and the potential for the possible incorporation of alternative tests into regulatory procedures. The participants, all experts in vaccine quality control or rabies disease, came from international regulatory or government organisations, national control laboratories, vaccine manufacturers and academia. They reviewed the current status of various types of in vitro tests and their potential uses, and made recommendations about the best ways forward.

The outcome of the discussions and the recommendations agreed by the workshop participants were published in a report available from ECVAM (ECVAM Workshop Report 48; http://ecvam.jrc.it). The most important issues are summarised in this poster presentation.

Dodet B, Schudel A, Pastoret PP, Lombard M (eds): Rabies in Europe.
Dev Biol (Basel). Basel, Karger, 2006, vol 125, p 243.

SESSION VI

Bat Rabies

Chairperson: *T. Müller* (FLI, Germany)
Rapporteur: *A. Fooks* (VLA, United Kingdom)

Dodet B, Schudel A, Pastoret PP, Lombard M (eds): Rabies in Europe.
Dev Biol (Basel). Basel, Karger, 2006, vol 125, pp 245-254.

Bat Rabies in Europe: a Review

P.H.C. Lina[1], *A.M. Hutson*[2]

[1] National Museum of Natural History "Naturalis", Leiden, the Netherlands
[2] The Bat Conservation Trust, London United Kingdom

Abstract: Bats are legally protected in most European countries under some international treaties and national nature conservation legislations that prohibit deliberate capture and killing of bats except under permit from the competent authorities. However, bat rabies research is necessary to gain insight into whether bat rabies is a real problem for public health and whether bat conservation efforts are in conflict with public health interests. It is also important to know the incidence of rabies in different bat species. Thus far, passive surveillance of bat rabies seems to be a sufficient mean of obtaining information about the occurrence of bat rabies that is not in conflict with bat conservation. Knowledge about the occurrence of bat rabies, the prevalence of rabies in particular species of bats, and the possible risk for public and animal health is also important for improving public awareness for bat conservation in conjunction with public health. There should, therefore, be good cooperation between bat conservationists and rabies research bodies.

INTRODUCTION

There have been four, possibly only three, recorded deaths in humans in Europe from bites by rabies-infected bats. The first two cases concerned two girls in Ukraine in 1977 and in Russia in 1985; there remains some doubt about the source of infection and the virus involved in the first case [1]. The third case was a biologist working on bats in Finland who died from bat rabies in autumn 1985, and the fourth case was a Scottish amateur bat conservationist who was probably bitten by a Daubenton's bat *(Myotis daubentonii)* and died in November 2002 [2,3].

The death of the biologist in Finland [4,5] had a very negative impact on public opinion towards bats at the time. The most publicised death was that of the Scottish bat worker. The impact of this incident on public opinion was very high. It highlighted the importance of the issue for bat conservation in conjunction with public health awareness and the need to collect good information for the authorities and the public. The Scottish case raised lots of questions pertaining to a variety of issues. Many bat workers had no contact with rabies researchers and were unaware of any national policy to prevent infection.

In the past 20 years rabies related viruses in bats in Europe have been identified as two distinct viruses, European Bat Lyssavirus 1 (EBLV-1) and European Bat Lyssavirus 2 (EBLV-2). Each of these has been subdivided into two variants

(EBLV1a and 1b, and EBLV2a and 2b) [2,6,7]. Advances have been made in understanding their occurrence, incidence, hosts and epidemiology [8,9], but further coordinated action is needed.

Bat Workers and Rabies Exposure

Two of the four human deaths from EBLV thus far have been bat workers. Bat workers form the highest risk group for encountering rabies infected bats. Before, most bat research work in the field involving the handling of bats, e.g. for marking, measuring, and collecting parasites, had been carried out by institutional bat workers. During the last three decades, however, there has been an increasing interest in bat studies and conservation by amateur naturalists across Europe [10]. A number of these naturalists also do field work on bats, involving catching them with mist-nets and other traps for inventories, marking or other scientific purposes, activities where bats are taken in the hand. Another, relatively small number of bat workers keep sick and wounded bats in captivity for rehabilitation. Both groups run a risk of being exposed to rabies-infected bats. The majority of bat workers is, however, involved in activities where the handling of bats is not necessary, such as the use of ultrasonic receivers for inventories or other field studies, and doing visual observations for monitoring bat populations in winter and summer roosts.

Most European bat species are quite small and many bat workers have difficulty with handling these bats with gloved hands. Therefore, on many occasions, bats are still handled with ungloved hands, despite the risk of being bitten. After the two fatal cases in Finland and Scotland, an increasing number of bat workers have received pre-exposure rabies vaccination and are receiving re-vaccination at pre-agreed intervals or subject to rabies titre level tests. There are still numerous bat workers in Europe, however, professionals as well as amateurs, who handle bats from time to time and have not yet received rabies vaccination, who do not consider the risk of exposure to bat rabies high enough to be of significant concern, or who cannot afford to receive vaccination treatment [11].

Domestic Predators of Bats

In Europe, domestic cats are the main predators of bats, especially in spring, summer and autumn. They mostly catch individuals of bat species that roost in houses and other buildings, such as the brown long-eared bat (*Plecotus auritus*), the common pipistrelle *(Pipistrellus pipistrellus)* and the serotine bat *(Eptesicus serotinus)*. The latter species is the main carrier of one of the European bat lyssaviruses, genotype 5 (EBLV-1), in Europe. Bat species that roost in trees are much less likely to fall victim to cat predation.

In some countries, cat owners who have seen their cat carrying a bat are recommended to give their cat a post-exposure vaccination. However, cat owners rarely see their cat carrying a bat. This means that most cats that have caught one or more bats do not get vaccination treatment. Thus far, bat lyssaviruses have not been isolated from domestic cats; there is only one preliminary report of antibodies to EBLV1 being found in a cat [12]. Cats might have a low prevalence for EBLVs or the virus concentration in the bats' saliva may be too low for effective contamination. Cats are, however, usually dexterous enough to not let themselves be bitten by their prey. Cats might have more risk of contact with rabies virus if their victims have spread virus with saliva on their fur during grooming .

Wildlife Mammalian Predators of Bats

The record of EBLV-1 in a stone marten *(Martes foina)* in Germany [13,14] is not a complete surprise. Stone martens often dwell in spaces such as cavity walls and attics where bats may also dwell. The possibility for stone martens to meet serotine bats, which are mainly building-dwelling, is quite high. Serotine bats usually roost in wall cavities and, less often, in attics [15]. The latter are generally more accessible for stone martens than cavity walls. Stone martens are, however, excellent climbers and true "cat-burglars" and can quite easily reach the access slits of bat roosts to catch emerging and arriving bats. Domestic cats sometimes use a similar hunting strategy. Either animals may also find grounded bats that may be suffering from disease. Stone martens therefore have a good chance to meet serotine bats suffering from rabies. However, the case in Germany is the only EBLV-1 positive one found so far. This might indicate that stone martens have a low susceptibility to bat lyssaviruses.

From time to time stone martens are observed in winter roosts of bats, such as caves, subterranean quarries and cellars. Claw marks on limestone walls in subterranean quarries indicate that stone martens have tried to climb up to take hibernating bats. There are also reports of bat remains in the faeces of stone martens. The chance of a stone marten encountering a rabid bat in these winter roosts is quite low since rabies has not yet been found, or is fairly rare, in most bat species that hibernate in such winter roosts. Records of hibernating serotine bats in this type of winter roost are very rare.

Bat Rabies in Cattle

The isolation of EBLV-1 in three sheep in Denmark is still a mystery [16]. Transmission from serotine bats to sheep does not conform to the behaviour of this species, not even with the aberrant behaviour that rabid serotine bats sometimes show. Rabid serotine bats rarely show an aggressive or attacking behaviour, although their flight can be uncontrolled as a result of disordered sonar emission and paralysis (although note that *M. daubentonii* carrying EBLV2 may show aggressive behaviour [e.g. 17]).

Misunderstandings

Bats are often considered as a homogeneous group, whereas the reality suggests that some of the 47 European species of bat are the main carriers of EBLVs while others show no or less evidence of infection. EBLVs are also more specific than generally perceived, in that in Europe there are two distinct genotypes associated with different hosts. Further, EBLVs are often associated, by the general public, with sylvatic (classic) rabies, when in fact the impact of EBLVs to public and animal health is much lower.

Bat Colonies and Rabies

The approach to bat rabies cases and colonies in which the presence of rabies is suspected differs from country to country. In some countries bat lyssavirus-positive colonies are destroyed, either as a recommendation or through legislation. However, is it not possible for people to live together with such colonies?

In the Netherlands, the policy is not to destroy or exclude colonies with infected individuals from their roosts. Monitoring for over 25 years has shown that there is no change in numbers of females over and above natural fluctuations. Colonies should not be destroyed because many bats survive contact with the virus and over time colonies can build up persistence to the disease. Exclusion of colonies may disperse the colonies (and the virus). As long as there is physical separation between tenants of the house and the place where the bats are roosting there is not much risk of virus transmission from bats to humans. There is frequent suggestion of aerosol transmission, but the only evidence of aerosol contamination in wildlife has come from two incidents about 50 years ago on the North American continent in a cave with about 30 million bats and is associated with serotype 1 virus [18].

The experience from the Netherlands is that it is possible to convince people not to remove or exclude colonies, as long as they are satisfied that there is a low risk or no risk of contact with the bats. Physical separation between the house occupants and a bat colony is an important issue.

Experience from the Bat Conservation Trust in the United Kingdom shows that if advice given includes being open about the risks involved then most people are happy to continue living with their bat colonies. The Bat Conservation Trust received over 50 calls a day on its bat helpline during the summer of 2003 and did not notice a backlash as a result of the human case with EBLV-2 in Scotland in 2002 and felt this was the result of effective public education on the subject [19].

In a fact sheet on bat rabies in Europe, issued in 1986 by the WHO Collaborating Centre for Rabies Surveillance and Research the following statement was made: "It should be stated that the recent bat rabies cases may only be of concern to a very small group of people. Scientists as well as medical authorities are being asked to initiate awareness on the problem rather than create hysteria in the press and amongst the general public, especially with those people that have bats living in their houses. Otherwise, efforts to conserve these animals would be more difficult."

Rabies in bats will never be eradicated because of the nature of the infection, unlike classical rabies (serotype 1) in other terrestrial mammals, which can be eradicated using a vaccination programme [20]. It is therefore something people must learn to live with.

In some bat species, like the serotine bat, rabies is a part of their ecological mechanism, just as predators are.

European Bat Rabies Workshops

In 1986 a small informal workshop was held in Germany to discuss EBLV, but there has been no European exchange of information since then.

The Agreement on the Conservation of Populations of European Bats (EUROBATS) is a regional Agreement under the Bonn Convention (the Convention on the Conservation of Migratory Species of Wild Animals, 1979) which aims to encourage international cooperation on bat conservation. Currently (June 2005) there are 31 Parties to the Agreement and interest from many other Non-Party Range States. The Agreement operates through its fundamental obligations and Resolutions passed by Parties and delivered through the work of the Secretariat, based with the United Nations in Bonn, and an international Advisory Committee that meets annually. Every three years a Session of the Meeting of Parties is held. This meeting is the decision-making body of the Agreement [21].

In December 2003, the Secretariat of the Agreement distributed a questionnaire to all Range States recognized as within the geographical scope of EUROBATS, that is Europe east to the Caucasian States and the Russian Federation to 50° E, Turkey and the Mediterranean States of Cyprus and Malta. This encompasses 48 States, although the questionnaire was not circulated to a few small States, such as Andorra and San Marino.

As of June 1, 2005 responses have been received from 35 States. The responses to the questionnaire suggest that it would take a few more years to establish a good EBLV surveillance in Europe. The collection of EBLV data was very varied, with some countries carrying out routine testing, others adopting occasional testing and others (ten) not doing any testing of bats. Most countries have an identified focal point for testing of material and reporting on bat rabies data.

As a follow-up to the questionnaire, on 16 May 2004 a European workshop on bat rabies was held in Vilnius (Lithuania) in conjunction with the 9th Meeting of the Advisory Committee to UNEP/EUROBATS [9]. This workshop was considered to be highly beneficial since the outcome of the questionnaire clearly identified deficits in the handling of bat rabies cases in many European countries. This concerned the awareness of and information to bat workers, public health authorities, rabies researchers and the general public. It also concerned data collection relating to the testing of bats and test results, national and international reporting of bat rabies, as well as vaccination procedures. The workshop provided the first opportunity for bat workers and rabies epidemiologists at a European level to exchange knowledge and was the starting point for international cooperation. The aim of the Vilnius workshop was to improve data collection and research reporting methods to get a better picture of the actual situation and trends of bat rabies in Europe, clarify recommendations for vaccination procedures and develop informational material. The results of the questionnaire had identified a number of desired objectives for the workshop.

The objectives that were discussed at the workshop were:

- The harmonization of data collection.
- The use of a standard form for data collection.
- To confirm that reporting of negative cases is just as important as reporting of positive cases
- Sharing technology and facilities.
- Standardisation of testing procedures.
- Second opinion tests on bat species that normally do not show rabies.
- The identification of examined bats by qualified bat experts.
- Setting up standard national databases with minimum standards.

- The identification of high risk groups.
- Recommendations for vaccination procedures for high risk groups.
- Recommendations for post-exposure treatment.
- Reporting data to national and international authorities (national focal points on rabies and bat conservation and the World Health Organization).
- Development of information such as leaflets and manuals on bat rabies for high-risk groups, public health and veterinary authorities, medical doctors and veterinarians, and the general public.

The workshop was attended by a group of bat rabies experts and by administrative and scientific focal points of Parties and Non-Party Range States to EUROBATS.

Conclusions and Recommendations of the Vilnius Workshop

The conclusions and recommendations of the workshop were as follows.

Passive surveillance should be encouraged, but the constraints of testing capacity in some states was recognized. Countries that do not have the capacity for testing should be able to send bats to other countries that have the necessary laboratories to do so. Training should be provided in order to support countries that do not have the capacity for testing. The aim should be to get a good overview of the distribution and hosts of each virus in Europe. [There is also a need for passive surveillance to see how the virus is distributed by host]. Data on serotine bats that have tested positive for EBLV1 in the Netherlands since the 1980s as well as data from Denmark, suggested that there had been an EBLV1 epidemic or outbreak in serotine bat populations in the late 1980s. However, comparison of the number of serotine bats tested each year against the positive results shows that the percentage of positives remains fairly constant. There was in fact no outbreak of bat rabies in the late 1980s, but rather an "outbreak" of surveillance in some European countries following the death from bat rabies of the bat scientist in Finland, and the finding of a rabies positive serotine bat in a school yard in Denmark in autumn 1985 followed by more positive cases in this species. The relatively high number of lyssavirus records in serotine bats in some countries, such as Denmark and the Netherlands, is likely to reflect more extensive surveillance in these countries rather than major differences in epidemiology.

Only dead bats can be tested for rabies under such passive surveillance. In some countries only bats involved in bite incidents are tested, in most all submitted bats are tested, although some countries are more active in the encouragement to submit. Six countries have tested more than 1000 bats.

The meeting recognised that full identification of tested bats (negative and positive) is important, noting constraints that in some countries positive bats must be destroyed and that in other countries all bats (positive and negative cases) that have been in a rabies laboratory unit must be destroyed.

The questionnaire showed that identification of the different species is very incomplete. Over half of the respondents to the EUROBATS questionnaire do not consistently get bat identification verified. Even in some well-established laboratories bat identification is not carried out or verified, although without identification test data are of limited value. A further problem is that, in some countries, laboratories rarely get bats for testing.

Bat species verification is very important and there is a need to have one agreed national (or regional) authority responsible for bat identification, because there has been publication of misidentifications, of positives with no host data, contaminations and false positives for the viruses.

Other information on specimens, e.g. sex, age, locality and date should also be collected to assess the incidence of the virus and also the degree of representation of the test samples. Specimens should be preserved for future reference and because they have value for other purposes. Most are preserved in alcohol or frozen, and some countries use formalin.

Therefore, the engagement of bat specialists in surveillance is very important, and not just for identification, but also for general advice to medical and veterinary colleagues, interpretation of data and sampling.

It is also important to record negative cases as well as positives. Laboratories in general seem to be much more interested in positive than in negative cases but recording of only positive cases can give misleading information on epidemiology. Often negative cases are not reported to the WHO, although they should be.

The situation concerning submission forms in the different countries was discussed. It was recommended that a submission form with minimum standards should be developed for the European region. The forms developed in the United Kingdom and the Netherlands can be used as models with some modifications. Positive cases are reported to WHO, but it is not always clear when the bats were collected so statistics relating to date, including year, of occurrence, are not always correct. The use of a common submission form can improve the data collecting of tested bats.

The United Kingdom database of bat and testing data works well and more or less conforms to databases established in some other countries, such as the Netherlands. There should be a national central database where possible.

In some countries negative specimens are passed to national or other museums. Positives may have to remain in the investigating laboratory, or be destroyed. Particularly in these circumstances tissues samples should be taken to confirm identification with DNA testing, especially when the identification of sibling species from morphological characteristics alone may be difficult.

Following a human biting incident, it was considered that post-exposure treatment should be started immediately, including washing the wound, vaccination and rabies immunoglobulin (RIG) where appropriate. If laboratory results from the "suspect" bat are negative by fluorescent antibody test (FAT) (4 hrs) and rabies tissue culture isolation test (RTCIT) (24 hrs) further treatment is not necessary.

FAT on brain smears should be the primary diagnostic tool for rabies "suspects". Additional OIE-recommended tests should include the rabies tissue culture isolation test (RTCIT). In some circumstances when RTCIT is not available the mouse inoculation test (MIT) can be used. Molecular tools (principally RTPCR) can be used for rapid confirmatory diagnosis and in further sequence analysis and genotyping.

All rabid suspected bats, regardless of species, should be submitted to a national or regional rabies reference laboratory for lyssavirus testing. For testing rare bat species, brain sample collection using a biopsy needle through the orbit of the eye socket can be used to cause minimal disruption to the bat skull. The bat can then be archived as a museum specimen.

Two virus typing techniques can be used: serotyping using monoclonal antibody reactivity patterns and genotyping using EBLV-specific primers or lyssavirus generic primers. For any diagnostic laboratory that detects a FAT positive bat, the virus should be typed from original brain material. Confirmation can be conducted in collaboration with a number of specialised rabies laboratories, OIE reference laboratories and WHO Collaborating Centres responsible for rabies. A Med-Vet-Net project is looking at ways of improving collaboration in testing and molecular epidemiology.

Regarding passive surveillance for lyssaviruses in bats, the meeting sought to encourage all countries to implement the following:

Lyssavirus surveillance of any bat following a biting/scratching incident in humans.

Lyssavirus surveillance of fresh dead and sick bats. This includes all bat species. (Negative diagnostic results are as important as positive results for our understanding of variant/host adaptation).

Active surveillance is also recommended in all European countries in order to improve our understanding of lyssavirus dynamics, the epidemiology and the pathogenesis in different bat species. This approach can be 'targeted' to specific species of bats ensuring that statistically significant numbers are caught and tested. Research is required to understand which bat species are the main reservoirs for EBLVs and also to identify the species (either anthropophilic or not) that constitute the greater risk to public health.

The questionnaire showed that about one third of the countries responding had published the results of their bat rabies investigation and others planned to do so. Many reported intentions to carry out a range of research activities or identified research that they considered would help with their situation.

Rabies vaccination should be compulsory or at least highly recommended for all people working with bats. Human tissue culture derived vaccines are recognised by the WHO to elicit the best protection. Vaccine elicited antibodies will neutralise both EBLV type-1 and type-2. Individual follow-up of EBLV specific neutralising antibodies should be considered.

Lyssaviruses in bats pose an extremely low but significant risk. Members of the general public should be aware of the risk and be advised what they should do if bitten by a bat and who to contact when confronted with a "grounded" bat. Advice is required for other animals (especially companion animals) that are bitten by a bat. Some countries like France and the United Kingdom have issued leaflets with information about bat rabies and the risk of the disease to humans. Other countries should follow these examples.

To increase overall public health awareness of bat rabies as well as the public's awareness of bat conservation efforts, it is necessary to improve our knowledge about the prevalence of bat lyssaviruses in European bat species and the actual level of risk of bat rabies for public health. This requires a Europe-wide research program and collaboration between the public health community on the one hand and the bat conservation community on the other hand. At present the occurrence of bat rabies across Europe might be under-reported as prevalence is routinely reported only in countries that have a regular surveillance programme.

Thus, the bat conservation community has made the first steps forward in this direction with the initiative by EUROBATS to organise the European bat rabies workshop in Vilnius. It has used the results of that workshop to draw up a draft Resolution on Bats and Rabies in Europe that will be submitted for governmental adoption at the 5th Session of the Meeting of Parties to the EUROBATS Agreement to be held in 2006.

This resolution contains the recommendation of the Vilnius Rabies Workshop and is an instrument to improve the public awareness of bat rabies and the surveillance of bat rabies across Europe. At the same time, some of these areas of concern are being developed through a Med-Vet Net programme to improve collaboration on the sequencing of bat-associated viruses, the establishment of databases of viral isolates and the use of such data in human risk assessment.

References

1 Kuzmin IV, Botvinkin AD, Poleschuk EM, Orciari LA, Smith JS, Rupprecht CE: Bat rabies surveillance in the former Soviet Union, in Dodet B, Schudel A, Pastoret PP, Lombard M (eds): Rabies in Europe. Dev Biol (Basel). Basel, Karger, 2006, vol 125, pp 273-282.

2 Fooks AR, McElhinney LM, Pounder DJ, Finnegan CJ, Mansfield K, Johnson N, Brookes SM, Parsons G, White K, McIntyre PG, Nathwani D: Case report: Isolation of a European Bat Lyssavirus Type 2a from a fatal human case of rabies encephalitis. J Med Virol 2003; 71: 281-289.

3 Fooks AR, Brookes SM, Johnson N, McElhinney LM, Hutson AM: Review article: European bat lyssaviruses: an emerging zoonosis. Epidemiol Infect 2003:131: 1029-1039.

4 Lumio J, Hillbom M, Roine R, Ketonen L, Haltia M, Valle M, Neuvonen E, Lahdevirta J: Human rabies of bat origin in Europe. Lancet 1986; i: 378.

5 Roine RO, Hillbom M, Valle M, Haltia M, Ketonen L, Neuvonen E, Lumio J, Lahdevirta J: Fatal encephalitis caused by a bat-borne rabies-related virus; clinical findings. Brain 1988; 111: 1505-1516.

6 Amengual B, Whitby JE, King A, Serra Cobo J, Bourhy H: Evolution of bat Lyssaviruses. J Gen Virol 1997; 78: 2319-2328.

7 King AA, Fooks AR, Aubert M, Wandeler AI: Historical perspective of rabies in Europe and the Mediterranean Basin. OIE, Paris, 2004, 359 p.

8 Hutson AM: Occurrence, distribution and incidence of lyssavirus in bats, in Racey PA, Raynor R, Prichard S (eds): A review of European Bat Lyssavirus (EBLV) and the status of bats in Scotland. Scottish Heritage Commissioned Report No. 63 (ROAME No. FO3AC318), 2004, pp 40-70.

9 Brookes SM: The epidemiology of rabies and other lyssaviruses, in Racey PA, Raynor R, Prichard S (eds): A review of European Bat Lyssavirus (EBLV) and the status of bats in Scotland. Scottish Heritage Commissioned Report No. 63 (ROAME No. FO3AC318), 2004, pp 71-95.

10 Hutson AM, Mickleburgh SP, Racey PA (compilers): Microchiropteran bats: global status survey and conservation action plan. IUCN, Gland, Switzerland & Cambridge, UK 2001; 1-258.

11 Anon: European Workshop on Bat Rabies, Vilnius, Lithuania, 16 May 2004. EUROBATS Bat Rabies Workshop Report 2004; 1-33.

12 Tjørnehøj K, Rønsholt L, Fooks AR: Antibodies to EBLV-1 in a domestic cat in Denmark. Vet Rec 2003; (October): 571-572.

13 Müller T, Cox J, Peter W, Schäfer R, Bodamer P, Wulle U, Burow J, Müller W: Infection of a stone marten with European bat lyssa virus (EBL1). Rabies Bull Europe 2001; 25 (3): 9-11.

14 Müller T, Cox J, Peter W, Schäfer R, Johnson N, McElhinney LM, Geue JL, Tjornehoj K, Fooks AR: Spill-over of European Bat Lyssavirus Type 1 into a stone marten (*Martes foina*) in Germany. J Vet Med B Infect Dis Vet Public Health 2004; 51: 49-54.

15 Baagøe HJ: *Eptesicus serotinus (Schreber, 1774) – Breitflugelfledermaus,* in Krapp F (ed): *Handbuch der Säugetiere Europas*, Band 4: Fledertiere, Teil I: Chiroptera 1: Rhinolophidae, Vespertilionidae I. AULA-Verlag, Wiesbaden, 2001, pp 519-559, 603 p.

16 Rønsholt L: New case of European Bat Lyssavirus (EBL) infection in Danish sheep. Rabies Bull Europe 2002; 26 (2): 15.

17 Johnson N, Selden D, Parsons G, Healy D, Brookes SM, McElhinney LM, Hutson AM, Fooks AR: Isolation of a European bat lyssavirus type 2 from a Daubenton's bat in the United Kingdom. Vet Rec 2003; 152: 383-387.

18 Brass DA: Rabies in Bats: natural history and public health implications. Livia Press, Ridgefield, Connecticut, 1994, 335 p.

19 Bat Conservation Trust, pers. comm. 2005.

20 Tordo N, Bahloul C, Jacob Y, Jallet C, Perrin P, Badrane H: Rabies: Epidemiological tendencies and control tools, in Dodet B, Schudel A, Pastoret PP, Lombard M (eds): Rabies in Europe. Dev Biol (Basel). Basel, Karger, 2006, vol 125, pp 3-13.

21 Hutson AM: Transboundary movements and the conservation of bats in Europe, in UNEP/CMS (ed): Proceedings of the CMS Symposium on Animal Migration (Gland, Switzerland, 13 April 1997), CMS Technical Series Publication 1999; 2:51-58.

P.H.C. Lina, National Museum of Natural History "Naturalis", P.O. Box 835, NL-2300 AV Leiden, the Netherlands.
E-mail: phc.lina@tiscali.nl

Dodet B, Schudel A, Pastoret PP, Lombard M (eds): Rabies in Europe.
Dev Biol (Basel). Basel, Karger, 2006, vol 125, p 255.

The Evolution and Origin of European Bat Lyssaviruses

P.L. Davis[1], F. Larrous[2], W. Alonso[1], E.C. Holmes[1], H. Bourhy[2]

[1] Department of Zoology, University of Oxford, South Parks Road, Oxford, UK

[2] Rabies Laboratory, WHO collaborating centre for reference and research on rabies, Institut Pasteur, Paris, France

Abstract: European bat lyssaviruses (EBLVs) are widespread in Europe. However, information concerning the evolution of EBLV is scarce. Herein we provide a comprehensive analysis of the evolutionary history of these viruses. Sixty-six EBLV isolates were sequenced and maximum likelihood and Bayesian methods used to analyse selection pressures, rates of nucleotide substitution, time of the most recent common ancestor (MRCA) and rates of population growth. A Mantel-test-based approach was also used to track the geographical movement of strains. The study encompassed data from 10 countries, over a time-span of 36 years and focused on the glycoprotein (G) and nucleoprotein (N) genes, as well as a 527-base-long noncoding region. The results confirmed the known geographic distribution of EBLV-1 and EBLV-2 and there was clear evidence of the existence of two subtypes of EBLV-1 (EBLV-1a and EBLV-1b). Notably, we found that EBLV-1a and EBLV-1b have different patterns of geographical spread and possibly have different points of introduction into Europe. EBLV-1a appears to have spread along a north-south axis in the west of Europe, while EBLV-1a has clearly spread along an east-west axis in Northern Europe. The ratio of non-synonymous to synonymous substitutions (d_N: d_S) was extremely low for EBLV, indicating that the virus is subject to strong selective constraints. However, d_N: d_S is lower in EBLV-1 (0.088 in G and 0.049 in N) than EBLV-2 (0.097 in G and 0.068 in N) and lower in EBLV-1b (0.079 in G and 0.034 N) than EBLV-1a (0.096 in G and 0.065 in N). Our Bayesian analysis revealed that a model of exponential population growth was the best fit to the data and from this we inferred the substitution rate for EBLV-1 to be 5.10×10^{-5} and 6.11×10^{-5} substitutions per site, per year for the G and N genes, respectively. These rates are some of the lowest ever reported for RNA viruses. This low rate of evolutionary change suggests that the virus has reached an adaptative peak, so that most amino acid changes reduce fitness and are therefore eventually removed through selection pressures. It also implies that the current genetic diversity in the virus arose 500 to 750 years ago. Finally, although the population sizes of EBLV in European bats are increasing, the measured growth rates are very low, suggesting that the virus exists in a near-equilibrium state in many bat species.

For more information on this study please see:

Amengual B, Whitby JE, King A, Serra-Cobo J, Bourhy H: Evolution of European bat *Lyssavirus*es. J Gen Virol 1997; 78: 2319-2328.

Davis PL, Holmes EC, Larrous F, Van der Poel WH, Tjornehoj K, Alonso WJ, Bourhy H: Phylogeography, population dynamics, and molecular evolution of European bat lyssaviruses. J Virol 2005; 79 (16): 10487-10497.

Dodet B, Schudel A, Pastoret PP, Lombard M (eds): Rabies in Europe.
Dev Biol (Basel). Basel, Karger, 2006, vol 125, pp 257-261.

EBLV1 Circulation in Natural Bat Colonies of *Eptesicus serotinus*: a Six Year Survey

S. Vázquez[1], C. Ibáñez[2], J. Juste[2], J.E. Echevarria[1]

[1] Centro Nacional de Microbiología, Instituto de salud Carlos III, Ctra. Majadahonda-Pozuelo s/n, Majadahonda, Madrid, Spain

[2] Estación Biológica de Doñana, CSIC, Avda de Maria Luisa s/n, Seville, Andalusia, Spain

Abstract: The serotine bat *(Eptesicus serotinus)* accounts for 95 % of cases of human exposition to EBLV1. The aim of this study was to focus on the epidemiology and pathogenesis of EBLV1 infection in the serotine bat. Our first objective was the development of an RT-PCR technique for the specific detection of EBLV1 RNA in oro-pharyngeal swabs. This technique showed better performance than the classical immunofluorescence (IF) on brain in detecting EBLV1 in healthy flying bats. We have used this technique together with antibody detection by the fluorescent focus inhibition test (FFIT) to investigate EBLV1 circulation in 19 natural colonies of serotine bats in Andalusia (Spain) from 1998 to 2003. The survey was based on 1223 different captures of 1080 individuals that were ring banded, sampled and released. Individuals that were repeatedly captured were always found in the same colony even though some colonies were less than five Km apart. Viral circulation was detected in nine colonies either by RT-PCR, serology or both. Each colony showed a different temporal pattern of viral circulation suggesting independent endemic circulation. Some positive individuals were captured healthy in following campaigns evidencing survival after viral infection.

INTRODUCTION

Rabies is caused by different rhabdoviruses included within the genus Lyssavirus. Land mammals are infected worldwide by the classical rabies virus (RABV) or serotype 1, as well as bats in America. This virus causes nearly all the human cases in the world. A few African land mammals have been found to be infected by a different lyssavirus, the Mokola virus (serotype 3, MOKV). The hosts for the remaining lyssaviruses are non-American bats: Lagos bat virus (serotype 2, LBV) and Duvenhage virus (serotype 4, DUVV) in Africa, the Australian bat lyssavirus (genotype 7, ABLV) in Australia, the European bat lyssavirus type 1 (EBLV1), and European bat lyssvirus type 2 (EBLV2) in Europe [1]. More than 700 infected bats have been found in Europe after the first case was found in 1957 [2] and more than 95 % of the bats correctly identified were serotines, presumably infected by EBLV1 [2].

Most of the remaining bats were pond bats infected by EBLV2. According to this data from passive surveillance, the serotine bat (*Eptesicus serotinus*) has been considered the reservoir of EBLV1, while EBLV2 has been found so far in two species of the genus *Myotis (M. dasycneme* and *M. daubentonii*). However, a recent study using active surveillance in bat colonies [3] shows extensive circulation of EBLV1 in other bat species that live mostly in wild areas and consequently rarely act as vectors for transmission to humans, but perhaps constitute an important natural reservoir. The study shows how passive surveillance is biased to bat species linked to inhabited areas, such as the serotine bat, because it places the focus on cases of interaction between bats and humans. Consequently, active surveillance is fundamental for the complete study of the epidemiology and pathogenesis of lyssavirus infection in bats.

Despite the fact that most human exposure to bat lyssaviruses in Europe is to EBLV1, the first human case in 1985 [4], as well as the last one in Scotland in 2002 [5] involved EBLV2. Both were habitual bat handlers who did not receive post exposure prophylaxis after being bitten. The remaining two known cases involved EBLV1, in Ukraine in 1977 and Russia in 1985 both cases being people without professional contact with bats. All four human cases were fatal. Hundreds of Europeans have been exposed to rabid bats since 1985 [2] but all have received post-exposure prophylaxis and none have been infected.

Rapid diagnosis of lyssavirus infection should be made on the animal brain after any human exposure. Direct antigen detection by IF is the most widespread screening method [6]. Results are usually confirmed by the mouse inoculation test or by viral isolation on murine neuroblastoma cells [6]. More recently, RNA detection by reverse transcription-polymerase chain reaction (RT-PCR) has been proposed as a rapid and sensitive alternative. However, as RT-PCR is not faster than IF, and rabid animal brains usually contain high amounts of virus, very few laboratories have adopted this technique. On the other hand, direct sequencing of RT-PCR products is the most common technique for virus identification and in molecular epidemiology studies.

Most European bats are protected species [7] and thus the brain cannot be used for the screening of active lyssavirus infection in natural bat populations. For this reason, most studies have been based exclusively on serology [8,9], however, total antibody presence merely reflects past exposure to the virus and does not demonstrate active infection. Moreover, conclusive identification of the lyssavirus involved, based on serological techniques, is not possible due to cross reactivity.

The first lyssavirus infection in Spain was diagnosed in 1987 in a bat that bit a child in El Saler (Valencia, eastern Spain). This same year a similar case was reported in Granada (Andalusia, southern Spain). Both viruses were classified as Duvenhage virus (genotype 4) (at this time EBLV1 and EBLV2 had still not been described and European bat lyssaviruses were included in genotype 4). Additional cases of human exposure to positive bats were reported again in Granada in 1994, Seville (Andalusia) in 1999 and in Murcia (south-eastern Spain) in 1999 and 2002. In all four cases, the bat species involved was *Eptesicus serotinus* and the virus was EBLV1. In 1989, five EBLV1 infections were described in serotine bats found dead during a zoologic survey in natural colonies in Huelva (Andalusia). Serosurveillance in these colonies with FFIT using the EBLV1 isolate obtained from the dead bats [8] showed prevalences of up to 20 % among completely healthy individuals. As bats were identified with rings and released after sampling, some of the positive individuals could be captured one year later providing for the first time direct evidence of long term survival of *Eptesicus serotinus* after EBLV1 infection. Some years later we decided to resume surveillance in this area, complementing the serology with direct detection by RT-PCR with an oropharyngeal swab. The colony involved in the case of human exposure in 1999 in Seville provided an excellent opportunity for the evaluation of this last technique [10]. We review here the experience of the evaluation of this technique together with some preliminary conclusions based on the currently available results of continuing studies that started in1998 on additional bat colonies.

Materials and Methods

Samples

1,080 serotine bats (*Eptesicus serotinus)* from 19 colonies located in Huelva, Seville and Granada provinces (Andalusia, Spain). The distance between colonies varies from 0.5 to 317 km. Three colonies were sampled every year from 1998 to 2003, two were sampled on five different years, two on four years, five on three years, three on two years and four only in one year. As some individuals were captured several times, the total number of captures was 1,223. Bats were mist-netted at the exits used by the animals for leaving the shelters for night feeding. After capture, each animal was assessed for age and sex, measured, weighed and identified by its ring. Oropharyngeal samples were taken as described previously [10]. Bats were usually released after sampling. For 619 captures, blood samples were also taken and processed to be used for antibody detection.

Analytical methods

Total nucleic acids were extracted from oropharyngeal swabs by guanidium thyocianate treatment and alcohol precipitation. Extracts were tested for lyssavirus RNA by RT-PCR designed to target a conserved region and capable of detecting RNA from the seven rabies related lyssaviruses, optimised for EBLV1 detection [10].

The presence of EBLV1-specific antibodies was determined with a modified, previously published, FFIT [8], using an EBLV1 isolate obtained in 1989 from the geographical area of the study.

Results

The frequency of repeated captures was variable but increased with the number of campaigns, reaching 43 % among the individuals belonging to colonies that were sampled in all six years of the study. Within this group of colonies, no single bat was captured for all six campaigns, but 6.4 % of the individuals were captured on five different years. Subsequent captures of the same individual were always made within the same colony, with not a single case of translocation observed.

Nine colonies showed positive results. The virus was detected either by RT-PCR or antibody detection from 1998 to 2002, but not in 2003. The temporal pattern of circulation was completely different for each colony. Some of them showed continuous circulation from 1998 to 2002, while viral infection markers were detected intermittently or sporadically in others. Sporadic results in different colonies occurred in different years. One individual PCR positive bat plus another five antibody positive bats were captured healthy in the following campaigns. Only one individual was found simultaneously positive both by PCR and antibodies.

Discussion

Our previous results [10] showed that the presence of EBLV1 RNA in the oropharyngeal cavity is a marker of the presence of EBLV1 infection in serotine bats and can be used together with antibody detection for the active surveillance of natural bat colonies. For this reason, we decided to carry out active surveillance on 19 colonies from a geographical area where several infected bats had been found as a result of passive surveillance.

The breeding colonies of *Eptesicus serotinus* behave as close communities whose members are very linked with no interchange of individuals. Data on viral detection is independent for each colony as a result of this apparent isolation suggesting a pattern of independent endemic viral circulation. However, some degree of viral transmission among individuals of different breeding colonies should occur, although at which moment remains unknown, perhaps during mating or hibernation. On the other hand, some mechanism of viral persistence or latency seems to be necessary to ensure viral survival during the hibernation period. In any case, all this data makes it difficult to imagine a pattern of epidemiological circulation based on periodical epidemic waves of fast viral spreading.

Most bats seem to survive after the infection, according to the EBLV1 specific antibody prevalence in some colonies. Some positive individuals could be captured healthy one year later. RT-PCR positive bats were captured flying while showing viral RNA in the oral cavity. Similar facts have been observed in fruit bats (*Rousettus aegyptiacus*) from a zoo in The Netherlands several months after an outbreak of EBLV1 in this captive colony [11]. In consequence, clinical rabies does not seem to be the most common event after EBLV1 infection in *Eptesicus serotinus* and viral circulation seems to occur without important consequences for the health of the bats. Nevertheless, as observed in the study area in 1989, stressful conditions can lead to an increase in neurological disease induced by EBLV1 and increased mortality. Additional work should be done in order to establish whether EBLV1 RNA presence in the oral cavity is associated with excretion of live virus as well as to establish the impact of this asymptomatic excretion in spill-over to other animal species [12] or even in the transmission to humans.

Conclusions

Natural breeding colonies of *Eptesicus serotinus* behave as close communities with independent EBLV1 circulation. This data suggests a pattern of endemic circulation.

The usual clinical expression of the EBLV1 infection in *Eptesicus serotinus* seems to be asymptomatic or mild disease without important consequences for the health of bat populations. Nevertheless, local outbreaks of neurological disease are possible under stressful conditions.

The presence of viral RNA in the oral cavity of healthy individuals strongly suggests asymptomatic viral excretion with unknown epidemiological implications.

References

1 Rupprecht CE, Hanlon C, Hemachudha T: Rabies re-examined. Lancet Infect Dis 2002; 2: 327-343.

2 Pötzsch CJ, Müller TH, Kramer M: Summarizing the rabies situation in Europe 1990-2004 from the Rabies Bulletin Europe. Rabies Bulletin Europe 2004; 4.

3 Serra-Cobo J, Amengual B, Abellán C, Bourhy H: European bat lyssavirus infections in Spanish bat populations. Emerg Infect Dis 2002; 8 (4): 413-420.

4 Lumio J, Hillbom M, Roine R, Ketonen L, Haltia M, Velle M, Neuvonen E, Lahdevirta J: Human rabies of bat origin in Europe. Lancet 1986; i (8477): 378.

5 Nathwani D, McIntyre PG, White K, Shearer AJ, Reynolds N, Walker D, Orange GV, Fooks AR: Fatal human rabies caused by European bat lyssavirus type 2a infection in Scotland. Clin Infect Dis 2003; 37: 598-601.

6 Meslin FX, Kaplan MM: An overview of laboratory techniques in the diagnosis and prevention of rabies and in rabies research, in Laboratory techniques in rabies, fourth edition. WHO, 1996, Geneva.

7 Council directive 92/43/EEC of 21 May, 1992 on the conservation of natural habitats and wild fauna and flora. Official Journal of the Council of the European Communities L206, 22/07/1992, pp 7-50.

8 Pérez-Jordá JL, Ibáñez C, Muñoz-Cervera M, Téllez A: Lyssavirus in *Eptesicus serotinus* (Chiroptera, Vespertilionidae). J Wildl Dis 1995; 31: 372-377.

9 Steece R, Altenbach JS: Prevalence of rabies specific antibodies in the Mexican free tailed-bat (*Tadarida brasiliensis mexicana*) at Lava cave, New Mexico. J Wildl Dis 1989; 25: 490-496.

10 Echevarría JE, Avellón A, Juste J, Vera M, Ibáñez C: Screening of active lyssavirus infection in wild bat populations by viral RNA on oropharyngeal swabs. J Clin Microbiol 2001; 39 (10): 3678-3683.

11 Wellenberg GJ, Audry L, Ronsholt L, van der Poel WH, Bruschke CJ, Bourhy H: Presence of European bat lyssavirus RNas in apparently healthy Rousettus aegyptiacus bats. Arch Virol 2002; 147 (2): 349-361.

12 Müller T, Cox J, Peter W, Schäfer R, Johnson N, McElhinney LM, Geue JL, Tjørnehøj K, Fooks AR: Spill-over of European Bat Lyssavirus Type 1 into a Stone Marten (Martes foina) in Germany. J Vet Med B Infect Dis Vet Public Health 2004; 51 (2): 49-54.

Dr. J.E. Echevarría, Centro Nacional de Microbiología, Instituto de Salud Carlos III, Ctra. Majadahonda-Pozuelo s/n, ES-28220 Majadahonda, Madrid, Spain.
E-mail: jeecheva@isciii.es

Dodet B, Schudel A, Pastoret PP, Lombard M (eds): Rabies in Europe.
Dev Biol (Basel). Basel, Karger, 2006, vol 125, p 263.

Distribution of European Bat Lyssaviruses in Native Bats in the Netherlands

J.A. Kramps[1], R. van der Heide[2], E.R.A.M. Verstraten[1], K. Takumi[2], P.H.C. Lina[3], W.H.M. van der Poel[2]

[1] Central Institute for Animal Disease Control-Lelystad, Lelystad, The Netherlands

[2] Microbiological Laboratory for Health Protection, National Institute for Public Health and the Environment, Bilthoven, The Netherlands

[3] Naturalis Leiden, The Netherlands

Aim

In the Netherlands, lyssaviruses are often detected in bats and presumed to constitute a public health hazard. To study the epidemiology of European bat lyssavirus (EBLV), native bats have been tested for rabies since 1984.

Materials and Methods

As of 1991, all bats involved in contact incidents have been tested for rabies. For all collected bats, data including species, age, gender and place found have been documented and analysed. To molecularly characterize the prevalent lyssaviruses in these native bats, lyssavirus RNA of 48 EBLV-positive samples was amplified by RT-PCR and subsequently the virus nucleoprotein encoding region was directly sequenced and analysed phylogenetically.

Results

The serotine bat (*Eptesicus serotinus*) appeared to be the most important bat reservoir of EBLV. Of 1,218 serotine bats tested, 251 (21 %) were found to be rabies-positive. Only a few EBLV detections were observed in pond bats (*Myotis dasycneme*): 5 out 115 bats were found to be EBLV-positive (4 %). The most common bat (*Pipistrellus pipistrellus*) was never found to be positive for EBLV (number investigated: > 2,000).

All serotine bat specimens clustered with virus genotype 5 (EBL type 1) sequences and included both EBL1a and EBL1b sequences. Homology within sub-genotypes were high.

At least 4 of 5 isolates from *Myotis* sp. from the Netherlands were found by others to belong to genotype 6 (EBL2).

Conclusions

Our findings indicate that EBLV of genotype 5 is endemic in serotine bats in the Netherlands (prevalence ~20 %). A much lower lyssavirus prevalence of ~4 % was found in pond bats. Since EBLV can cause fatal infections, it is indicated to test all serotine and pond bats involved in contact incidents in order to determine if the victim was exposed to potentially fatal EBLV.

For more information on this study please see:

Van der Poel VHM, Van der Heide R, Verstaten ERAM, Takumi K, Lina PHC, Kramps JA: European Bat Lyssaviruses, the Netherlands. Emerg Infect Dis 2005; 11 (12) 1854-1859.

Dodet B, Schudel A, Pastoret PP, Lombard M (eds): Rabies in Europe.
Dev Biol (Basel). Basel, Karger, 2006, vol 125, pp 265-271.

EBLV-2 Prevalence in the United Kingdom as Determined by Surveillance Testing

G.C. Smith[1], S.M. Brookes[2], S.L. Harris[2,3], J.N. Aegerter[1], G. Jones[3], A.R. Fooks[2]

[1] Central Science Laboratory, York, UK

[2] Veterinary Laboratory Agency, Addlestone, Surrey, UK

[3] School of Biological Sciences, University of Bristol, Bristol, UK

Abstract: Five cases of EBLV-2 have been detected in the UK since 1996, with all wildlife cases in the Daubenton's bat: one on the south coast in Sussex in 1996, one in Lancashire in 2002, another in 2003, one in Surrey in 2004 and a human fatality in Angus, Scotland, in 2002. As a result of the human case, a seroprevalence study, aimed primarily at the Daubenton's bat was conducted in 2003 in Scotland and at some sites in England. In Scotland, 198 Daubenton's, 20 Natterer's and 6 pipistrelles were caught at 19 sites and analysed, while in England 67 Daubenton, 2 Brandts/Whiskered and 4 pipistrelle bats were analysed from four sites in Lancashire. Analysis of blood was performed by a modified fluorescent antibody virus neutralisation test (mFAVN) to determine antibody titre to EBLV-2. Ignoring those sites where we had a priori reason to expect infected bats, the overall seroprevalence was between 0.7-5.1 % (95 % confidence interval), with a maximum likelihood estimate of 2.2 %. Mouth swabs were taken and tested for virus genome by RT-PCR and live virus by tissue culture isolation. All of the PCR and isolation results were negative suggesting that none of the bats sampled were actively excreting virus. This suggests a low level of active infection in Britain and raises the possibility that bats may recover following exposure to EBLV-2.

Introduction

Two Lyssaviruses circulate in European bats: European Bat Lyssavirus 1 (EBLV-1) and European Bat Lyssavirus 2 (EBLV-2). To date over 758 cases of bat rabies have been recorded in Europe [1]. Nearly all of these are EBLV-1, and over 95 % of those cases where the species was recorded occurred in the Serotine bat, *Eptesicus serotinus,* in Northern Europe [2]. Spill-over cases, all of EBLV-1, into terrestrial mammals are rare, with three recorded events in sheep [3-5], one in a stone marten [6] and one report of antibodies to EBLV-1 in a cat [7]. EBLV-1 has also been recorded in one confirmed human death and is suspected in a second case, although the virus was not genotyped [8]. As a comparison, Table 1 shows there have been only 18 confirmed cases of EBLV-2, including two human fatalities [1], six cases in the

Table 1: The distribution, year and host, of all 18 confirmed samples positive for EBLV-2. A further suspected EBLV-2 case from Ukraine is likely to have been caused by contamination, or other error [9].

Country	Year	Host	Variant
Denmark	1986	*M. dasycneme*	?
	1986	*M. daubentonii*	?
	1987	*M. daubentonii*	?
Finland	1985	Human	2b
Germany	1986	*M. daubentonii*	?
Netherlands	1987 x 3	*M. dasycneme*	2a
	1989	*M. dasycneme*	2a
	1993	*M. dasycneme*	2a
Switzerland	1992 x 2	*M. daubentonii*	2b
	2002	*M. daubentonii*	?
United Kingdom	1996	*M. daubentonii*	2a
	2002	*M. daubentonii*	2a
	2002	Human	2a
	2003	*M. daubentonii*	2a
	2004	*M. daubentonii*	2a

pond bat, *Myotis dasycneme*, and ten in Daubenton's bats *M. daubentonii*. In addition one possible case has been reported in a Noctule bat, *Nyctalus noctula*. The small number of cases of EBLV-2 are widely distributed across Central and Northern Europe. Despite the occurrence of EBLV-2 in the UK, Denmark, The Netherlands, Germany and Switzerland, all recorded bat cases in France have been EBLV-1 [9]. The first recorded case of human bat rabies in Western Europe was in 1985 in a bat worker who died in Finland, and this sparked a massive increase in the number of submissions of bats, and thus the number of detected cases of rabies in bats.

Passive Surveillance in the UK

Between 1987 and 1995, 882 bats, including 23 *M. daubentonii*, were submitted to the Veterinary Laboratory Agency (VLA) as part of a newly established passive surveillance scheme and all were negative for Lyssaviruses [10]. In May 1996, a sick adult female *M. daubentonii* was recovered from the cellar of a public house in Newhaven, near the south coast of England and was euthanized four days later [11]. Despite searching, no *M. daubentonii* roosts were detected in the area, and because of local wind conditions it was generally concluded that the individual had been blown across the English Channel [11]. During 1996 there was a large increase in the number of bats submitted to the VLA. This included an additional 23 *M. daubentonii* by 2001. All these bats were also negative for EBLVs. Then in July 2002 a juvenile female *M. daubentonii* was caught by a cat in Lancashire, Northwest England. During recovery in a bat sanctuary it began to show signs of aggression after seven weeks. These signs persisted and the bat was killed humanely three and a half weeks later, and submitted for rabies testing. It was positive for EBLV-2 [12]. In November of the same year a bat conservationist was admitted to hospital in Scotland with acute haematemesis. He gave a 5-day history of pain and paraesthesia in the left arm followed by increasing weakness of his limbs with evidence of evolving encephalitis with cerebellar involvement. The patient had never been vaccinated against rabies, and had not received post exposure prophylaxis. EBLV-2 was later identified [13] and infection was presumed to result from contact with local *M. daubentonii*. As a result of the human death, the number of bats submitted to the passive surveillance scheme increased dramatically. In September 2003, a member of the public observed an adult male *M. daubentonii* bat, in daylight, flying into a tree and falling to the ground. The site at which the bat was found (Near Bury, Lancashire) was within 45 miles of the previous EBLV-2 positive case in Lancashire in 2002 (although in a different water catchment area). The bat was rescued and died a week later in captivity, but remained in a freezer for a year before being submitted and confirmed as EBLV-2 positive [14]. During the interim, in September 2004, a juvenile female *M. daubentonii* bat was observed by a member of the public, in close proximity to the Thames River in central Staines, Surrey. It was moved to some nearby undergrowth and remained there for several days before being taken into care by local bat workers to attempt rehabilitation. The bat died a week later and EBLV-2 was confirmed [15]. These later cases are not necessarily due to any increase in disease prevalence or geographical spread, as insufficient *M. daubentonii* have been submitted to determine any change in disease prevalence over time with statistical confidence. To the end of 2004 a total of 113 *M. daubentonii* were submitted to the passive surveillance scheme, giving an overall prevalence of 3.5 %.

It is unlikely that these bats were detected as soon as signs began, but in two cases it appears that the bats were behaving strangely for at least a week before death. In the second bat case, it is possible that the stress of injury and captivity helped to bring on symptomatic rabies, and it is interesting to note that it survived for three weeks before being euthanised. Terrestrial wild mammals suffering from classical rabies (RABV) are rarely symptomatic for more than four or five days [16].

Active Surveillance in the UK

The University of Bristol and the VLA were awarded a studentship to begin active surveillance of bats in 2002. However, government interest in conducting active surveillance in bats in the UK increased following the human death in Scotland in late 2002. The UK Department for Environment, Food and Rural Affairs (Defra) began funding active surveillance in England and Wales, and Scottish Natural Heritage (SNH) began funding active surveillance in Scotland. Due to the human fatality occurring in Scotland, most bat sampling was performed in and around the suspected location of the incident, resulting in many more samples from Scotland than England. During 2003 the Central Science Laboratory (CSL), York, and the VLA organised and conducted the bat sampling in Scotland. This involved the capture of a total of 230 bats on 22 nights at 19 locations (Fig. 1). Each bat was assessed for health, sex, age, and reproductive status and ringed. Mouth swabs were then taken and the bat bled by puncture from the antebrachial or uropatagial veins

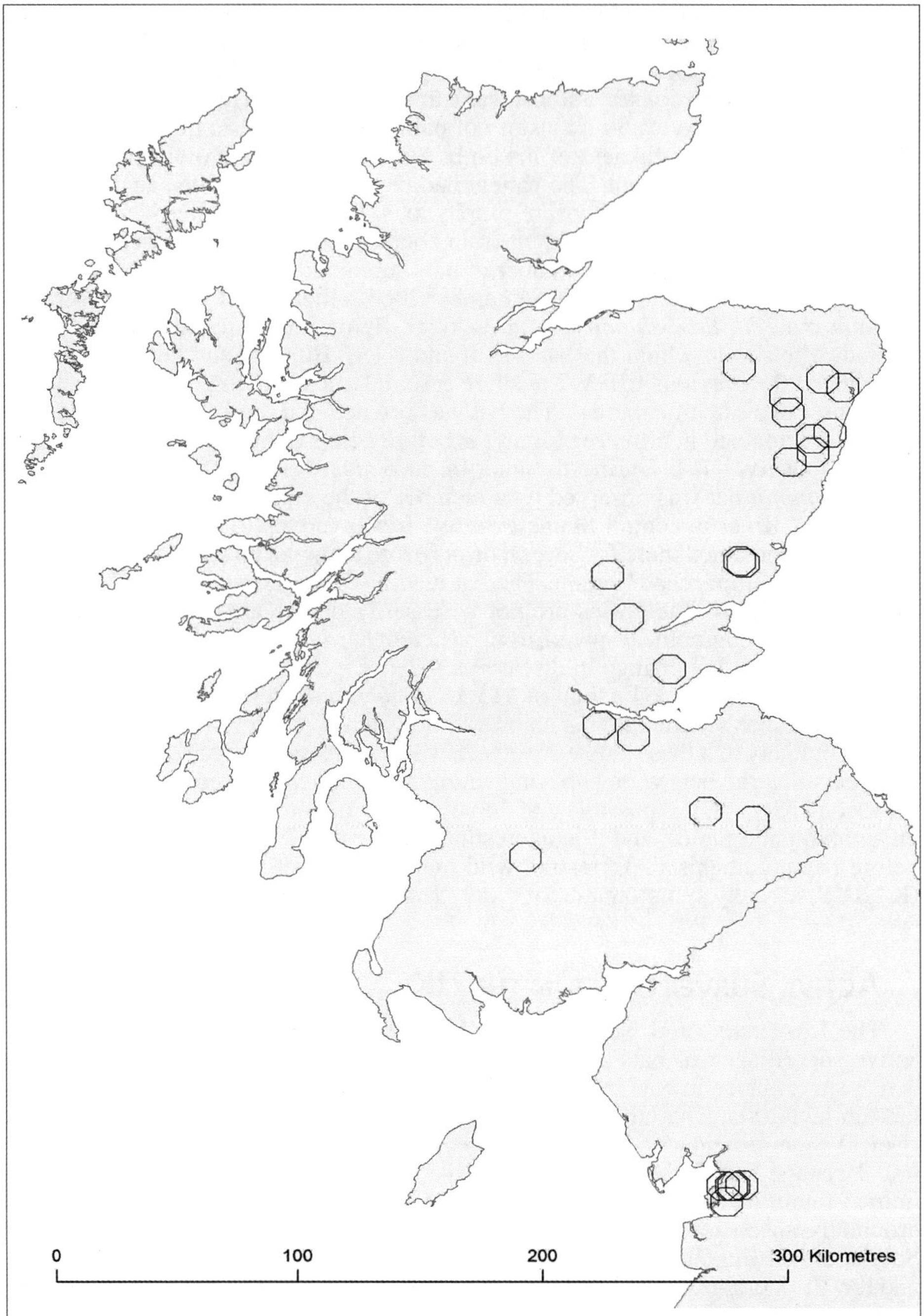

Fig. 1: The distribution of sites in Scotland and northern England sampled during the active surveillance in Great Britain during 2003.

using 10 to 50 μL heparinised glass capillary tubes. Early sampling was problematic partly due to limited experience, which necessitated pooling blood samples from the same species at the same site for analysis. Blood samples were subjected to a modified fluorescent antibody virus neutralisation (mFAVN) test to measure antibodies to EBLV-2 [17]. A reciprocal titre ≥ 27 was used as a positive cut-off in all samples. At the site where we had a priori suspicion of finding infected bats (one where the human case was believed to have occurred and one roost next to the Lancashire bat case of 2002), a total of 69 Daubenton's bats were analysed, and the 95 % confidence interval (CI) for the seroprevalence was from 2.9-16.3 %. We assumed that all other sites were effectively located at random, and thus represented a better estimate of the national levels of seroprevalence in *M. daubentonii*. The 115 *M. daubentonii* analysed from these sites gave a 95 % CI from 0.05-3.8 % [17]. The presence of virus and viral RNA was determined by rabies tissue culture infection test (RTCIT) and reverse transcriptase-polymerase chain reaction (RT-PCR), but no virus or viral RNA was found. In addition to the *M. daubentonii*, 20 Natterer (*M. nattereri*) and 6 pipistrelle (*Pipistrellus pipistrelle/pygmaeus*) bats were analysed and found to be negative for EBLV-2 and antibodies to this virus.

Sampling in England in 2003 comprised the collection and analysis of 67 *M. daubentonii* at 4 sites. Again, there was an a priori site in Lancashire where the presence of infected bats was likely. At this site a 95 % CI seroprevalence of 4.9-31.6 % was determined, whereas at the other (random) sites the 95 % CI was 1.2-11.6 %. Two Brandts/Whiskered (*M. branti/M. mystacinus*) and four pipistrelle (*Pipistrellus pipistrelles/pygmaeus*) bats were also caught and analysed, but were found to be negative for EBLV-2.

Combining all samples from the "random" sites yielded an overall seroprevalence of about 2.2 % (95 % CI: 0.7 – 5.1 %) in *M. daubentonii* [18].

Discussion

Overall, the active surveillance work in Britain in 2003 suggests a national seroprevalence of between 1 and 5 % in *M. daubentonii*, with insufficient evidence to determine whether or not this varies nationally or regionally within the UK. At roost sites where infection has been present, seroprevalence levels are between 3-16 %. With classical rabies (RABV), animals and people are rarely seropositive until the last few days before death [19]. In the active seroprevalence study, the seropositive bats were all apparently healthy, suggesting that bats may either recover from EBLV-2 infection, or they may mount an immune response following challenge (indicating they did not suffer from disease).

These seroprevalence levels may be higher than the true level of disease prevalence, as bats may survive challenge by EBLVs. Further sampling is required at sites where bats positive for antibodies to EBLV-2 have been identified to determine how seroprevalence varies with time. More dispersed regional sampling is also required to determine how widespread the disease currently is within the United Kingdom. Given the low seroprevalence rate in *M. daubentonii*, insufficient individuals of other species were analysed to have any confidence that spillover infection was absent. In any event, if *M. daubentonii* or *Myotis* bats in general were the main host species, spillover prevalence levels in other species would be expected to be much lower, and thus much larger numbers of other bat species would need to be tested. We therefore recommend that for EBLV-2, non-*Myotis* bats are preferentially analysed from roosts close to infected *Myotis* roosts to first determine if spillover occurs.

Passive surveillance suggested a prevalence of about 3.5 %. This is likely to be an overestimate, since bats that are moribund or behaving strangely are more likely to be submitted, and all bats that tested positive for infection had a history of unusual behaviour. Nonetheless, prevalence levels determined from active and passive surveillance are similar.

All wildlife records of EBLV-2 in the United Kingdom are in *M. daubentonii*, however, the pond bat *M. dasycneme* is not generally found in the UK. Therefore the information collected in the UK does not help to determine whether *M. daubentonii* is the main reservoir species, or whether the disease cycles in a broader range of *Myotis* species.

Conclusions

Current findings indicate that there is a low level of EBLV-2 distributed throughout the United Kingdom in *M. daubentonii*, and potentially other *Myotis* bats. The inability to find live virus or viral RNA in bat saliva in both seropositive and seronegative individuals suggests that further work is required to understand the relationship between infection, immune response and viral excretion. There may be a differential response to infection with EBLV-1 and EBLV-2 in bats. It is therefore imperative that the species of bat is identified and tissue is retained for genetic typing, in all cases, and that the genotype of lyssavirus is identified.

Acknowledgements

The authors thank Scottish Natural Heritage and the Department for Environment, Food and Rural Affairs for funding, Steve Langton and the Bat Conservation Trust, and the BBSRC for funding SH.

References

1 Harris SL, Brookes SM, Jones G, Hutson AM, Racey P, Aegerter J, et al: Viruses in bats: rabies virus. Biol Conserv 2006, in press.

2 Müller WW: Review of reported rabies case data in Europe to the WHO collaborating centre Tübingen from 1977 to 2000. Rabies Bulletin Europe 2000; 24 (4): 11-19.

3 Stougaard E, Ammendrup S: Rabies in individual countries: Denmark. Rabies Bulletin Europe 1998; 22 (4): 6.

4 Stougaard E, Ammendrup S: Rabies in individual countries: Denmark. Rabies Bulletin Europe 1998; 22 (3): 5.

5 Ronsholt L: A new case of European Bat Lyssavirus (EBL) infection in Danish sheep. Rabies Bulletin Europe 2002; 26 (2), [available online http://www.who-rabies-bulletin.org/q2_2002/startq2_02.html].

6 Müller T, Cox J, Peter W, Schäfer R, Bodamer P, Wulle U, et al: Infection of a stone marten with European Bat Lyssavirus (EBL1). Rabies Bulletin Europe 2001; 25 (3), [available on line http://www.who-rabies-bulletin.org/q3_2001/frame3_01.html].

7 Tjørnehoj K, Rønsholt L, Fooks AR: Antobodies to EBLV-1 in a domestic cat in Denmark. Vet Rec 2004; 155 (18): 571-572.

8 Vos A, Müller T, Cox J, Neubert L, Fooks AR: Susceptibility of ferrets (*Mustela putorius furo*) to experimentally induced rabies with European Bat Lyssaviruses (EBLV). J Vet Med B Infect Dis Vet Public Health 2004: 55-60.

9 Kuzmin IV, Botvinkin AD, Poleschuk EM, Orciari LA, Rupprecht CE: Bat rabies surveillance in the Former Soviet Union, in Dodet B, Schudel A, Pastoret PP, Lombard M (eds): Rabies in Europe. Dev Biol (Basel). Basel, Karger, 2006, vol 125, pp 273-282.

10 Picard-Meyer E, Barrat J, Wasniewski M, Wandeler A, Nadin-Davis S, Lowings JP, et al: Epidemiology of rabid bats in France, 1989 to 2002. Vet Rec 2004; 155 (24): 774-777.

11 Whitby JE, Johnstone P, Parsons G, King AA, Hutson AM: Ten-year survey of British bats for the existence of rabies. Vet Rec 1996; 139: 491-493.

12 Whitby JE, Heaton PR, Black EM, Wooldridge M, McElhinney LM, Johnstone P: First isolation of a rabies-related virus from a Daubenton's bat in the United Kingdom. Vet Rec 2000; 147 (14): 385-388.

13 Johnson N, Selden D, Parsons G, Healy D, Brookes SM, McElhinney LM, et al: Isolation of a European bat lyssavirus type 2 from a Daubenton's bat in the United Kingdom. Vet Rec 2003; 152 (13): 383-387.

14 Fooks AR, McElhinney LM, Pounder DJ, Finnegan CJ, Mansfield K, Johnson N, et al: Case report: Isolation of a European bat lyssavirus type 2a from a fatal human case of rabies encephalitis. J Med Virol 2003; 71: 281-289.

15 Fooks AR, Selden D, Brookes SM, Johnson N, Marston DA, Jolliffe TA, et al: Identification of a European bat lyssavirus type 2 in a Daubenton's bat found in Lancashire. Vet Rec 2004; 155 (19): 606-607.

16 Fooks AR, McElhinney LM, Marston DA, Selden D, Jolliffe TA, Wakeley PR, et al: Identification of a European bat lyssavirus type 2 in a Daubenton's bat found in Staines, Surrey, UK. Vet Rec 2004; 155 (14): 434-435.

17 Blancou J, Aubert MFA, Artois M: Fox rabies, in Baer GM (ed): The natural history of rabies. 2nd ed Boston, CRC Press, 1991, pp 257-290.

18 Brookes SM, Aegerter J, Smith GC, Healy DM, Jolliffe TA, Swift SM, et al: European Bat Lyssavirus in Scottish bats. Emerg Infect Dis 2005; 11, [online http://www.cdc.gov/ncidod/eid/vol11no04/pdfs/04-0920.pdf].

19 Fooks AR, Brookes SM, Healy D, Smith GC, Aegerter J, Harris S, et al: Detection of antibodies to European bat lyssavirus type-2 in Daubenton's bats in the United Kingdom. Vet Rec 2004; 154 (8): 245-246.

20 Fishbein DB: Rabies in humans, in Baer GM (ed): The natural history of rabies. 2nd ed Boston, CRC Press, 1991, pp 519-549.

Dr. G.C. Smith, Central Science Laboratory, Sand Hutton, York, YO41 1LZ, U.K.
E-mail: g.smith@csl.gov.uk

Dodet B, Schudel A, Pastoret PP, Lombard M (eds): Rabies in Europe.
Dev Biol (Basel). Basel, Karger, 2006, vol 125, pp 273-282.

Bat Rabies Surveillance in the Former Soviet Union

I.V. Kuzmin[1,2], A.D. Botvinkin[3], E.M. Poleschuk[2], L.A. Orciari[1], C.E. Rupprecht[1]

1 Centers for Disease Control and Prevention, Atlanta, GA, USA
2 Institute for Natural Foci Infections, Omsk, Russia
3 State Medical University, Irkutsk, Russia

Abstract: More than 3,000 bats were examined for lyssaviruses in the territory of the Former Soviet Union (FSU) over the past 41 years (1964-2004). European bat lyssavirus type 1 (EBLV-1) was registered in the Ukraine and the European part of Russia. Lyssaviruses Aravan (ARAV, Kyrgyzstan, 1991), Khujand (KHUV, Tajikistan, 2001), Irkut (IRKV, Irkutsk region, 2002) and West Caucasian Bat virus (WCBV, Krasnodar region, 2002) were proposed as new lyssavirus genotypes. All reports on rabies virus (RABV; serotype/genotype 1) isolation from bats to date are questionable and must be corroborated. Two human rabies cases of bat origin were registered in the town of Voroshilovgrad, the Ukraine (1977) and the town of Belgorod, Russia (1985). The second case was confirmed as EBLV-1, whereas the first case was not identified. At least five lyssaviruses, different from RABV and from each other, were recognized in the territory of the FSU, and their potential significance for veterinary and public health should not be underestimated.

INTRODUCTION

Bats maintain circulation of all known lyssavirus "genotypes" (or more correctly termed "species", as recognized by the International Committee on Virus Taxonomy, ICTV) except Mokola virus (MOKV). However, the ecology and epidemiology of MOKV has not been studied sufficiently and it is not possible to determine a principal host range and the circulation properties of this particular virus.

In the New World, bats maintain circulation of different lineages of rabies virus (RABV), whereas in the Old World, members of the Chiroptera maintain circulation of such non-RABV lyssaviruses as Lagos bat virus (LBV), Duvenhage virus (DUVV), European bat lyssavirus, type 1 (EBLV-1) and type 2 (EBLV-2), and Australian bat lyssavirus (ABLV, genotype 7). While LBV and DUVV have been found only in Africa, EBLV-1 is broadly distributed in Europe, from Spain to the European part of the former Soviet Union (FSU), and EBLV-2 circulates predominantly in Northern and Northwestern Europe. Both EBLVs have caused human rabies cases after bat exposure [1].

Very limited information on bat lyssaviruses is available from Asia. This situation is not due to the absence of these viruses in Asian bats, but rather to a lack of appropriate surveillance. A few records reported "RABV" of bat origin in India and Thailand, but these were not confirmed by further identification. The presence of antibodies to lyssaviruses was detected in bat sera from several countries in tropical Asia, as reviewed recently [2].

Four lyssaviruses, considered as potentially new genotypes of the genus, were discovered in the FSU: Aravan virus (ARAV) and Khujand virus (KHUV) originated from Central Asia [3], Irkut virus (IRKV) from Eastern Siberia and West Caucasian bat virus (WCBV) from the Black Sea region [4]. Additionally, some cases of EBLV-1 and RABV infection were reported from the territory of the FSU, including human rabies of bat origin [5-13]. After further examination, these records were re-assessed, and other claims require substantiation. The objective of this paper is to review the literature on bat rabies occurrence in the FSU, to track the history of available isolates and the results of their characterization, and to present unpublished data from our archives.

Material and Methods

Data included active surveillance of 1,424 bats of 26 species, carried out from 1979 to 2003 (Table 1). The bats were collected in different regions of Russia, Kazakhstan, Kyrgyzstan, Uzbekistan and Tajikistan. Field sampling and processing were performed as previously described [4]. The direct fluorescent antibody test (DFAT), enzyme-linked immunosorbent assay, and mouse inoculation test were conducted according to standard recommendations [14]. Anti-nucleocapsid monoclonal antibody (N-mAb) typing of the isolates obtained in our study was performed as previously described [15]. RNA extraction, reverse transcriptase – polymerase chain reaction (RT-PCR), direct sequencing and further phylogenetic analysis of the isolates had been previously described [3].

To accomplish a comprehensive historical and geographical description of bat rabies surveillance, data available in the Russian literature, as well as international reports, were joined with our own records. The data were compared in terms of apparent reliability and comments to this effect are provided in the text.

Results

Bat rabies surveillance did not attract great scientific or public attention in the FSU. Almost all available information for the period covering the past 41 years is summarized in Figure 1 and Table 1.

Additionally, only a few bat rabies cases were recorded by local veterinary laboratories, without species identification. For example, one rabid bat was recorded in Russia during 2004 [16].

The first lyssavirus isolate was yielded from a serotine bat (*Eptesicus serotinus*) in Kiev, Ukraine in 1964 [5]. The virus was called "rabies virus" due to the lack of identification capabilities available at that time, and from the observation that the general biological properties of the isolate were similar to RABV. The virus was not stored for further investigation. Shortly after that case, a rabies surveillance study was carried out on 517 bats in Moldavia, but all results were negative [17].

Nevertheless, a human rabies case of bat origin was registered in the city of Voroshilovgrad (currently Lugansk), Ukraine, in 1977. A 15-year-old girl was attacked by a bat during the daytime and bitten on a finger. The bat was not examined, and the patient did not apply for rabies prophylaxis. Approximately 35 days later, the patient developed typical rabies symptoms, and the diagnosis was confirmed postmortem [7]. This virus was not stored for further investigation.

Table 1 : Information on bat rabies surveillance in the territory of the FSU (cf. also Fig. 1).

Number on the map (Fig. 1)	Bat species and number (if applicable)	Total number, the isolate name in parentheses (if applicable)	References
1	*Eptesicus serotinus*	1/1*	[5]
2	*Myotis daubentonii, M. blythi, Plecotus auritus, Rhinolophus hipposideros*	517/0	[17]
3	*Nyctalus noctula, Vespertillio murinus, M. blythi, M. daubentonii, M. mystacinus*	5/2 (UB-1 and UB-2 ; 9443UKR)	[10]
4	Unknown**	1/1	[7]
5	Unknown**	1/1 (Yuli, or 9397RUS)	[9]
6	*M. myotis*	300/0	After [8]
7	*N. noctula, V. murinus*	5/0	This paper
8	*Rh. ferrumequinum* – 6, *M. blythi* – 10, *M. daubentonii* – 43, *M. emarginatus* – 4, *Pipistrellus kuhlii* – 9, *P. pipistrellus* – 2, *Barbastella barbastellus* – 3, *N. noctula* – 28, *Miniopterus schreibersi* – 24	129/1 (WCBV)	[4]
9	*Myotis dasicneme* – 110, *E. serotinus* – 147, *V. murinus* – 3	260/0	This paper
10	Unknown	15/0	After [8]
11	*P. auritus*	2/0	This paper
12	*Otonycteris hemprichi*	1/0	This paper
13	*N. noctula, P. pipistrellus, E. serotinus* and other unknown species	527/6	[6]
14	*Rh. ferrumequinum* – 59, *M. blythi* – 16	75/0	This paper
15	*Rh. ferrumequinum* – 15, *Rh. hipposideros* – 2, *M. blythi* – 58, *M. mystacinus* – 1, *P. austriacus* – 27, *B. leucomelas* – 5	108/1 (KHUV)	[3]
16	*Rh. ferrumequinum* -18, *Rh. bocharicus* – 1, *Rh. hipposideros* – 6, *M. blythi* – 95, *M. emarginatus* – 2, *E. serotinus* – 103, *E. bottae* – 3, *P. pipistrellus* – 26, *Hypsugo savii* – 5, *P. austriacus* – 1, *B. leucomelas* – 5, *O. hemprichi* – 1, *Tadarida teniotis* – 3	269/1 (ARAV)	[3]
17	*N. noctula*	452/0	[24]
18	*P. pipistrellus* – 1, *M. blythi* – 26	27/0	This paper

Table 1 : (continued)

19	*V. murinus*- 31, *M. daubentonii* -22	53/1 (Omsk Bat, or 1150)	[8] with additions
20	*M. blythi* – 72, *M. daubentonii* – 13, *P. auritus* – 1	82/0	This paper
21	*M. dasycneme* – 5, *M. daubentonii* – 94, *M. brandtii* – 11, *P. auritus* – 2, *Murina leucogaster* – 18	130/1 (Novosibirsk bat, or 1157)	[8] with additions
22	*M. daubentonii* – 55, *M. brandtii* – 3, *M. ikonnikovi* – 2, *P. auritus* – 22, *E. nilssoni* – 26, *V. murinus* – 1, *M. leucogaster* – 1	110/1 (IRKV)	[4]
23	*M. daubentonii* – 8	8/0	This paper
24	*E. nilssoni* – 3, *V. murinus* – 79, *Vespertilio sp.* – 18	100/0	After [8]
25	*E. nilssoni*	4/1 (Olekma)	[11]
26	*M. daubentonii* – 27, *V. murinus* – 1	28/0	After [8]
27	*M. cappaccini* – 3, *M. shreibersi* – 34	37/0	After [8]
28	*M. daubentonii, M. brandtii, P. auritus, M. leucogaster*	88/24	[12]
	Total	**3335/40**	

* Numerator – number tested, denominator – number positive.

** Viruses isolated from human infection acquired from bats.

Eight years later, in 1985, a second case (and the last registered in the territory of the FSU) of bat-transmitted human rabies occurred in Russia, close to the Ukrainian border, in the town of Belgorod. The story was similar to the 1977 case: an 11-year-old girl was attacked and bitten on her upper lip by a bat. No diagnosis was performed because the bat escaped and the species was not determined. The girl did not apply for rabies prophylaxis and developed the disease after approximately three weeks. The virus was studied with panels of N-mAbs, and was found to be representative of EBLV-1 [9]. The isolate was referred to as Yuli virus or 9397RUS in a number of publications.

In 1988, five carcasses of noctule (*Nyctalus noctula*) and parti-coloured (*Vespertilio murinus*) bats were collected in Western Ukraine, and two lyssavirus isolates were obtained (one from each bat species). Both viruses were described as EBLV-1 representatives. Their antigenic patterns were identical to each other and to those of the Yuli isolate [10,18]. The viruses were referred to as Ukrainian Bat virus 1 and 2 (UB-1 and UB-2). UB-2 was sequenced and submitted to GenBank as 9443UKR (U89465).

The UB-1 isolate was later sequenced at the Veterinary Laboratories Agency in the United Kingdom, and the EBLV-2 sequence was obtained [19]: GenBank record RV264 (AY212119). Quite likely, given the geographical location of this isolate (which is quite distinct from other EBLV-2 records), the isolation circumstances, the

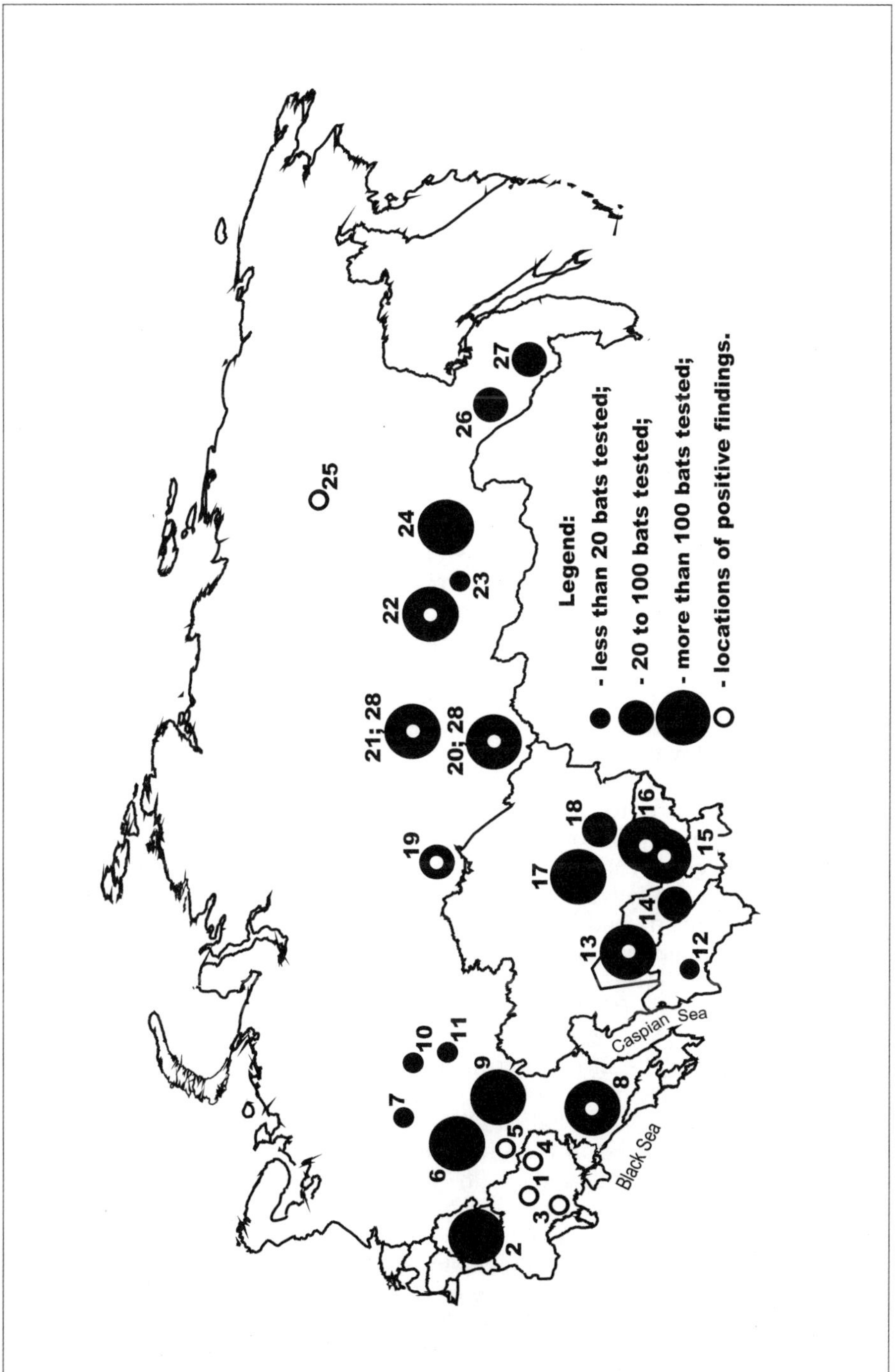

Fig. 1: The map of bat surveillance as described in the text and Table 1.

bat species, the initial antigenic typing with N-mAbs, and the further history of transfer from one laboratory to another with subsequent passages, either this virus was contaminated before sequencing, or an error of database transcription occurred.

Other limited surveillance in the European part of the FSU yielded negative results, except for the isolation of WCBV in 2002. This virus was obtained from the brain of an apparently healthy Schreibers's bat (*Miniopterus schreibersi*) during a field survey [4].

In the Asian part of the FSU, the first data on bat rabies was reported from Uzbekistan in 1976 [6]. However, this communication is considered questionable, because the author did not describe the isolation and identification methods. Moreover, rabies was reported in a wide variety of mammals (including rodents), with rather high prevalence, and not confirmed by further studies. The viruses reported were not conserved for further study.

In 1981, a lyssavirus was isolated from the Daubenton's bat (*Myotis daubentoni*) captured in a cave in the south of Western Siberia (Novosibirsk province) at the end of the hibernation period [8]. The virus was isolated in mice from a portion of bat brain, with an incubation period of 9-15 days. The virus was re-isolated from another portion of the brain in a different laboratory. Positive fluorescence with typical lyssavirus inclusions was detected in the mouse brain impressions. Additionally, the virus was neutralized with commercial polyclonal anti-rabies globulin, and was considered to be RABV. The isolate was referred to as 1157, or Novosibirsk Bat virus. However, sequencing of the virus N gene identified only the presence of a fixed laboratory rabies virus strain (CVS). Thus, it is not possible to determine whether the isolation was a primary laboratory mistake, or whether the original virus was contaminated by CVS during further mouse passages.

A similar situation occurred with another isolate obtained from the particoloured bat in the town of Omsk, Western Siberia [8]. In October 1984, the bat entered an administrative building, was captured and placed in a refrigerator for hibernation. After transfer to ambient conditions during spring, the animal was fed by insects and appeared well for a few days. Thereafter, it became weak and died. The virus was isolated repeatedly from two portions of the brain and from the spinal cord, and the presence of lyssavirus antigen was demonstrated in suspensions of the bat brain, salivary glands and brown fat. From the first mice passages, the virus demonstrated a short incubation period of between five and seven days. The isolate was referred to as 1150, or Omsk Bat virus. However, as in the previous case, N gene sequencing revealed RNA of the CVS strain. It was impossible to determine whether results of N-mAb identification were obtained from the original isolate or the contaminated sample [8,20]. Experimental inoculations of bats were performed with the contaminated specimen of 1150 [21,22].

A third Siberian bat isolate, called Olekma, was obtained from a northern bat (*Eptesicus nillsoni*) captured in a mine in the Olekma district of Yakutia at the beginning of the hibernation period in 1987 [11]. The bat specimens were delivered and processed together with a collection of Arctic fox (*Alopex lagopus*) samples, some of which were identifed as positive for RABV (Arctic virus variant). The virus was isolated from one of five inoculated mice and demonstrated properties of Arctic RABV circulating in the same region among terrestrial mammals, including a positive reaction with N-MAb P-41. The isolate was lost quickly, and it was impossible to say whether it was a primary error, further cross-contamination, or an original bat isolate. The original brain was not tested by other methods.

In summary, it is not possible to confirm the presumed bat lyssavirus isolates obtained from the Asian part of the FSU prior to 1991, and no original or low-passage samples are available for further investigation.

Two interesting lyssaviruses were discovered during the course of an active bat survey in Central Asia. The first, ARAV, was isolated in Southern Kyrgyzstan during 1991 from the lesser mouse-eared bat (*Myotis blythi*). The second virus, KHUV, was obtained in Northern Tajikistan in 2001 from the whiskered bat (*Myotis mystacinus*). Although the isolation site of KHUV was only 260 km from that of ARAV, these viruses demonstrated quite different antigenic patterns and phylogenetic relations. Implementation of different phylogenetic methods to distinct genome fragments suggested that KHUV was mainly related to EBLV-2. In contrast, ARAV, was related to KHUV, but demonstrated moderate similarity to DUVV, EBLV-1 and EBLV-2. According to previous deliberation and present classification criteria, both viruses should be considered as new putative genotypes of the genus [3]. Both viruses were isolated from apparently healthy bats. This finding may be related to the end of an incubation period or the very beginning of clinical disease manifestations. The only suggestion of abnormal behaviour in the bat which was the KHUV source was that it did not attempt to escape when captured by hand on the wall of a house. No carcasses were found in the bat roosts during field surveys.

Another surprising finding occurred in 2002 in the town of Irkutsk (Eastern Siberia). A male of the greater tube-nosed bat (*Murina leucogaster*) entered an apartment building, was captured and maintained in captivity. No abnormal behaviour was noted at first, and the bat consumed insects and water. Thereafter it became sluggish, rejected food and water, and died, approximately 10 days after capture, with signs of generalized weakness. The brain appeared positive for lyssavirus antigen, and further isolation in mice was also successful. Genetic sequencing suggested that the virus, named IRKV, was related to DUVV and EBLV-1. The amount of genetic diversity suggested that IRKV should be considered as another new lyssavirus genotype [4]. Remarkably, the Irkutsk province was believed to be rabies-free for at least 35 years prior to the IRKV isolation. Previous bat rabies surveillance, sporadically performed since 1979 (Table 1) revealed negative results, although "suspicious", sick or dead bats were predominantly sacrificed for virological studies.

Unusual communications on bat rabies in Western Siberia appeared in ProMed mail in 2003 (Archive # 20030525.1291). Of 18 *Myotis daubentonii* collected in the caves of the province of Novosibirsk and the Altay region, six (33 %) were reported as positive for lyssavirus antigen detection in the brain, by fluorescent antibody test. The viruses were preliminarily described as RABV representatives. This report was extended further. In total, the authors collected 88 hibernating bats. The brains of 24 (27.3 %) were positive for lyssavirus antigen, and 17 (19.3 %) were positive by RT-PCR performed using internal N gene primers. Mouse inoculation revealed encephalitic signs in a limited number of animals (such as bristled fur, humped back and lack of coordination). The authors observed lyssavirus antigen in the mouse brain impressions examined by DFAT, but RT-PCR tests of mouse brains, performed using the same primers, were negative. During the next intracerebral passages the number of mice demonstrating encephalitic signs was reduced, and all isolates except one were eliminated [12].

A partial N gene sequence was obtained for seven isolates (positions 319 to 856 according to the Pasteur virus genome). At least for one of them (BAT-BN1) the sequence was compared with other RABVs, originating from different regions of the world and belonging to different phylogenetic lineages. The bat isolate was clearly placed within the clade of terrestrial RABVs in the surrounding territory of Western Siberia, including samples obtained from small canids, a badger, a cat and a human (exposed to a fox). This clade subsequently belonged to the generic 'dog-fox' RABV cluster circulating worldwide, and was quite distinguishable from the American RABV lineages. The authors proposed that bats in Western Siberia maintain circulation of the same RABVs that persist among terrestrial mammals, and virus transmission between those hosts may be realized via the food chain [13].

Discussion

Bat rabies is not common, and is not easily documented without adequate modern laboratory-based surveillance. Passive surveillance of abnormal bats, or bats involved in human exposure, is performed infrequently by the local veterinary laboratories of the FSU. This system of passive surveillance allows neither for extensive identification of lyssavirus isolates by local veterinary laboratories nor for identification of bat species. The transfer of positive samples to specialized research laboratories, where such studies can be performed, is not readily supported due to a number of legal limitations. For this reason, veterinary records are difficult to obtain for verification and interpretation.

Active surveillance has been performed sporadically by some research teams. In most cases, virus prevalence in bat populations has been found to be limited. For example, our tests of 1,424 bats yielded only four (0.28 %) to 6 (0.42 %) isolates (depending on assessments of the isolates 1150 and 1157, as a primary mistake or further contamination). A number of surveys yielded no isolates at all (Table 1). In this regard, the records of ~ 27.3 % rabid bats from Western Siberia [12,13], with inconsistent results of virus isolation and RNA detection, and with sequencing of the fox RABV variant from the bat sample, need to be corroborated.

Four new lyssaviruses, ARAV, KHUV, IRKV and WCBV, are the only representatives confirmed to date. There is no information about their host range, distribution and circulation properties, because only a single isolate of each virus is available. Serological testing of bat sera is useful for establishing the baseline distribution of lyssaviruses. However, this survey should be performed carefully, taking into account cross-antigenic reactivity of different lyssaviruses. For example, low titres of antibody to EBLVs, ARAV, KHUV and IRKV may be easily missed if RABV or another heterologous virus is used as a target for detection. The WCBV demonstrated no neutralizing cross-reactivity with other lyssaviruses [23]. Hence, to determine antibody against this virus, it alone should be used for comparison. We do not know what amount of cross-reactivity one may expect if encountering antibody to some other undescribed lyssavirus.

Another lesson from the discovery of new lyssaviruses addresses the dilemma of appropriate surveillance using PCR-based methods only, as practised in a number of European countries during the past few years. Without universal molecular diagnostic reagents, one can never be sure that the design of primers is adequate, and whether or not they will react with new viruses. If divergent representatives, such as WCBV, are present in a field sample, they may be missed. Virus isolation accompanied by further diagnostic identification is an important consideration for such surveillance. Also, given the example of IRKV isolation, it is not possible to consider any territory truly rabies-free, based only on the apparent absence of infection in other mammals.

Two human rabies cases of bat origin were registered, and one of them (Belgorod, 1985) was identified as EBLV-1 [9]. It is incorrect to describe the other case (Voroshilovgrad, 1977) as EBLV [1], because the isolate was not subjected to typing. For example, this case could be WCBV (since the isolation point of this virus lies close to Voroshilovgrad) or another lyssavirus, yet to be described. Indeed, some human cases may be misdiagnosed for a number of reasons [3].

To date, the investigations on bat rabies performed in the FSU have not been adequate. Further passive and active surveillance should be undertaken, recruiting the experience and strategies developed elsewhere in Europe and abroad, and introducing the most suitable methods for new lyssavirus detection. The monitoring of encephalitis with unknown aetiology should be established in humans and veterinary species for enhanced pathogen discovery.

Acknowledgements

The authors thank J.S. Smith (CDC, Atlanta, GA, U.S.A.), L.M. McElhinney, N. Johnson (VLA, Waybridge, U.K.), Y.T. Arai (National Institute for Infectious Diseases, Tokyo, Japan) for independent sequencing of the 1150 and 1157 isolates to confirm the presence of CVS RABV strain. We appreciate the help of our colleagues and the numerous staff members of the local sanitary-epidemiological and veterinary institutions, during our field trips and laboratory trials. This study was supported in part by the Russian Foundation for Basic Research (project 00-04-48004) and the Association of Public Health Laboratories (International EID fellowship, 2002-2005). We thank OIE for the opportunity to present our data at this conference.

References

1 Fooks AR, Brookes SM, Johnson N, McElhinney LM, Hutson AM: European bat lyssaviruses: an emerging zoonosis. Epidemiol Infect 2003; 131: 1029-1039.

2 Kuzmin IV, Niezgoda M, Carroll DS, Keeler N, Hossain MJ, Breiman RF, Ksiazek TG, Rupprecht CE: Lyssavirus surveillance in bats from Bangladesh. Emerg Infect Dis 2006; 12: 486-488.

3 Kuzmin IV, Orciari LA, Arai YT, Smith JS, Hanlon CA, Kameoka Y, Rupprecht CE: Bat lyssaviruses (Aravan and Khujand) from Central Asia: phylogenetic relationships according to N, P and G gene sequences. Virus Res 2003; 97: 65-79.

4 Botvinkin AD, Poleschuk EM, Kuzmin IV, Borisova TI, Gazaryan SV, Yager P, Rupprecht CE: Novel lyssavirus isolated from bats in Russia. Emerg Infect Dis 2003; 9 (12): 1623-1625.

5 Ryaboshapka AP, Krolevetskaia NM: Investigation of biological properties of the rabies virus isolated from insectivorous bat, in Proceedings of session 13 of the Polio Institute meeting on the actual problems of virology and specific prophylaxis of viral diseases. Polio Institute. Moscow, 1967, pp 80-81 (in Russ).

6 Mamatov NM: Virological surveillance of wild and domestic animals on rabies in different landscape zones of Uzbekistan, Jubilee conference for the 50th anniversary of the Uzbek Scientific Research Veterinary Institute. Abstracts. Tayliak, 1976, vol 1, pp 174-176 (in Russ).

7 Scherbak YuN: Epidemiology of natural rabies. Thesis dissertation for D Sc degree, Kiev, 1982, 38 p (in Russ).

8 Botvinkin AD: The results of a study on the role of bats in the circulation of rabies in the USSR, in Chiroptera. Morphology, ecology, echolocation, parazites, protection. Proceedings of the USSR seminar. Kiev, Naukova Dumka, 1988, pp 138-141 (in Russ).

9 Selimov MA, Tatarov AG, Botvinkin AD, Klueva EV, Kulikova LG, Khismatullina NA: Rabies-related Yuli-virus; identification with a panel of monoclonal antibodies. Acta Virol 1989; 33: 542-545.

10 Selimov MA, Smechov AM, Antonova LA, Klueva EV, Kulikova LG: New strains of rabies-related viruses isolated from bats in the Ukraine. Acta Virol 1991; 35: 226-231.

11 Khozinski VV, Selimov MA, Botvinkin AD, King AA, Antonova LA, Smekhov AM, Shablovskaia EA, Klueva EV, Aksenova TA: Rabies virus of bat origin in the USSR. Rabies Bulletin Europe 1991; 14:10-11.

12 Zaikovskaia AI, Ternovoy VA, Tomilenko AA, Rassadkin YuV, Aksenov VI, Shestopalov AM: Lyssaviruses of bats inhabiting the south of Western Siberia. J Infectious Pathology 2004; 11: 70-73 (in Russ).

13 Zaikovskaia AV, Ternovo VA, Aksenov VI, Rassadkin IuN, Shestopalov AM: Molecular genetic characterization of rabies virus, isolated in Western Siberia. Vestnik Rossiyskoy Akademii Medicinskih Nauk 2005; 2:30-35.

14 Meslin F-X, Kaplan MM, Koprowski H (eds): Laboratory techniques in rabies. Geneva, World Health Organization, 1996, 476 p.

15 Wiktor TJ, Koprowski H: Monoclonal antibodies against rabies virus produced by somatic cell hybridization: detection of antigenic variants. Proc Natl Acad Sci USA 1978; 75: 3938-3942.

16 Distribution of rabies in Europe. Rabies Bulletin Europe 2004; 28: 11-24.

17 Anina-Radchenko ND, Korchmar ND, Glushko LV: Rabies of wild animals. Veterinary 1970; 10: 64-65 (in Russ).

18 King AA: Monoclonal antibody studies on rabies-related viruses. Onderstepoort J Vet Res 1993; 60: 283: 287.

19 Johnson N, Selden D, Parsons G, Healy D, Brookes SM, McElhinney LM, Hutson AM, Fooks AR: Isolation of a European bat lyssavirus type 2 from a Daubenton's bat in the United Kingdom. Vet Rec 2003; 152: 383-387.

20 King A, Davies P, Lawrie A: The rabies viruses of bats. Vet Microbiol 1990; 23: 165-174.

21 Botvinkin AD, Kuzmin IV, Chernov SM: Experimental inoculation of bats with lyssaviruses serotypes 1 and 4. Voprosy Virusologii 1994; 4: 215-218 (in Russ).

22 Kuzmin IV, Botvinkin AD: The behaviour of bats *Pipistrellus pipistrellus* after experimental inoculation with rabies and rabies-like viruses and some aspects of pathogenesis. Myotis 1996; 34: 93-99.

23 Hanlon CA, Kuzmin IV, Blanton JD, Weldon WC, Manangan JS, Rupprecht CE: Efficacy of rabies biologics against new lyssaviruses from Eurasia. Virus Res 2005; 111: 44-54.

24 Sansyzbaev BK: Nozoareal and structure of the rabies natural focus in Kazakhstan, in Problems of medical geography of Kazakhstan. Materials of action of medical geography of the 1st Congress of geographers of Kazakhstan, April 14-16, 1980. Alma-Ata, 1980, pp 55-60 (in Russ).

Dr. I. Kuzmin, Centers for Disease Control and Prevention, 1600 Clifton Rd, Bldg 17, MS G-33, Atlanta, GA 30333, USA.
E-mail: ikuzmin@cdc.gov

Dodet B, Schudel A, Pastoret PP, Lombard M (eds): Rabies in Europe.
Dev Biol (Basel). Basel, Karger, 2006, vol 125, pp 283-288.

Bat Rabies Surveillance in France, from 1989 through May 2005

E. Picard-Meyer, J. Barrat, E. Tissot, A. Verdot, C. Patron, M.J. Barrat, F. Cliquet

Laboratory of Research on Rabies and Wildlife Diseases, OIE, World Health Organization Collaborating Centre for Research and management in Zoonoses Control, Community Reference Institute for Rabies Serology, AFSSA Nancy, Laboratoire d'études et de recherches sur la rage et la pathologie des animaux sauvages, Malzéville, France

Key words: Rabies, lyssavirus, bat.

Abstract: In France, the passive surveillance of lyssaviruses in bats started in 1989, with the first positive case found in the East of the country. In 2000, the French bat rabies surveillance network in France was improved on the basis of the one used for the surveillance of fox rabies. The objectives of this network are to improve bat rabies surveillance by increasing the number of specimens and to provide an estimation of rabies incidence in bat populations across the country. The surveillance network is principally constituted by the network of local Veterinary Services and by the National Bat Conservationists Network (French Society for the Study and Protection of Mammals).
From 1989 to through 2004, 21 autochtonous rabies cases were diagnosed out of the 934 French bat cadavers found. The laboratory techniques used for diagnosis, recommended by WHO and OIE, were fluorescent antibody test (FAT), rabies tissue culture infection test (RTCIT) on murine neuroblastoma cells, and the mouse inoculation test (MIT). All 21 cases were diagnosed in serotine bats *(Eptesicus serotinus)* and were due to European bat lyssavirus type 1 (EBLV-1), genotype 5, infection.

The genus *Lyssavirus* within the family *Rhabdoviridae* is subdivided into seven genotypes comprised of classical rabies virus (RV, genotype 1) and rabies-related viruses (RRVs, genotypes 2 to 7) [1]. Recently, four additional RRVs isolated from bats in Eurasia have been proposed as new members of the genus *Lyssavirus* [2,3].

In Europe, bat rabies is caused by two specific virus genotypes, EBLV-1 (genotype 5) and EBLV-2 (genotype 6) [1], identified in several European bat species. From 1957 to 2004, more than 700 infected bats were found in Europe and more than 95 % of the rabid bats were identified as *Eptesicus serotinus*. All infection in *Eptesicus serotinus* was caused by EBLV-1 [4], while EBLV-2 appears to infect only *Myotis* species. Infected bats have been reported throughout Europe, from Russia to Spain, particularly in coastal regions, in The Netherlands, Germany, Denmark, Poland, Spain, The United Kingdom, Switzerland, Ukraine, and France. In France, the first case of a bat infected by EBLV-1 was found in 1989.

The passive surveillance of bat rabies in France was enhanced in 2000 following the request of the Direction Générale de l'Alimentation (French Ministry of Agriculture). The ultimate objective of this program consists of estimating public health risks linked to the infection of autochthonous bats by lyssavirus and consists of the following activities:

1 to increase the number of bat rabies tests performed to improve surveillance of rabies in all parts of the country,

2 to estimate the prevalence of rabies disease in the sub-population of French bat cadavers analysed at the Agence Française de Sécurité Sanitaire des Aliments – Laboratoire d'Etudes et de Recherches sur la Rage et la Pathologie des Animaux Sauvages (AFSSA-LERRPAS) and Pasteur Institute, Paris, and

3 to provide biological samples for the study of lyssavirus pathogenicity.

The bat rabies surveillance network is an adaptation of the general system for fox rabies surveillance which has been in place since the 1970s. This network is passive, based on a collection of bat cadavers found in human environments, as well as other animals that have been in contact with humans. This network regroups the French Departmental Directions of Veterinary Services (DDSV) and associative network of volunteer bat handlers within the French Society for the Study and the Protection of Mammals (SFEPM). In case of human contamination (bite, scratch or licking), bat cadavers are sent by the DDSV to the Pasteur Institute (National Reference Centre for Rabies), Paris, for rabies testing. In all other cases, they are submitted by the SFEPM or DDSV to AFSSA (National Reference Laboratory for Rabies Epidemiology) for rabies testing.

Three methods of laboratory diagnosis of rabies, standardised and recommended by the the World Health Organisation (WHO) [5] and the World Organisation for Animal Health (OIE) [6] are routinely used at AFSSA: the fluorescent antibody test (FAT), the rabies tissue culture infection test (RTCIT) and the mouse inoculation test (MIT). As a complement to these three techniques, hemi-nested reverse transcriptase-polymerase chain reaction (hnRT-PCR) is used to detect viral RNA in each bat brain. and RT-PCR is carried out, as described previously [7], with universal primers described by Heaton et al [8] which are able to detect the RNA of all seven genotypes of RV and RRVs. The second PCR is performed with specific primers JW12 and Jebl1 and specifically detects the two isoforms a and b of EBLV-1 [7]. In case of positive diagnosis, the RT-PCR method is followed by the sequencing of amplified products for RV or RRV typing. Necessary safety measures are applied to prevent any cross-contamination and false positive results when using PCR.

From 1989 through May 2005, 21 out of a total of 968 found bat cadavers were diagnosed rabid both by AFSSA and the Institute Pasteur, Paris. All were identified as serotine bats and shown infected by the two isoforms EBLV-1 a and b.

From January 1st, 2001 the first year following the improvement of national bat rabies surveillance), until the end of May 2005, a total of 821 dead bats were submitted to AFSSA for rabies testing. Out of 821 bats collected, 33 were exotic (especially *Rousettus sp*) and 788 autochthonous. For this period, classical rabies detection methods were not performed on 157 out the 788 autochthonous bats cadavers received by AFSSA, due principally to the high level of decomposition of the carcasses. A total of nine out of 622 autochthonous bat cadavers were found to be infected with EBLV-1 ; all cases were isolated in *Eptesicus serotinus*. Over the same period, 133 autochthonous bat cadavers sent to Pasteur Institute, Paris, were investigated for rabies diagnosis: 126 were found negative, and 3 serotine bats were shown to be EBLV-1 positive by referenced techniques.

Recently, on May 18, 2005, one bat rabies case was reported, by the Pasteur Institute, Paris, in a serotine bat, shown to be infected with EBLV-1 isoform b. Studies were conducted on the bat, three days before its death, in close collaboration between two bat handlers of the SFEPM and AFSSA. Molecular biology techniques (hnRT-PCR followed by the sequencing of amplified products) and referenced rabies diagnostic methods (RTCIT, MIT) were performed on the saliva sample. Virus isolation on Neuro2a cells and MIT gave negative results while hnRT-PCR showed the presence of EBLV-1b nucleoprotein RNA in the saliva (unpublished data).

From 2001 through May 2005, 24 bat species were submitted to AFSSA for rabies testing. The 24 species collected represent the three families of Chiropteras: *Molossidae* (n = 4), *Rhinolophidae* (n = 24) and *Vespertilionidae* (n = 760 collected with 74 serotine bats). No case of rabies was found in *Pipistrellus pipistrellus.* Out of 338 common pipistrelle cadavers received, 259 tested negative, and 80 were not diagnosed due to the high decomposition of cadavers.

The 812 bat cadavers sent to AFSSA-Nancy since 2001 have come from all 22 regions of France, with high variability between regions. Before the bat rabies surveillance system was improved (from 1998 to 2000), only 57 bat cadavers from 16 different regions had been submitted for diagnosis to AFSSA.

The number of bat cadavers sent to the two French laboratories distinctly increased between January 2001 and December 2004 (Fig. 1). The number of autochthonous bat cadavers submitted increased ten-fold (from 1989 to 2000 about twenty animals were tested *vs* 218 in 2004) (Figure 1). It is important to note that the increase of autochthonous bat cadavers submitted to AFSSA for rabies testing was also accompanied by an increase in putrefied bats, which could not be analysed in 2002 and 2003 (about 20 % per year). Twenty-four out of the 33 species reported in France were submitted for analysis between 2001 and 2004. The increase of autochthonous bat cadavers submitted for rabies testing between 2001 and 2004 is not accompanied by an increase in the submission of *Eptesicus serotinus* or *Myotis daubentonii* (only 9 out of 12 bat cadavers were analysed in this study), species which are predominantly associated with EBLV-1 and EBLV-2 isolates, respectively. It is also necessary to note that the passive surveillance is biased and may lack sensitivity. Indeed, the proportion of serotine bats as well as *Myotis* sp. submitted for diagnosis is under-represented compared with the estimation of bat populations in France.

Rabies in bats and in mammals has a long history, the oldest recorded descriptions of the disease were found in Mesopotamia over 4,300 years ago. Molecular studies have estimated that lyssaviruses may have originated from an insect rhabdovirus which bats contracted from insects some 7,080 to 11,631 years ago and that lyssaviruses moved from the order *Chiroptera* to the order *Carnivora* between 888 and 1459 years ago [9]. Though bat rabies is widespread in Europe with hundreds of positive cases recorded in several European countries (17 countries between 1954 and 2001 reported bat rabies cases [10,4]), it is rarely transmitted to terrestrial mammals. EBLV-1 was isolated from several Danish sheep between 1998 and 2002 [11] and from a German stone marten [12]. So far, between 1977 and 2002, four fatal human cases have been reported [13]. Our knowledge of EBLV transmission

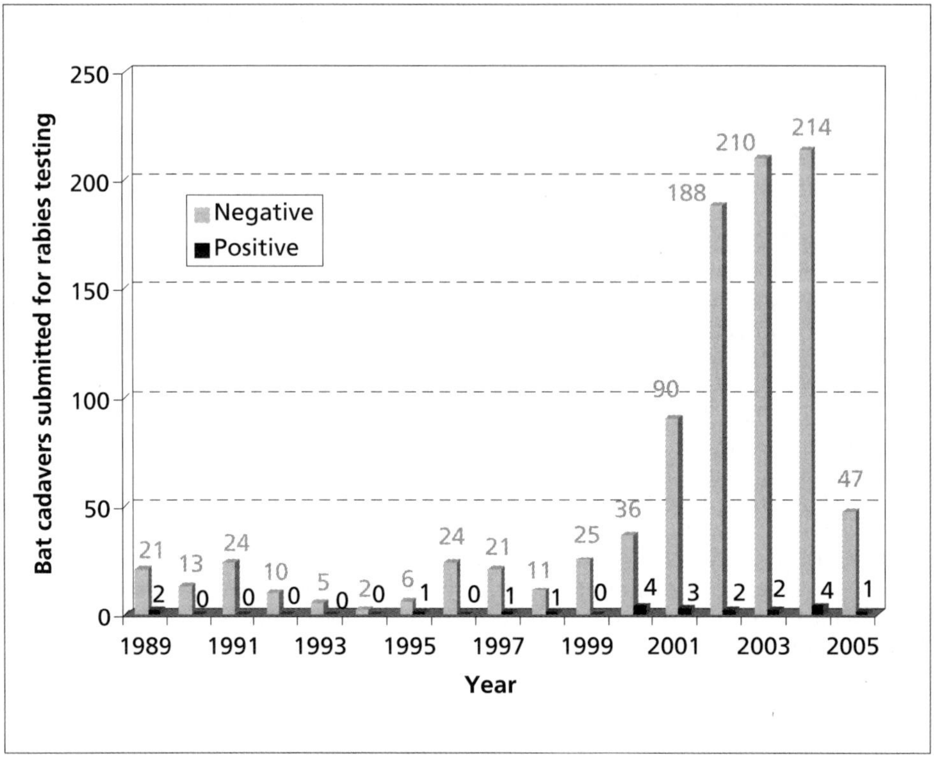

Fig. 1: Evolution of the number of autochthonous bat cadavers submitted to AFSSA and Pasteur Institute, Paris, for rabies testing from September 1989 through May, 2005.

between bats and the spill-over infections in terrestrial mammals is limited. At the present time, few investigations have been conducted in European bats. The Netherlands is one of the few countries to actively survey infected bat cadavers: between 1986 and 2001, 250 positive cases were reported in this country [10]. Continuing passive surveillance of rabies in bats, with closer collaboration between bat biologists and rabies scientists, is necessary to trace spill-over transmission from reservoir species to non-reservoir animals. Active "surveillance" should be initiated to complement passive surveillance in close collaboration between bat handlers and laboratory scientists. The final objective of active surveillance, with the collection of oropharyngeal samples and micro-samples of blood, is to fully assess the prevalence and the epidemiology of EBLV-1 in bat populations.

EBLV-1 is the only lyssavirus that has been detected in France, with the first reported case in 1989. Twenty-one cases of infection with EBLV-1 have been reported, all occurring in *Eptesicus serotinus*. An additional case was recorded in May 1999 on a tropical bat, *Rousettus aegyptiacus*. This exotic bat, that was imported from Africa via Belgium and sold in a pet shop in Bordeaux, was shown to be infected by Lagos bat virus genotype 2 [14,15] (Fig. 2).

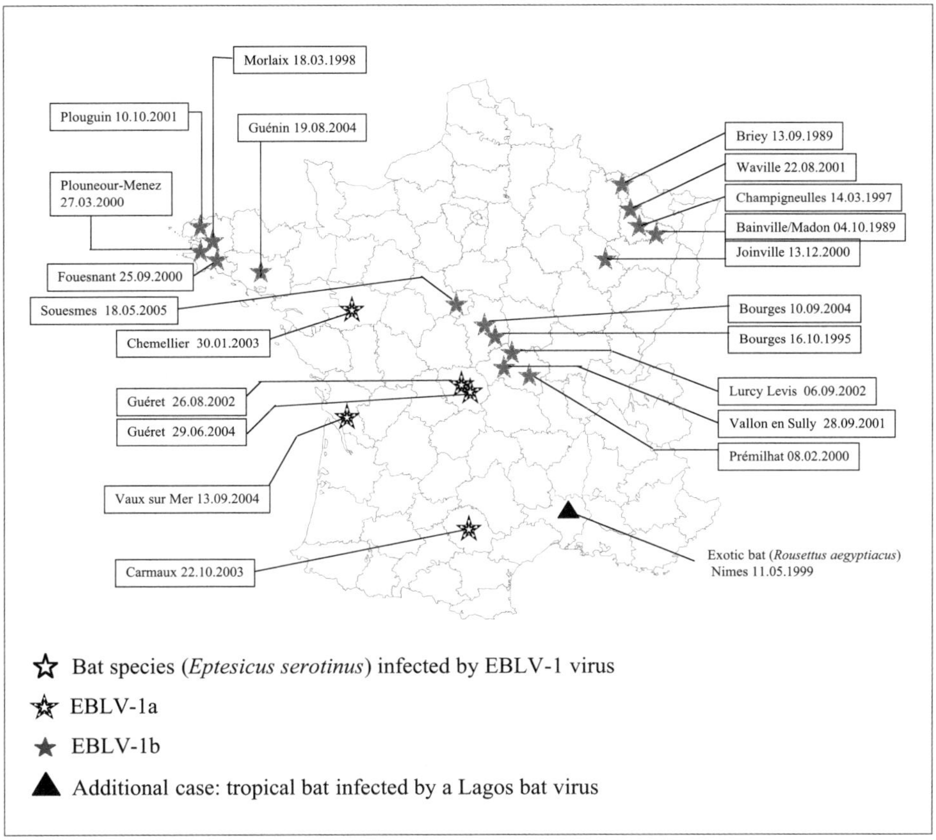

Fig. 2: Geographical distribution of rabies in bats in France: 21 cases of rabies were identified in autochthonous bats from 1989 through May 2005.
Since 1989, 21 *Eptesicus serotinus'* have been found infected by European Bat Lyssavirus type 1 in France. Isoforms a and b of EBLV-1, still called genotype 5, were identified using molecular biology techniques [7] in all isolated, rabies positive, French bats. EBLV-1a was first identified in August 2002 in France, in the region of Limousin [16], then in January and October, 2003, in two distinct regions, the Loire and Midi Pyrénées, respectively, and in June and September, 2004, in Limousin and Poitou Charente. More recently, on May 22, a serotine bat, isolated in Souesmes (a city located in the Centre of France) was diagnosed as positive with an EBLV-1b isolate by the Pasteur Institute, Paris.

Acknowledgements

We thank the Société Française pour l'Etude et la Protection des Mammifères, groupe Chiroptères for supplying bat cadaver specimens and the local Directions of Veterinary Services. We especially thank Laurent Arthur, François Moutou, Michèle Lemaire and François Schwaab for their active collaboration in this study.

We also thank Josiane Ambert, Claudine Bujack, Marie José Duchêne and Nathalie Stroucken.

We thank the Direction Générale de l'Alimentation of the French Ministry of Agriculture for their financial support of this work.

References

1 Bourhy H, Kissi B, Tordo N: Molecular diversity of the lyssavirus genus. Virology 1993; 194: 70-81.

2 Arai Y, Kuzmin I, Kameoka Y, Botvinkin A: New lyssavirus genotype for the lesser Mouse-Eared bat (Myotis blythi), Kyrghystan. Emerg Infec Dis 2003; 9: 333-337.

3 Kuzmin IV, Orciari LA, Arai YT, Smith JS, Hanlon CA, Kameoka Y, Rupprecht CE: Bat *Lyssaviruses* (Aravan and Khujand) from Central Asia: phylogenetic relationships according to N, P and G gene sequences. Virus Res. 2003; 97: 65-79.

4 Müller WW: Review of reported rabies case data in Europe to the WHO Collaborating Centre Tübingen from 1977 to 2000. Rabies Bulletin Europe 2000; 24: 11-19

5 WHO Expert Committee on Rabies, Technical Report Series. Eight Report, N°824. Geneva: World Health Organization 1992, 84 pages.

6 Cliquet F, Barrat J: Rabies, in Manual of Diagnostics Tests and Vaccines for Terrestrial Animals (mammals, birds and bees). Paris, Fifth edition, World Organisation for Animal Health, 2004, vol 1, pp 328-346.

7 Picard E, Bruyere V, Barrat J, Tissot E, Barrat MJ, Cliquet F: Development of a hemi nested RT-PCR method for the specific determination of European Bat *Lyssavirus* 1. Comparison with other rabies diagnostic methods. Vaccine 2004; 22: 1921-1929.

8 Heaton P, Johnstone P, Mc Elhinney L, Cowley R, O'Sullivan, E, Whitby J: Heminested PCR assay for detection of six genotypes of rabies and rabies related viruses. J Clin Microbiol 1997; 35: 2762-2766.

9 Badrane H Bahloul C, Perrin P, Tordo N: Evidence of two lyssavirus phylogroups with distinct pathogenicity and immunogenicity. J Virol 2001; 75: 3268-3276.

10 King AA, Haagsma J, Kappeler A: Lyssavirus infections in European bats, in King AA, Fooks AR, Aubert M, Wandeler AI (eds): Historical Perspective of Rabies in Europe and the Mediterranean Basin. Office Internationale des Epizooties, 2004, Chapter 17, pp 221-242.

11 Ronsholt L: A new case of European bat *Lyssavirus* (EBL) infection in Danish sheep. Rabies Bulletin Europe 2002; 26: 9.

12 Müller T, Cox J, Peter W, Bodamer P, Wulle U, Burow J, Müller W: Infection of a stone marten with European bat *Lyssavirus* (EBL1). Rabies Bulletin Europe 2001; 25: 9-11.

13 Fooks AR, Brookes SM, Johnson N, Mc Elhinney LM, Hutson AM: European bat lyssaviruses: an emergent zoonosis. Epidemiol Infect 2003; 131: 1029-1039.

14 Aubert M, Lemarignier O, Gibon C, Alvado-Brette M, Brie P, Rosenthal F: Un cas de rage dans le Gard sur une Roussette d'Egypte considérée comme animal familier. Bulletin Epidémiologique Mensuel de la Rage Animale en France, 1999; 29: 1-17.

15 Picard E, Barrat J, Wasniewski M, Wandeler A, Nadin Davis S, Lowings JP, Fooks AR, Mc Elhinney L, Bruyere V, Cliquet F: Epidemiology of rabid bats in France, 1989 to 2002. Vet Rec 2004; 155: 774-777.

16 Picard E, Barrat J, Bruyere V, Barrat MJ, Cliquet F: Genetic analysis of European bat *Lyssavirus* Type 1 isolates from France. Vet Rec 2004; 154: 589-595.

Dr. E. Picard-Meyer, Laboratory of Research on Rabies and Wildlife Diseases, AFSSA Nancy, Laboratoire d'études et de recherches sur la rage et la pathologie des animaux sauvages, BP 9, FR-54220 Malzéville, France.
E-mail: e.picard@nancy.afssa.fr

Dodet B, Schudel A, Pastoret PP, Lombard M (eds): Rabies in Europe.
Dev Biol (Basel). Basel, Karger, 2006, vol 125, p 289.

Conclusions and Recommendations

Dodet B, Schudel A, Pastoret PP, Lombard M (eds): Rabies in Europe.
Dev Biol (Basel). Basel, Karger, 2006, vol 125, pp 291-296.

The Prevention, Control and Eradication of Rabies in Europe

First International Conference "Rabies in Europe"
Kiev, Ukraine, 15-18 June 2005

CONSIDERING THAT

The World Health Organization (WHO) recommendations and requirements and the World Organisation for Animal Health (OIE) standards are relevant tools for the control of rabies in humans and animals and should be continually updated.

During the past few years, Europe has witnessed the re-emergence of several infectious animal diseases, including rabies, in some regions that have had a major impact on animal and human health.

New scientific and technological knowledge for the prevention and detection of rabies could contribute to the development of safer and more efficacious vaccines, diagnostic tests and preventive and control methods.

For ethical, ecological and economical reasons, it is no longer acceptable to control and eradicate disease outbreaks mainly through the mass slaughtering of animals.

The OIE, as well as the WHO, the European Union (EU) and other national administrations and organizations have recognized the important threat posed by the presence of rabies in Europe.

The International Conference in Kiev provided information on the valuable experience, gained through combating the re-emergence of rabies in some parts of Europe, in the control and elimination of rabies and other significant animal diseases and zoonoses through the use of appropriate strategies and standardized recommended diagnostic tests and vaccines with a strong and close partnership between veterinary and public health authorities.

The most important aim of this Conference was to bring together veterinarians, scientists, wildlife experts, clinicians and public health officials to share their experience in modern rabies control, to agree on the best strategies for the prevention and control of the disease in reservoir animal species, and to examine the threat posed by classical rabies virus and the emerging bat lyssaviruses.

The Conference was also an opportunity to evaluate and improve the current OIE standards and guidelines for better control of rabies.

For this event, the OIE acted in collaboration with the WHO, the EU, the French Food Safety Agency (AFSSA), together with the Veterinary Service of Ukraine, and the participation of stakeholders and the International Association for Biologicals (IABs). It brought together representatives of all the key rabies control and research groups from around the world including the OIE Reference Laboratories and the WHO Collaborating Centres.

CONFERENCE ATTENDEES OF THE OIE INTERNATIONAL CONFERENCE "RABIES IN EUROPE" RECOMMEND THE FOLLOWING:

Session I: Epidemiology

1. Rabies surveillance is still inadequate in many European countries and this deficit should be addressed by national authorities, with the technical support of international agencies (OIE/WHO) and with the support of the EU.
2. An effective surveillance system to collect epidemiological data on rabies in healthy "suspected" and confirmed animals must be established in each country to confirm free status. Wild animals shot during hunting or night shooting operations are not the main relevant source for disease surveillance.
3. Surveillance should be managed with a focus on laboratory confirmation and effective reporting of definite human and animal rabies cases and by examining "suspected" sick or dead animals.
4. Epidemiological data should be collected, processed, analysed and disseminated rapidly between sectors and different administrative levels (veterinary and health ministries in each country must share data systems). This work should be undertaken in designated and well-equipped provincial, national or regional laboratories. An effective surveillance network should be available to transport specimens rapidly from the field to the diagnostic laboratory, without presenting a risk for the shipment company workers. Each country should establish **one** national rabies data collection centre.
5. Reliable data reporting on the epidemiology of rabies in animals across Europe is inconsistent. In addition to OIE information systems, the *Rabies Bulletin Europe* (RBE), sponsored by WHO, is considered a pivotal source of information and decision support for rabies control. All countries should be encouraged to submit data to RBE. Support for its future existence and modernisation should continue.
6. More research programmes should be conducted concerning the epidemiology of rabies in recognised reservoir species specifically domestic dogs, foxes, raccoon dogs and bats.
7. Increased research is necessary to clarify host/virus adaptation.
8. Uncontrolled translocation of susceptible animals from rabies endemic areas should be avoided.
9. There is a need for the harmonisation of control measures between neighbouring countries.
10. The definition of the rabies status of countries should be clarified by the OIE and WHO in relation to the epidemiological situation.

Session II: Rabies diagnosis

1. Clinical diagnosis of rabies is **not** reliable. A definitive diagnosis can only be made by laboratory investigations. **Each country should establish one national rabies reference laboratory.**
2. Routine rabies laboratory diagnosis should be undertaken using only the techniques as specified by OIE and WHO. The 5th edition of the OIE *Terrestrial Manual* and the 4th edition of the "Laboratory Techniques in Rabies" (WHO) must be available to each national and provincial laboratory.
3. The recommended primary diagnostic test for rabies is the fluorescent antibody test (FAT).
4. Confirmatory diagnosis, where required, should be undertaken using the rabies tissue culture inoculation test (RTCIT). The mouse inoculation test (MIT) should only be used if tissue culture is not available.
5. Methods for rabies diagnosis in animals should be harmonised across Europe. The techniques should be standardised using regular inter-laboratory tests in compliance with OIE standards.
6. The use of the polymerase chain reaction (PCR) and other amplification techniques is **not** currently recommended for the routine diagnosis of rabies. These molecular techniques, however, can be applied to epidemiological surveys and for confirmatory diagnosis in specific circumstances and under strict quality control in national reference laboratories that routinely work with these techniques.
7. Attempts should be made to isolate viruses for the characterization of prevalent strains. The strains should be typed and compared with isolates from neighbouring countries. The data should be rapidly exchanged and the original isolates submitted to an independent laboratory for further characterisation and stored in an archive.
8. Positive samples should be shared for further characterisation.
9. Serological methods should **not** be used for routine rabies diagnosis. These tests are indirect, demonstrate past-exposure to virus only and are applicable to sero-prevalence surveys and vaccine control.
10. An infrastructure for training of personnel from national diagnostic laboratories and the exchange of personnel between reference laboratories should be established.
11. There is a need for rapid and accurate serological methods (i.e. ELISA tests) to replace currently used virus neutralisation tests (FAVN/RFFIT) for both follow-up investigations of oral vaccination campaigns and analysis of serum from vaccinated domestic carnivores in the context of international animal movements.

Session III: Animal rabies control

1. An understanding of the epidemiological situation of rabies in each country is a pre-requisite for animal rabies control measures.
2. A long-term and consistent rabies control strategy must be prepared and revised at regular intervals. This strategy should explicitly state the necessary steps for

a national rabies elimination programme in animals. This strategy should be published and copies made freely available to the general public.

3. This requires national political willingness with the assistance of international agencies (OIE/WHO) and the EU. These agencies should demonstrate a fully co-operative and integrated approach.
4. An integrated international approach, which includes when necessary appropriate financial support for rabies control in animals should be a high priority.
5. Canine rabies can be eliminated, as has been demonstrated in specific regions using mass parenteral vaccination programmes. Stray dog destruction alone is **not** fully effective in rabies eradication.
6. Further research should be undertaken on the use of oral vaccines for domestic species. Under specific circumstances, oral vaccination campaigns should be also considered as complementary measures for interrupting the rabies infectious cycle in stray animals.
7. Currently, wildlife rabies control can only be effectively undertaken using oral vaccination of reservoir species. Vaccination should be the principal method of rabies control in animals. Culling reservoir species alone is not effective.
8. The selected vaccines should meet all the efficacy and safety requirements according to procedures recommended for veterinary use and according to international standards and guidelines.
9. The bait should include a biomarker to monitor bait uptake.
10. Wherever possible, rabies control in animals should be undertaken as prescribed in currently available documents by the OIE/WHO and the EU (http://europa.eu.int/comm/food/fs/sc/scah/out80_en.pdf).
11. The success of rabies control strategies must be further monitored by follow-up investigations. The biomarker detection method is the preferred option if only a single test is available in rabies negative/susceptible animals.
12. There is an urgent requirement to finance rabies research aimed at improved control.
13. Public information needs to be improved concerning the risks of rabies.
14. Awareness of rabies should be raised among health and veterinary professionals in rabies-free countries.
15. Monitoring of reservoir species should be strengthened in countries where there is a risk of re-emergence.
16. Research aimed at the development of new biological tools should be encouraged, i.e. specific contraceptive vaccines for reservoir species.
17. There is a critical need for the establishment of an oral vaccine bank for emergency use.
18. A need exists for the development of oral vaccines/baits/delivery systems for use in all terrestrial animals.

Session IV: Human rabies prevention

1. Rabies prophylaxis in humans should be undertaken as prescribed in the WHO Expert Consultation on Rabies (series 931; 1st report, 2005, www.who.int).
2. As rabies remains a "neglected" disease, an increased awareness of human infection is needed among the medical community, as demonstrated by the recent cases of rabies following organ transplantation.
3. Additional research is required to understand the pathogenesis of rabies in humans.
4. Exchange of information and cooperation between medical and veterinary authorities must be considered a priority.
5. The production of an alternative to rabies immune globulin for passive immunization (such as monoclonal antibodies) is urgently required.
6. There is a need for clear harmonised guidelines for vaccine prophylaxis for people at high risk of rabies-related virus infection.
7. Although, post-exposure prophylaxis is considered fully effective when administered properly; cross-neutralisation/protection profiles for conventional human vaccines should be assessed against all members of the lyssavirus genus.
8. Training of personnel in rabies diagnosis in humans is needed.

Session V: Vaccinology and immunology

1. Rabies vaccines for human and animal use should meet WHO, OIE, the European Directorate for the Quality of Medicines (EDQM) and European Pharmacopoeia requirements for production and control of rabies vaccines.
2. Post-vaccination serological monitoring of vaccinees should be considered as an alternative to lifelong repeat vaccination.
3. The risk of sarcoma in cats following vaccination should be considered.
4. The immune response during infection and/or the response to vaccination in animals and humans should be studied in detail.
5. Attempts to correlate the minimum measurable VNA titre of 0.5 IU/ml with protective immunity should be considered.
6. The immunogenicity testing of vaccines should use appropriate challenge strains.
7. Consideration for the need of broad spectrum vaccines for animal/human use is highly required.
8. Recombinant (live vector) vaccines for parenteral vaccination of domestic animals should be considered for rabies control purposes as equivalent to inactivated vaccines.
9. Disease control authorities must pay attention to the vaccine and immunoglobulin supply chain to avoid shortages.
10. Manufacturers and regulatory bodies are recommended to follow the principle of the three R's (reduction, refinement, replacement) taking into account the outputs of the European Centre for the Validation of Alternative Methods (ECVAM) workshop (http://ecvam.jrc.cec.eu.int).

11. Research should be undertaken to standardise antigenic mass determination in place of in vivo tests.

Session VI: Bat rabies

1. In considering the protected status of all bats in Europe, a national bat rabies surveillance network should be established in all European countries in close collaboration with bat specialists, including international bat agencies.
2. This network should be based on a passive surveillance programme (collection of sick or dead bats of all species present in the country). Active surveillance with micro-samples of blood and saliva (capture of bats, bats maintained in wildlife hospitals) is also recommended. The active capture of bats should target high risk species.
3. A database is required to register submission details and sequence data for bat lyssavirus isolate sequences and archive bat lyssavirus isolates from countries throughout Europe.
4. Epidemiological data available so far show that the destruction of an infected bat colony is ineffective and must be avoided. This strategy will disturb the balance of the metacolony and should be avoided as much as possible as it may induce the unpredictable dispersion of infected animals. It is preferable to monitor the known positive colonies (using salivary excretion and serological survey with marking of sampled bats belonging to the colony), and to collect all sick or dead bats.
5. Laboratory and sampling techniques for bat rabies should be harmonised throughout Europe.
6. All bat handlers should be vaccinated.
7. All negative samples should be reported.
8. All bat cadavers (regardless of species) should be submitted to the National Rabies Reference Laboratory for lyssavirus testing. Brain sample collection using a needle through the orbit of the eye socket can be used to cause minimal disruption to the bat skull and allow species identification. The bat can then be archived as a specimen.
9. Research is required to understand the dynamics, epidemiology and pathogenesis of these viruses and their distribution, hosts and incidence in European bat species.
10. Research is needed on the ability of lyssaviruses to spillover between host bat species and other relevant domestic/wildlife species.

General recommendation

To hold a Second OIE International Conference on "Rabies in Europe" in two years (2007)

Adopted by the OIE First International Conference on "Rabies in Europe"
Kiev, (Ukraine), 15-18 June 2005

Dodet B, Schudel A, Pastoret PP, Lombard M (eds): Rabies in Europe.
Dev Biol (Basel). Basel, Karger, 2006, vol 125, p 297.

Poster Session

Dodet B, Schudel A, Pastoret PP, Lombard M (eds): Rabies in Europe.
Dev Biol (Basel). Basel, Karger, 2006, vol 125, p 299.

Evolution of the Rabies Epidemic in the Vladimir and Nizhny-Novgorod Regions in 1998-2004

A.A. Egorov, S.S. Rybakov, A.E. Metlin, A.V. Chepurkin, E. Neuvonen

FGI Federal Centre for Animal Health, Yurevetz, Vladimir, Russian Federation

The goal of the research was to study peculiarities of the rabies epidemic situation in the Nizhny-Novgorod and Vladimir regions during the period from 1998 to June 2004. These regions have a common border, their area is 105,900 km^2, and coniferous woods occupy 46,900 km^2.

The analysis of the evolution of the epidemic situation was carried out on the basis of data obtained from the Federal Service for Veterinary and Phytosanitary Surveillance of the Ministry of Agriculture of the Russian Federation, as well as the results of a diagnostic study of animal brain samples, obtained from the Vladimir and Nizhny-Novgorod regions, carried out at the FGI Federal Centre for Animal Health.

In the centre of the European part of Russia, the rabies epidemic has been spreading in recent years to the north and northeast. In the Vladimir region, rabies occurred in 1998 (5 cases), in 1999 (3 cases), in 2000 (9 cases) and in 2001 (13 cases). At the end of 2001, the first four rabies cases were registered in the Nizhny-Novgorod region. In 2002, there were 35 rabies cases in the Vladimir region, 27 cases in the Nizhny-Novgorod region. In 2003, there were 24 cases in the Vladimir region and 113 cases in the Nizhny-Novgorod region.

In all, 139 brain samples from red foxes were tested during the period from January 2002 to June 2004; 109 (78 %) samples were positive. The peak of the epidemic among foxes was observed in 2003 – 39 positive samples out of 41 tested in January – March, and 35 positive samples out of 37 tested in April – June. Among wild animals of other species, one case of rabies was diagnosed in a badger in 2003.

During the same period, 26 rabies cases were diagnosed in dogs as a result of testing 108 brain samples and 22 rabies cases were diagnosed in cats as a result of testing 100 samples. The peak of the rabies epidemic in dogs coincided with the peak of the rabies epidemic in foxes; there were 10 positive samples out of 26 tested in January-March 2003 and 4 positive samples out of 16 tested in April-June. There were no pronounced peaks in the cat population. Out of 22 tested samples of bovine brains, 9 were positive. One rabies case was registered in a pig, one in a horse and one in a rat.

The results show that in the Vladimir and Nizhny-Novgorod regions the major rabies carrier is the red fox.

Dodet B, Schudel A, Pastoret PP, Lombard M (eds): Rabies in Europe.
Dev Biol (Basel). Basel, Karger, 2006, vol 125, p 300.

Phylogenetic Analysis of Some Street Rabies Virus Strains Isolated From Foxes in Slovakia

A. Ondrejková, R. Ondrejka, J. Süli, Z. Beníšek, Š. Švrček

University of Veterinary Medicine, Department of Infectious and Parasitic Diseases, Košice, Slovak Republic

Aims

Phylogenetic analysis of autochtonous epizootic « fox strains » of rabies virus isolated from foxes in Slovak territory.

Materials and Methods

Samples : Isolates from brain of common foxes hunted within the framework of monitoring of oral rabies vaccination of foxes.

Rabies antigen detection :

• fluorescence antibody test (FAT) in brain impression smears ;

• mouse inoculation test.

Reverse transcriptase polymerase chain reaction (RT-PCR) : performed according to the procedure recommended by WHO, partially modified in our laboratory.

Electrophoresis : in 2 % agarose gel.

Sequencing of amplified products : Applied Biosystem 373A.

Phylogenetic analysis : Comparison with strains from other European States (GeneBank), Clustal W 1.60 program.

Results

A direct sequencing of the amplification product of nRT-PCR from the region of genome that codes for nucleoprotein with subsequent analysis of sequenced fragments and comparison with strains from other European States allowed us to type the fox strains isolated in our laboratory as genotype 1 ; they were very similar to strains isolated abroad.

Conclusions

The isolated strains belong among the first strains from the Slovak territory, sequenced, included in the phylogenetic tree, and compared with strains from other European countries. According to the phylogenetic analysis, these strains are part of the sylvatic terrestrial « fox » rabies cycle.

Acknowledgements

This work was supported by projects SP 51/0280800/0280803, VEGA 1/9010/02 and APVT-20-043902 (Slovak Republic).

Dodet B, Schudel A, Pastoret PP, Lombard M (eds): Rabies in Europe.
Dev Biol (Basel). Basel, Karger, 2006, vol 125, p 301.

Molecular Analysis of Rabies Virus Circulating in Terrestrial Animals in the Slovak Republic

R. Franka[1,2], M. Mojzis[2], I. Kuzmin[1], A. Velasco Villa[1], P. Yager[1], C.E. Rupprecht[1]

[1] Centers for Disease Control and Prevention, Atlanta, GA, USA
[2] State Veterinary Institut Zvolen, Zvolen, Slovak Republic

Rabies of terrestrial mammals remains a problem in eastern Europe despite active oral vaccination campaigns. To date, the red fox (*Vulpes vulpes*) and the raccoon dog (*Nyctereutes procyonoides*) are the main reservoirs of rabies virus (RABV) in Europe. In this preliminary study, we sequenced the nucleoprotein (N) and glycoprotein (G) genes of RABV, obtained from 22 red foxes, 6 cats, 1 wild cat, 4 dogs, 2 lynxes, 1 goat, 4 stone martens, 1 polecat and 1 badger collected during the period from 2000 to 2003 in the Slovak Republic. A phylogenetic analysis was undertaken, using for comparison RABV sequences originating from terrestrial animal species from other European countries, which were available from GenBank. Sequences were edited using BioEdit software, and multiple alignments were carried out using the Clustal X package. Neighbour joining analysis for 1000 bootstrap replicates was performed using MEGA version 2.1. Also, monoclonal antibody typing was performed using a panel of 13 anti-nucleocapsid monoclonal antibodies (N-Mabs) from the Centers for Disease Control and Prevention (Atlanta, GA, USA). Analysis of results revealed that 96 % of RABV samples belonged to one clade and were joined to a lineage with the variants previously described as the "Eastern Europe" group, and 4 % of the samples were joined to the lineage described as the "Central Europe" group. We have not found any significant associations according to the year of occurrence, host species, or a particular geographical location. Moreover, we did not detect any evidence in support of a reversal of virulence of the RABV vaccination strain used in the Slovak Republic during the oral vaccination campaigns. According to the patterns obtained using the limited N-Mab panels, European RABV samples were not easily distinguishable from each other, but were clearly different from RABV variants in the United States.

Dodet B, Schudel A, Pastoret PP, Lombard M (eds): Rabies in Europe.
Dev Biol (Basel). Basel, Karger, 2006, vol 125, p 302.

PLATELIA RABIES II: A New Elisa Kit for the Detection of Rabies Antibodies in Animal or Human Serum or Plasma

M. Feyssaguet, J.L. Morize, V. Todorova, J.P. Bourgeois

Bio-Rad, FSD Division, Marne-la-Coquette, France

A new microplate assay, PLATELIA RABIES II, for the detection of anti-rabies antibodies in human or animal serum or plasma has been developed by Bio-Rad. Reagents were optimised to improve specificity and practicability and facilitate automation with microplate processors. Here we show the results of sensitivity and specificity assays performed on human and animal samples.

PLATELIA RABIES II is based on the ELISA technique with an inactivated and purified solid phase antigen and uses Protein A-POD conjugate. Enzymatic revelation is done with TMB chromogen. Quantification standards are included in each test for rabies antibody titrations.

Preliminary data for validation of sensitivity and specificity were obtained by testing serum samples from naïve (n = 51) and vaccinated dogs with negative (n = 58) or very low (n = 50) FAVN titres. For human samples, sera from negative blood donors (n = 439) and from vaccinated people (n = 50) were also tested and compared to the RFFIT test.

Using a cut-off value of 0.50 UI/ml for fluorescent and ELISA techniques, the results show 100 % specificity on negative samples from vaccinated or naïve dogs and 99.8 % specificity on negative samples from human blood donors. No discrepant results were observed on the 50 human positive samples with high RFFIT titres but 13 dog samples on the 0.50-0.87 IU/ml FAVN titre range were found in the 0.30-0.48 IU/ml ELISA titre range.

PLATELIA RABIES II represents a promising tool for titration of anti-rabies antibodies in human or animal sera.

Dodet B, Schudel A, Pastoret PP, Lombard M (eds): Rabies in Europe.
Dev Biol (Basel). Basel, Karger, 2006, vol 125, p 303.

The Development of a System for Laboratory Diagnosis of Rabies

V. Nedosekov

All Russian Scientific and Research Institute of veterinary virology and microbiology, Pokrov, Russia

An analysis of both the prevalence and occurrence of rabies during the last 10 years testifies to the fact that the epizootic situation is getting worse (Selimov M. A 1987; Vedernikov V.A. 2002). Against this background it is important to know that modern and reliable laboratory diagnosis of diseases plays a key role in modern conditions.

Materials and Methods

1,842 brain samples of wild and domestic animals from different natural climatic zones of Yakuti as well as the European zone of the Russian Federation and Commonwealth of Independent States (CIS) countries were used.

Results

Previously, in order to develop the means for the diagnosis of rabies, monoclonal and polyclonal immunoglobulins specific to major rabies virus polypeptide were produced. Based on the studies of these antibodies, a fluorescent antibody method, an enzyme-linked immunosorbent assay (ELISA) and an immunoperoxidase test were developed. To detect the genome of rabies virus a test system PCR using primer complementary to both rabies virus nucleoprotein and glycoprotein was developed.

Restriction endonucleases allowing the differentiation of the isolates of classical and arctic rabies were selected.

During the years 1996-2003 the tests were studied from a comparative aspect using the data of research on brain samples of 1,842 animals. A mouse inoculation test was used as the «gold standard». When conducting research on an isolate of classical rabies, a primary evaluation of the effectiveness of the developed test system was carried out. It was established that the result of the immunofluorescence test was 98 %, ELISA was 97 %, and PCR was 100 %. When studying the isolate of arctic rabies the diagnostic sensitivity of the immunofluorescence method and PCR was 98 and 99 %, respectively. The diagnostic sensitivity of ELISA was 64 %. Based on these methods, a universal scheme for the diagnosis of rabies allowing rabies diagnosis to be carried out in any situation was developed.

Conclusion

Modern methods for laboratory diagnosis were developed, and their sensitivity studied. This serves as the basis for including them in the scheme for laboratory diagnosis of rabies.

Dodet B, Schudel A, Pastoret PP, Lombard M (eds): Rabies in Europe.
Dev Biol (Basel). Basel, Karger, 2006, vol 125, p 304.

Development of a Real-Time, Differential, RT-PCR TaqMan Assay for Lyssavirus Genotypes 1, 5 and 6

P.R. Wakeley, N. Johnson, L.M. McElhinney, D. Marston, J. Sawyer, A.R. Fooks

Rabies Research and Diagnostic Group and the Technology Transfer Unit, Veterinary Laboratories Agency (Weybridge), Surrey, UK

A number of RT-PCR methods for the detection of lyssaviruses have been reported which invariably involve multiple transfers of nucleic acids between different tubes with the associated risk of contamination and production of false-positive results. In order to address this problem we have developed a single, closed tube, real time RT-PCR using TaqMan technology to detect and differentiate classical rabies virus and European bat lyssaviruses 1 and 2. Despite sequence heterogeneity within the N-gene between different genotypes, a universal forward and reverse primer set has been designed allowing simplification of our previously described assays. Four TaqMan probes, labelled with different fluorophores, were used to specify viral genotype and to identify an internal (host) gene transcript. The internal control assay uses β actin mRNA as the template and was included to assess the efficiency of the total RNA extraction process and subsequent reverse transcription. A set of 62 archival RNA samples, corresponding to lyssavirus genotypes 1, 5 and 6, were analysed using the new method and, with the exception of one isolate, all were typed correctly according to sequence data. The non-nested TaqMan RT-PCR performed equivalently to that of our original hemi-nested RT-PCR with respect to sensitivity. The host species from which the brain sample was taken did not apparently affect the detection or genotyping of the infecting virus. The TaqMan assay was shown to be rapid (approximately 2hr 10min), sensitive and specific.

Dodet B, Schudel A, Pastoret PP, Lombard M (eds): Rabies in Europe.
Dev Biol (Basel). Basel, Karger, 2006, vol 125, p 305.

Rabies in Lithuanian Wildlife – Epidemiology and Prevention

D. Zienius

Department of Virology, Veterinary Institute of the Lithuanian Veterinary Academy, Kaisiadorys, Lithuania

Aims/Objectives

To study the epidemiological situation and prevention of rabies in wildlife in Lithuania during the period 1993-2003.

Materials and Methods

The reports of the Lithuanian State Food and Veterinary Service and statistical data of the Lithuanian Ministries of Agriculture and the Environment were analysed. Monitoring of the oral rabies vaccination (ORV) programme in the target species included the following: testing for the presence of the biomarker (tetracycline); examining sera for rabies virus neutralizing Ab; analysing the incidence of rabies in wildlife before, during and after the ORV programme.

Results/Discussion/Conclusion

During the period 1993-2003, 3,182 cases of rabies were registered among wild animals. The majority of cases were registered in foxes (1,420-[44.6 %]) and raccoon dogs (1,400-[44.0 %]). Within the last 5 years, rabies among foxes and raccoon dogs increased significantly (9.7 and 26.6 times, respectively), compared with the period 1993-1997. During the period 1995-2000, 820,000 baits with SAG-1, Lysvulpen (1998) and Rabifox (1999-2000) vaccines were used for wildlife rabies prevention in Lithuania. Vaccines were distributed within an area of 9,550 km^2 (15-25 baits/per km^2) in 27 of 44 districts of Lithuania. During the ORV programme, 189 (59 positive) samples for OTS markers and 138 (75 positive) fox sera samples for IFA were investigated. That comprised 0.023 % (OTS) and 0.017 % (ELISA) of all vaccine baits distributed in that period only. The total cost of the rabies prevention campaign in wildlife was 746,730.9 EUR (28.3 EUR per 1 km^2).

The 1995-2000 ORV programme was unsuccessful. The number of investigations of OTS markers and serology by IFA was extremely low to evaluate the ORV programme.

Dodet B, Schudel A, Pastoret PP, Lombard M (eds): Rabies in Europe.
Dev Biol (Basel). Basel, Karger, 2006, vol 125, pp 306-307.

Elaboration of an Immuno-Enzyme Assay Test System for Control of Rabies Vaccinoprophylaxis Efficacy

N.A. Khismatullina[1], *T.A. Savitskya*[2], *A.N. Chernov*[3], *R.H. Yusupov*[1], *V.G. Gumerov*[1]

[1] Federal State Scientific Establishment « All-Russian Research Veterinary Institute », Kazan, Russia

[2] Federal State Establishment « The Centre of state Sanitary and Epidemiologic inspectorate in the Republic of Tatarstan », Kazan, Russia

[3] Chief Veterinary Administration of the Council of Ministers of the Republic of Tatarstan, Kazan, Russia

The Aim of our investigation was to elaborate an immuno-enzyme assay test system based on the rabies viral glycoprotein to control the immune status of humans and animals vaccinated against rabies, to carry out a comparative evaluation of its efficacy using the neutralization test (NT) and prolonged complement-fixing test (PCFT) under laboratory and production conditions.

Materials and Methods

Our investigations were carried out with the vaccine strain « Vnukovo-32", the production one – « Ovetchiy GNKI », and a standard one – CVS rabies virus. In our tests we investigated 507 samples of sera from sheep and rabbits infected with rabies virus, 296 samples of bovine sera from cattle vaccinated with an anti-rabies « Schelkovo-51 » strain vaccine, 216 sera of foxes and 32 of dog foxes from rabies-threatened territories in the Omsk region and Tatarstan, and 28 blood sera of people vaccinated by anti-rabies culture « Vnukovo-32" strain vaccine. Rabies viral glycoprotein was produced according to D. Dietzschold (1996). An immuno-enzyme test was performed in the indirect variant. As conjugate we used peroxidase-labelled diagnostic antibodies to human and animal Ig, A-protein (The Gamaleya Institute, RAMS) and peroxidase-labelled rabbit antibodies to fox Ig (I.V. Kuzmin et al, 2001). PCFT was performed according to E. Kuwert (1975) and NT according to P. Atanasiu (1973).

Results and Discussion

As a result of our investigation we obtained a specific antigen based on rabies viral glycoprotein, the strain « Ovetchiy GNKI » the activity of which in IET was

1 : 256 (K_{sp} = 2.1), while the protein concentration was 338 mcg/ml. On the basis of rabies viral glycoprotein we elaborated and approved an immuno-enzyme test system that ensures the detection of specific antibodies in blood sera of humans and animals vaccinated against rabies and the evaluation of vaccinoprophylaxis during 7-8 hours in rabies-threatened epizootic nidi.

A comparative investigation of 507 samples of blood sera in indirect IET, PCFT and NT on mice revealed a direct correlation of the results of blood sera titration using IET and NT methods ($r = 0.3$; $P < 0.05$) and a high degree of IET sensibility. In this case, IET sensibility surpassed that of PCFT by 100-200 times; as for the arrangement period, IET also surpassed NT on mice at 14 days and at 2 days.

The IET investigation of 296 samples of blood sera from the cattle vaccinated against rabies in different unfavourable areas of Tatarstan established a high quantity of specific antibodies, with a titre of 1 : 200 - 1 : 3200, during the first 6 months after vaccination. During the subsequent periods after vaccination we observed a decrease in the level of antibodies. In this connexion, considering the epizootic situation, we recommended the vaccination of all livestock during 2-3 years for the creation of stable immunological protection of farmed animals against rabies virus.

The elaborated test system was used for the screening evaluation of the immune status of foxes and dog foxes in natural nidi in the south of Western Siberia and the areas of oral vaccination in the Republic of Tatarstan.

A selective comparison of IET and NT results in white mice showed that the results coincided in 77.3 % of cases.

Conclusion

On the basis of rabies viral glycoprotein, we elaborated a highly sensitive specific immuno-enzyme test system that ensures the detection of antibodies to rabies virus in blood sera of humans and animals vaccinated against rabies. We established the possibility of using the elaborated test system for the screening evaluation of the immune status of the fox population in natural rabies nidi and areas of oral vaccination.

Dodet B, Schudel A, Pastoret PP, Lombard M (eds): Rabies in Europe.
Dev Biol (Basel). Basel, Karger, 2006, vol 125, p 308.

Current Problems of Control of Rabies and other Lissavirus Diseases

Š. Švrček, V. Bajová, Z. Beníšek, M. Čížek, R. Franka, V. Hipíková, M. Levkutová, J. Mojžišová, R. Ondrejka, A. Ondrejková, Š. Paulík, S. Pošiváková, J. Süli, Š. Vilček

University of Veterinary Medicine, Department of Infectious and Parasitic Diseases, Košice, Slovak Republic

A research project for improvement of immunoprophylaxis of rabies and rabies-related lyssavirus diseases of domestic and farm animals was developed, in accordance with current requirements of rabies control.

- The project was oriented towards the following problem areas: Feline AIDS (or infection of cats by FIV) from the point of view of immunoincompetence for rabies vaccination;
- Rationalisation and improvement of vaccination efficacy in domestic and farm animals; quantification of protective immunity (intradermal needle-less administration of vaccines, utilization of adjuvants, immunomodulation, elimination of suppressive factors, determination of immunocompetence and protection criteria, etc.); Efficacy of rabies vaccination in homotypic and heterotypic infections.

This work was supported by APVT (Slovak Republic) No. APVT-20-043902.

Dodet B, Schudel A, Pastoret PP, Lombard M (eds): Rabies in Europe.
Dev Biol (Basel). Basel, Karger, 2006, vol 125, pp 309-310.

Determination of the Level of Rabies Immunity and the Efficacy of Domestic Animal Vaccination in Russia

A.N. Panin[1], *I.L. Obukhov*[1], *V.V. Nedosekov*[2], *E.E. Davydova*[1]

[1] FGU « All-Russian Center on Quality and Standardization of Veterinary Medications and Feed » (VGNKI), Moscow, Russian Federation

[2] FGU « All-Russian Research Institute of Veterinary Virology and Microbiology », Pokrov, Vladimir Region, Russian Federation

In view of the absence of any marked decline in the incidence of rabies, prevention methods must be improved. Therefore, the European Parliament issued Regulation No. 998/2003, according to which animals (dogs, cats, polecats) imported into European Union countries must be tested for the presence of neutralising antibodies. The test may only be carried out by licensed laboratories. The laboratory of Molecular Diagnostics of FGU VGNKI has been participating in AFSSA Nancy proficiency testing since 2003.

Aims

To determine the level of rabies immunity and the efficacy of vaccination of domestic carnivores.

Materials and Methods

Rabies immunity was estimated based on the level of virus neutralizing antibodies in animal blood serum. The antibodies were detected using the FAVN technique, in accordance with the OIE *Manual of Diagnostic Tests and Vaccines for Terrestrial Animals.*

Results

The Veterinary Department of the Russian Ministry of Agriculture entrusted the carrying out of tests to FGU VGNKI (Directive No. 135-11/489). In the period from

2003 to August 2004 the Laboratory of Molecular Diagnostics of FGU VGNKI tested 105 dogs and 71 cats of various breeds. The animals had been vaccinated with Nobivac (Intervet, Holland), Hexadog, Quadricat, Rabisin (Merial, France). The average antibody titre was 1.29 IU/ml in the dogs and 1.48 IU/ml in the cats. However, 9 of the dog sera and 3 of the cat sera had titres of less than 0.5 IU/ml.

Controlling the efficacy of vaccination helps to break the links in the epizootic chain and prevent the development of the epizootic process.

Dodet B, Schudel A, Pastoret PP, Lombard M (eds): Rabies in Europe.
Dev Biol (Basel). Basel, Karger, 2006, vol 125, pp 311-312.

Rationalization, Objectivisation and Simplification of Rabies Vaccine Potency Testing

Z. Beníšek, J. Süli, Š. Švrček, R. Ondrejka, A. Ondrejková, J. Pošivák

University of Veterinary Medicine, Department of Infectious and Parasitic Diseases, Košice, Slovak Republic

Aims

To compare different vaccine administration routes of injected inactivated rabies vaccines corresponding to routine vaccination routes and different challenge methods corresponding to natural routes of exposure of target animal species (in vivo); to evaluate rabies vaccine potency in vitro bythe ELISA technique.

Materials and Methods

In vivo methods of vaccine efficacy evaluation:
- Immunogenic activity:

Vaccination	Challenge	Method
Intraperitoneal	Intracerebral	NIH
Subcutaneous	Subcutaneous	LPL
Intramuscular	Intramuscular	i.m./i.m.
Intradermal	Intramuscular	i.d./i.m.

- Antigenic activity: vaccination – 100 ED_{50} of tested rabies vaccine (administration i.p., s.c., i.m., i.d.), rabies antibody determination – ELISA method.

In vitro method of vaccine efficacy evaluation: quantification of antigenic value of live, inactivated and adjuvant (commercial) rabies vaccines by simplified ELISA method.

Results

In vivo: on testing by the NIH method we found a low correlation rate between the immunogenic and antigenic activity values of tested rabies vaccines; a high correlation rate was recorded using the LPL method. **In vitro:** there was a good correlation between the live and inactivated vaccines, but not between non-adjuvant and adjuvant vaccine.

Conclusions

In view of the low correlation rate between the immunogenic and antigenic activity values of rabies vaccines tested by the NIH method, we consider it as unobjective. Evaluation of rabies vaccine potency can alternatively be performed by in vitro techniques. For a sufficiently efficacious vaccine, we regard the antigenic value limit determined by the ELISA method to be 1.0 IU/cm^3.

This work was supported by projects VEGA 1/0572/03 and APVT-20-043902 (Slovak Republic).

Dodet B, Schudel A, Pastoret PP, Lombard M (eds): Rabies in Europe.
Dev Biol (Basel). Basel, Karger, 2006, vol 125, p 313.

A New Adjuvant Inactivated Rabies Vaccine

J. Süli, Z. Beníšek, A. Ondrejková, R. Ondrejka, Š. Švrček

University of Veterinary Medicine, Department of Infectious and Parasitic Diseases, Košice, Slovak Republic

Aims

Preparation of rabies inactivated vaccine with a lipoid squalene adjuvant (SA) in one step, at decreased temperature of emulsification (up to 37°C); testing of its effectiveness and harmlessness.

Materials and Methods

Composition of SA inactivated rabies vaccine: Suspension of inactivated rabies virus – 89 %; squalene – 5 %; emulsifiers – 6 % (Poloxamer 105 – 4 %, Abil-Care – 2 %).

Preparation of vaccine: Homogenisation: 35-37°C; 6,000 rpm; 5 min.

Verification of vaccine effectiveness: NIH method (mice); antigenic activity (guinea pigs); comparison of the inactivated SA rabies vaccine with adjuvant-free vaccine and aluminium hydroxide vaccine.

Verification of SA harmlessness: Study of possible sensitisation after the administration of the SA; pathomorphological determination of tissue reactivity after the administration of SA (guinea pigs); in vitro test of SA pyrogenicity.

Results

The SA increased the immunogenic activity of non-potentiated rabies vaccine approximately 1.8-fold, aluminium hydroxide only 1.08-fold. The antigenic activity was significantly increased by using both adjuvants; SA was more efficient than aluminium hydroxide. No significant differences were observed after sensitisation with SA and in control animals. Pathoanatomical, pathohistological and pyrogenicity tests confirmed the safety of SA.

Conclusions

The results obtained by testing the supportive effect and harmlessness of SA on the efficacy of rabies vaccine allow us to recommend the use of this adjuvant for veterinary rabies vaccines. Our laboratory focused on the preparation of adjuvant rabies vaccine but the use of this adjuvant may have much wider applications.

This work was supported by projects VEGA 1/0574/03 and APVT-20-043902 (Slovak Republic).

Dodet B, Schudel A, Pastoret PP, Lombard M (eds): Rabies in Europe.
Dev Biol (Basel). Basel, Karger, 2006, vol 125, p 314.

Development of a Modern System for the Control of Inactivated Anti Rabies Vaccines

V. Nedosekov

All Russian Scientific and Research Institute of Veterinary Virology and Microbiology
Pokrov, Russia

In worldwide practice since 1953, the NIH test is used for the detection of antirabies vaccines antigenic and immunogenic properties (Seligman E., 1973). However, this test has some drawbacks (waste of time, high cost, a great variability of the results, etc.). Against this background we have conducted research for the development of ELISA test systems using monoclonal antibodies.

Materials and Methods

In order to test the antigenic activity we used antirabies inactivated culture vaccines from the strains Shelkovo-51 and TC-80.

Results

The development of the ELISA test system was carried out using protective monoclonal antibodies, specific to antigenic determinant glycoprotein. In order to choose the optimal method for controlling the vaccine, both ELISA and the traditional method NIH were used for assessing the antigenic activity of the vaccines. It was then established that the best method remains sensitized plates with the mixed MA clones 14B 18.2, 17B 5.3, 19B 8.1, specific to three rabies virus antigenic determinant glycoproteins, and the detection of the bound protective antigen by polyclonal antibodies. Correlative analysis at a comparative evaluation of the antigenic activity of 13 serial vaccines, tested by both NIH and sandwich ELISA, has shown that the coefficient of correlation is 0.95. Based on these data, a scheme for testing vaccines at different technological production stages of antirabies vaccine was developed.

This scheme allows the control of liquid vaccines during 35 days and lyophilized vaccines during 6 days.

Conclusion

A system for the control of antigenic activity of liquid inactivated culture antirabies vaccines allowing the production of vaccines of high quality was developed.

Dodet B, Schudel A, Pastoret PP, Lombard M (eds): Rabies in Europe.
Dev Biol (Basel). Basel, Karger, 2006, vol 125, p 315.

Survey of Rabies in Bats in Sweden

G. Hallgren, L. Treiberg Berndtsson, B. Klingeborn, M. Nöremark

National Veterinary Institute (SVA), Uppsala, Sweden

A nationwide survey, granted by the Swedish Board of Agriculture, in which bats are examined for the presence of rabies virus, has been conducted in order to monitor the bat rabies situation in Sweden. For this purpose, dead bats and wounded euthanised bats, mainly from the southern parts of Sweden, are sent to the SVA for examination. Imprints from the brains are then analysed using a fluorescent antibody test, FAT. Between 1998 and 2003, more than 200 bats were examined. Sweden has had no cases of animal rabies since 1886. This favourable situation is threatened by the fact that bat rabies is frequently diagnosed in many of our neighbouring countries and rabies can be reintroduced to Sweden by bats. So far all the bats examined have been negative for rabies.

Dodet B, Schudel A, Pastoret PP, Lombard M (eds): Rabies in Europe.
Dev Biol (Basel). Basel, Karger, 2006, vol 125, p 316.

Lyssavirus Strain Isolated from a Bat in Slovakia

R. Ondrejka, A. Ondrejková, J. Süli, Z. Beníšek, Š. Švrček

University of Veterinary Medicine, Department of Infectious and Parasitic Diseases, Košice, Slovak Republic

Aims

Isolation and identification of a lyssavirus strain originating from a bat (*Eptesicus serotinus*) captured in Slovakia after contact with a human.

Materials and Methods

Sample: Isolate from brain of a bat captured in Slovakia.
Rabies antigen detection:

- fluorescence antibody test (FAT) in brain impression smears;
- mouse inoculation test.

Reverse transcriptase polymerase chain reaction (RT-PCR): performed according to the procedure recommended by WHO, partially modified in our laboratory.
Electrophoresis: in 2 % agarose gel.
Sequencing of amplified products: Applied Biosystem 373A.
Comparing of the sequences: Clustal W 1.60 program.

Results

Direct sequencing of the amplification product of nRT-PCR N-gene allowed us to isolate a bat strain classified as genotype 5 – EBL-1a.

Conclusions

The present isolation and identification of EBL-1a lyssavirus in Slovakia points to the potential existence of other rabies-infected bats in Slovakia and calls for maximum care in manipulation of bats.

This work was supported by projects VEGA 1/9010/02, SP 51/0280800/0280803 and APVT-20-043902 (Slovak Republic).

Dodet B, Schudel A, Pastoret PP, Lombard M (eds): Rabies in Europe.
Dev Biol (Basel). Basel, Karger, 2006, vol 125, p 317.

European Bat Lyssavirus Type-2a Isolated from a Fatal Human Case of Rabies Encephalitis in the United Kingdom

A.R. Fooks, L.M. McElhinney, N. Johnson, C.J. Finnegan, K. Mansfield, S.M. Brookes, G. Parsons

Rabies Research and Diagnostic Group, Veterinary Laboratories Agency (Weybridge), [WHO Collaborating Centre for the Characterisation of Rabies and Rabies-Related Viruses], Surrey, UK

In the past 25 years, the majority of emerging human pathogens have been zoonotic RNA viruses, including the rabies-related lyssaviruses. The detection of lyssaviruses from insectivorous, frugivorous and haematophagous bats indicates the diverse variety of bat species that act as hosts for these viruses and which continue to play a pivotal role in the global epidemiology of lyssaviruses. Since 1977, more than 700 cases of European bat lyssavirus (EBLV) infections have been confirmed in European bats, including two EBLV type-2a infections in Daubenton's bats in the UK, in Sussex (1996) and Lancashire (2002). In November 2002, a 55-year-old bat conservationist died, 19-days after the onset of clinical symptoms, following a suspected bite from an indigenous British bat. Both molecular and conventional diagnostic tests for rabies were used to confirm the isolate as EBLV type-2a. This was the first recorded case of indigenous human rabies in the UK for 100 years and represents only the fourth reported human case of rabies in Europe caused by a bat lyssavirus. The patient had never been vaccinated against rabies and did not receive post-exposure treatment (PET). This case re-emphasises that pre-immunisation against rabies should be mandatory for all licensed European bat handlers and that rabies PET is essential for anyone bitten by a bat. In addition, rabies testing should be included in the differential diagnosis of any patient with evidence of evolving viral encephalitis with cerebellar involvement following a known exposure with European bats, irrespective of travel history.

Dodet B, Schudel A, Pastoret PP, Lombard M (eds): Rabies in Europe.
Dev Biol (Basel). Basel, Karger, 2006, vol 125, p 318.

Adjuvant-Free Rabies Vaccines: Serological Immune Response in Cats

K. Duchow[1], *C. Kiefert*[2], *M. König*[3], *K. Cussler*[1]

[1] Paul-Ehrlich-Institut, Langen, Germany

[2] Max Planck Institute for Brain Research, Frankfurt, Germany

[3] Institute of Virology, Justus-Liebig-Universität Giessen, Giessen

Vaccination against rabies is of utmost importance in protecting both animals and humans against the disease. In Central Europe, it is common practice to use aluminium hydroxide adjuvanted vaccines in the veterinary field whereas adjuvant-free vaccines are used in humans.

In feline medicine, the use of adjuvanted vaccines is considered to be a major cause of the development of fibrosarcomas at sites usually used for the injection of medicines [1]. Especially rabies vaccines have been held responsible for inducing the disease [2]. The use of adjuvant-free rabies vaccines would obviously have major safety advantages in cats. For this reason, we started a laboratory trial in cats to compare the serological immune response between two commercial veterinary vaccines and two adjuvant-free rabies vaccines licensed for human use. The results for the time period of up to six months after vaccination are presented and discussed here.

1 Hendrick M, Goldschmidt MH: Do injection site reactions induce fibrosarcomas in cats? J Amer Vet Med Assn 1991; 199: 968.

2 Macy DW, Hendrick MJ: The potential role of inflammation in the development of postvaccinal sarcomas in cats. Vet Clin N Amer Small Anim 1996; 26: 103-103.

List of Participants

ABRAMOV Artur V., Central State Laboratory of Veterinary Medicine, 30, Donetska str., Kyiv 03151, Ukraine.

ÅKERSTEDT Johan, National Veterinary Institute, Virology and Serology, P.O. Box 8156 Dep., NO-0033 Oslo.

AKSIONOV Alexandr, Ministry of Agriculture and Food, 15 Kirov Street, 220050 Minsk, Belarus.

AMBROSINO Donna, University of Massachusetts Medical School, Massachusetts Biologic Laboratories, 305 South Street, Jamaica Plain, MA 02130, USA.

ARIC Tina, Veterinary Administration of the Republic of Slovenia, Parmova 53, SI-1000 Ljubljana, Slovenia.

ARTOIS Marc, OIE Working Group on Wildlife Diseases, Ecole Nationale Veterinaire de Lyon, Unité de Pathologie Infectieuse et épidémiologie, 1, avenue Bourgelat, FR-69280 Marcy l'Etoile, France.

AYLAN Orhan, Rabies Diagnosis Laboratory, Central Veterinary Control and Research Institute, Kolayl 305, Cad. No: 23 Etlik, Ankara 06020, Turkey.

BAETZA Hans-Joachim, Representative of the OIE Delegate, Ministry of Consumer Protection Food and Agriculture, Rochusstraße 1, DE-53123 Bonn, Germany.

BANKOVSKIY Denis, Pkrov Plant of Biopreparation, Volginskiy, Vladimir Region, Russia.

BARBOI Gheorghe, Institute for Diagnosis and Animal Health, 63, Dr. Staicovici Str., sector 5, Bucharest 050557, Romania.

BARRAT Jacques, Rabies Diagnosis, AFSSA Nancy, Domaine de Pixérécourt, BP 9, FR-54220 Malzéville, France.

BELEV Nikola, Bld Wasil Lewski 110, BG-1527 Sofia, Bulgaria.

BENISEK Zdenek, University of Veterinary Medicine, Department of Infectious Diseases, Komenskeho 73, Košice 04181, Slovak Republic.

BLANCHARD Irène, Group Product Manager, Bio-Rad, 3 bvd Raymond Poincaré, FR-92430 Marnes la Coquette, France.

BORISOV Alexey, FGI Federal Centre for Animal Health, RU-600901, Vladimir, Yur'evets, Russia.

BOTVINKIN Alexandr, Holder of the chair of Epidemiology, Irkutsk State Medical University, 1, Krasnogo Vosstania, RU-664003 Irkutsk, Russia.

BOURHY Hervé, Rabies Laboratory, Institut Pasteur, 25-28, rue du Dr Roux, FR-75724 Paris, Cedex 15, France.

BUSSI Beatrice, Food and Veterinary Office, European Commission, Grange, Dunsany, Co. Meath, Ireland.

CALISTRINI Paolo, Istituto Zooprofilattico Sperimentale dell'Abruzzo e del Molise, Via Campo Boario, IT-64100 Teramo, Italy.

CAPORALE Vincenzo, Istituto Zooprofilattico Sperimentale, dell'Abruzzo e del Molise «G. Caporale», Via Campo Boario, IT-64100 Teramo, Italy.

CEDERSMYG Maria, Swedish Board of Agriculture, SE-551 82 Jönköping, Sweden.

CHERKASSKIY Beniyamin, Zoonotic Laboratory, Central Research Institute of Epidemiology, Russian Ministry of Health, 3-A Novogireevskaya Str., RU-111123 Moscow, Russia.

CLIQUET Florence, AFSSA Nancy, Domaine de Pixérécourt, BP 9, FR-54220 Malzéville, France.

CROWCROFT Natasha, Immunisation Department, Centre for Infections, Health Protection Agency, 61 Colindale Avenue, London NW9 5EQ, U.K.

CUSSLER Klaus, Veterinary Pharmacovigilance and Animal Welfare, Paul-Ehrlich-Institut, Paul-Ehrlich-Str. 51-59, DE-63225 Langen, Germany.

DAINIUS Zienius, Veterinary Institute of Lithuanian Veterinary Academy, Instituto 2, LT – 56115 Kaisiadorys, Lithuania.

DANES Mihai, Societatea Nationala, Institutul Pasteur, Calea Giulestri Nr 333, RO-77862 Bucuresti, Romania.

DAVIS Rolan, Kansas State University, College of Veterinary Medicine, Mosier Hall 1800 Denison Ave, Manhattan, KS 66506, USA.

DE BENEDICTIS Paola, Istituto Zooprofilattico Sperimentale delle Venezie, Rabies National Reference Laboratory, Viale dell'Università 10, IT-35020 Legnaro (Padua), Italy.

DIDULEH Andrei, Intervet. Akzo Nobel Representativ Office BV, V. Vasilkivska Str., 9/2, Office 65, 01004 Kyiv, Ukraine.

DIRBAKOVA Zuzana, Laboratory for molecular biology, State veterinary institute Zvolen, Pod Drahami 918, Zvolen 96086, Slovak Republic.

DJURICIC Bosiljka, Faculty of veterinary medicine, Bul. JNA 18, Belgrade 11000, Serbia and Montenegro.

DOMSKI Igor, Russian Research Institute of Game Management and Fur Farming, 79 Engels Str, RU-610000 Kirov, Russia.

DUNDON William, Istituto Zooprofilattico Sperimentale delle Venezie, Laboratorio Virologia Viale dell'Università, 10, IT-35020 Legnaro (PD), Italy.

ECHEVARRÍA Juan, Centro Nacional de Microbiología, Instituto de Salud Carlos III, Ctra. Majadahonda-Pozuelo s/n, ES-28220 Madrid, Spain.

EDWARDS Steve, Veterinary Laboratory Agency, New Haw, Addlestone, Surrey KT15 3NB, U.K.

EVERT Victor, Intervet, V. Vasilkivska Str., 9/2, Office 65, 01004 Kyiv, Ukraine.

FAIZOU Tagir, All-Russian Research Veterinary Institute, Laboratory of Molecular-Genetic Research, Science ur., 2, RU-420075 Kazan, Russia.

FEVRIER Jacques, European Commission, DG Sanco E2, Rue Froissard 101, BE-1049 Bruxelles, Belgium.

FEYSSAGUET Muriel, Project Manager Bio-Rad, 3 bvd R. Poincaré, FR-92430 Marnes la Coquette, France.

FOOKS Anthony, Rabies Research and Diagnostics Group, Veterinary Laboratories Agency, Woodham Lane, New Haw, Addlestone, Surrey KT15 3NB, U.K.

FRANCHI Paola, Istituto Zooprofilattico Sperimentale, dell'Abruzzo e del Molise « G. Caporale », Via Campo Boario, IT-64100 Teramo, Italy.

GOLOVKO Anatoliy M., State Scientific Control Institute of Biotechnology and Microorganism Strains, 30, Donetska str., Kyiv 03151, Ukraine.

GREBENNIKOVA Tatyana, Molecular Biology Division, R & D NARVAC Ivanovski Virology Institute, 16 Gamalei st., RU-123098 Moscow, Russia.

GRUZDEV Konstantine, FGI Federal Centre for Animal Health, RU-600901 Yur'evets, Vladimir, Russia.

GUITTRÉ Caroline, AFSSA-ANMV, BP 90203, FR-35302 Fougères, France.

GUNILLA Hallgren, National Veterinary Institute (SVA), SE-751 89 Uppsala, Sweden.

HAMMARIN Anna-Lena, Swedish Institute for Infectious Disease Control, SE-171 82 Solna, Sweden.

HEIKO Rüdiger, IDT, Streetzer Weg 15a, DE-06862 Rodleben, Germany.

HOEFLECHNER Andrea, Division for Animal Health, Ministry for Health and Women, Radetzkystrasse 2, A-1030 Vienna, Austria.

HORZHEEV Volodimir M., State Department of Veterinary Medicine, Ministry of Agricultural Policy of Ukraine, 24, Khreshchatik str., Kyiv-01001, Ukraine.

HUIBERT Maurice, Ministry of Agriculture, Nature and Food Quality, Bezuidenhoutseweg 73, P.O. Box 20401, NL-2500 EK The Hague, The Netherlands.

HUTSON Anthony M., The Bat Conservation Trust, 15 Cloisters House, 8 Battersea Park Road, London SW8 4BG, U.K.

IASHVILI Konstantin, Veterinary Union of Tbilisi, Ministry of Agriculture, 41 Kostava Street, 0123 Tbilisi, Georgia.

IVARS Koloda, Veterinary Surveillance Division, Food and veterinary service, Republikas Square – 2, LV-1010 Riga, Latvia.

JEGERS Emils, Risk Management Division, Food and Veterinary Service, Republikas Square 2, LV-1010 Riga, Latvia.

KHISMATULLINA Nailya, Federal State Scientific Establishment, « All-Russian Research Veterinary Institute », Science ur., 2, RU-420075 Kazan, Russia.

KNEZEVIC Nikola, Virusol. lab., Veterinarski zavod Zemun, Batajnicki put 4, Belgrade-Zemun 11080, Serbia and Montenegro.

KRAMPS Johannes, CIDC Lelystad, Houtribweg 39, P.O. Box 2004, NL-8221 RA Lelystad, The Netherlands.

KUMOR Les, Veterinarian Disease Control, Canadian Food Inspection Agency-Canada, 2nd Floor West, 59 Camelot Drive, Ottawa, Ontario K1A OY9, Canada.

KUSHNEROV Oleg, FGI Federal Centre for Animal Health, RU-600901, Vladimir, Yur'evets, Russia.

KUZMIN Ivan, Centers for Disease Control and Prevention, 1600 Clifton Rd., Atlanta, GA 30333, USA.

LANDEG Fred, Dept for Environment, Food and Rural Affairs (Defra), Rm 302A, 1A Page Street, London SW1A 4PQ, U.K.

LELLI Rossella, Istituto Zooprofilattico Sperimentale Abruzzo & Molise, Via campo boario, IT-64100 Teramo, Italy.

LIKOR Nikolai Ivanov, National Veterinary Services, 15A Pencho Slaveikov Blvd., BG-1606 Sofia, Bulgaria.

LINA Peter H.C., P.O. Box 835, NL-2300 Av. Leiden, The Netherlands.

LISOVENKO Vasyl T., Corporation « Ukrzoovetprompostatch », 16, Vasylkivska str., Kyiv 03040, Ukraine.

LUKAUSKAS Kazimieras, OIE Delegate, State Food and Veterinary Service, Siesiku str. 19, LT-07170 Vilnius, 07170, Lithuania.

MACHITIDZE Tsezar, Epidemiological Department of the Veterinary Department of Georgia, Ministry of Agriculture, 41 Kostava Street, 0123 Tbilisi, Georgia.

MACIULSKIS Petras, State Food and Veterinary Service, Siesiku str. 19, LT-07170 Vilnius, Lithuania.

MAILLES Alexandra, Institut de Veille Sanitaire, 12 rue du Val d'Osne, FR-94410 Saint Maurice, France.

MAKI Joanne, Merial, 115 Trans Tech Dr, Athens GA 30601, USA.

MALERCZYK Claudius, Chiron Vaccines, Emil-von-Behring Straße 76, DE-35041 Marburg, Germany.

MALIK Peter, Central Veterinary Institute, Tabornok str 2., HU-1148 Budapest, Hungary.

MANGA Ivan Mohza, National Veterinary Services, 15A Pencho Slaveikov Blvd., BG-1606 Sofia, Bulgaria.

MANGANA-VOUGIOUKA Olga, Institute of Infectious and Parasitice Diseases, Ministry of Rural Development & Food, Rus Department 25, Neapoleos Street, GR-15310 Agia Paraskevi, Greece.

MANSFIELD Karen, Veterinary Laboratories Agency, Woodham Lane, New Haw, Addlestone, Surrey KT15 3NB, U.K.

MARTIN Victoria, Harvard University, 38 Glendower Street, Avon, MA 02322, USA.

MATOUCH Oldrich, State Veterinary Institute, National Reference Laboratory for Rabies, U Sila 1139, CZ-30 463 11 Liberec, Czech Republic.

MAURER WERNIG Jedrt, Official veterinarian, Animal Health Department, Veterinary Administration of the Republic of Slovenia, Parmova 53, SI-1000 Ljubljana, Slovenia.

MAZURKEVITCH Anatoliy I., UAAS Veterinary Medicine Sector, 12, Suvorova str., Kyiv 01010, Ukraine.

McELHINNEY Lorraine Marie, Rabies Research & Diagnostic Group, Veterinary Laboratories Agency, Woodham Lane, New Haw, Addlestone, Surrey KT15 3NB, U.K.

McLACHLAN Linda, British Embassy, FCO (KIEV), King Charles Street, London SW1A 2AH, U.K.

MESLIN François-Xavier, World Health Organization, 20, avenue Appia, CH-1211 Geneva, Switzerland.

METLIN Artem, FGI Federal Centre for Animal Health, RU-600901, Vladimir, Yur'evets, Russia.

MIRANDA Mary Elizabeth, Communicable Diseases Surveillance and Response, World Health Organization, Regional Office for the Western Pacific, P.O. Box 2932, 1000 Manila, Philippines.

MOJZIS Miroslav, State Veterinary Institute Zvolen, Pod Drahami 918, Zvolen 96086, Slovak Republic.

MONACO Federica, Istituto Zooprofilattico Sperimentale, dell'Abruzzo e del Molise, Via Campo Boario, IT-64100 Teramo, Italy.

MOORE Susan, Kansas State University, College of Veterinary Medicine, Mosier Hall 1800 Denison Ave, Manhattan, KS 66506, USA.

MORRIS Jill, Public Health Medicine, Centre for Infections, Health Protection Agency, 61 Colindale Avenue, London NW9 5HT, U.K.

MOSET MARTÍNEZ Sagrario, Sanitary Veterinary Alert Network Technician, Ministry of Agriculture, Fisheries and Food-Spain, ALfonso XII, 62, ES-28071 Madrid, Spain.

MUELLER Winfried, Pappelweg 1, DE-72076 Tübingen, Baden-Würtemberg, Germany.

MUKHARSKA Lyudmila M., Sanitary and Epidemiological Administration, Ministry of Public Health of Ukraine, 7, Grushevskogo str., Kyiv 01021, Ukraine.

MÜELLER Thomas, Friedrich-Loeffler-Institut, Federal Research Institute for Animal Health, Seestasse 55, DE-16868 Wusterhausen, Germany.

MUST Kylli, Virology-Serology Department, Estonian Veterinary and Food Laboratory, Kreutzwaldi 30, Tartu 51006, Estonia.

MUTINELLI Franco, National Reference Laboratory for Rabies, Istituto Zooprofilattico Sperimentale delle Venezie, Viale dell'Università, 10, IT-35020 Legnaro, Italy.

NADIN-DAVIS Susan, Canadian Food Inspection Agency, 3851 Fallowfield Rd, PO Box 11300, Station "H", Ottawa, Ontario K2H 8P9, Canada.

NEUVONEN Erkki, National Veterinary and Food Research Institute EELA, Department of Virology, P.O.Box 45, (Hämeentie 57), FI-00581 Helsinki, Finland.

NIIN Enel, Animal Health Department, Veterinary and Food Board of Estonia, Väike Paala Street 3, Tallinn 11415, Estonia.

OBRAZHEY Anatoliy F., UAAS Institute of Veterinary Medicine, 30, Donetska str., Kyiv 03151, Ukraine.

OLIYNYK Lyudmila V., The Kiev Veterinary Medicine Administration, 12, Volynska str., Kyiv 03151, Ukraine.

ONDREJKA Robert, University of Veterinary Medicine, Department of Infectious Diseases, Komenskeho 73, Košice 04181, Slovak Republic.

ONDREJKOVA Anna, University of Veterinary Medicine, Department of Infectious Diseases, Komenskeho 73, Košice 04181, Slovak Republic.

PASTORET Paul-Pierre, 7, rue de la Clissure, BE-4130 Fontin (Esneux), Belgium.

PATSYUK Mykola V., State Department of Veterinary Medicine, Ministry of Agricultural Policy of Ukraine, 24, Khreshchatik str., Kyiv-01001, Ukraine.

PICARD-MEYER Evelyne, Virology, AFSSA Nancy, WHO Coll Cent for Research and Management in Zoonoses Control, Domaine de Pixérécourt, BP 9, FR-54220 Malzéville, France.

PLAMADEALA Irina, Institute for Diagnosis and Animal Health, 63 Dr. Staicovici Str., Sector 5, Bucharest 050557, Romania.

POETZSCH Carsten J., Friedrich-Loeffler Institute, Seestr. 55, DE-16868 Wusterhausen, Germany.

PREDOI Gabriel, OIE Delegate, CVO, National Sanitary Veterinary and Food Safety Agency, Str. Negustori nr.1 Bis, sect.2, RO-7000 Bucharest, Romania.

ROTIVEL Yolande, CNE Rage, Institut Pasteur, 25, rue du Dr. Roux, FR-75724 Paris, Cedex 15, France.

RUPPRECHT Charles, Centres for Disease Control and Prevention, Rabies Section, Division of Viral and Rickettsial Diseases, Bldg 15, 55B6 11, 1600 Clifton Road, N.E., Mail Stop G 33, Atlanta, GA 30333, USA.

RYBAKOV Sergey, FGI Federal Centre for Animal Health, RU-600901 Vladimir, Yur'evets, Russia.

SABETA Claude, Agricultural Research Council, Onderstepoort Veterinary Institute, Virology Department, Rabies Unit, P Bag X05, Onderstepoort, Pretoria 0110, South Africa.

SANTRAC Violeta, Veterinary Institute RS Dr Vaso Butozan, Branka Radicevica 18, Banja Luka 51000, Bosnia and Herzegovina.

SCHONHOFF Susan, UMass Biologic Laboratory, 305 South Street, Jamaica Plain 02130, USA.

SCHUDEL Alejandro, Scientific and Technical Dept, World Organisation fo Animal Health, 12, rue de Prony, FR-75017 Paris, France.

SCHUMACHER Carolin, Grandes Prophylaxies Global Enterprise Merial, 29 avenue Tony Garnier, FR-69007 Lyon, France.

SELHORST Thomas, Friedrich-Loeffler Institut, Institut für Epidemiologie, Seestrasse 55, DE-16816 Wusterhausen, Germany.

SERVAT Alexandre, Immunology/CRL, AFSSA Nancy, Domaine de Pixérécourt, BP 9, FR-54220 Malzéville France.

SHADURA Mykola V., State Forestry Committee of Ukraine, 9-a, Shota Rustaveli str., Kyiv 01023, Ukraine.

SIHVONEN Liisa, Department of Virology, National Veterinary and Food Research Institute, P.O.Box 45, (Hämeentie 57), FI-00581 Helsinki, Finland.

SIMONOVIC Ljubisav, Veterinary Specialistic Institute, ul. Boska Jovica 8, 35 000 Jagodina, Serbia and Montenegro.

SKALKA Premysl, Laboratory for diagnostic of rabies, State Veterinary Institute Olomouc, Jakoubka ze Stribra, CZ-1 779 00 Olomouc, Czech Republic.

SLATE Dennis, U.S. Department of Agriculture, 59 Chenell Drive, Concord, NH 03301, USA.

SLAVOMÍR Jerg, NRL for Rabies, State Veterinary Institute Zvolen, Pod Drahami 918, Zvolen 96086, Slovak Republic.

SLIVKO Igor, R & D NARVAC Ivanovski Virology Institute, 16 Gamalei st., RU-123098 Moscow, Russia.

SMITH Graham, Central Science Laboratory, Sand Hutton, York YO41 1LZ, U.K.

SMRECZAK'S Marcin, National Veterinary Research Institute, Ul. Parrtyzantow 57, PL-24 100 Pulawy, Poland.

SOLODTCHUK Volodymyr L., Ukrvetprompostatch, Brovary, Kyiv Region 07403, Ukraine.

STANOJEVIC Slavoljub, Department for Veterinary Service, Ministry of Agriculture Forestry an Water Management, St. omladinskih brigada 1, SIV 3, office 92, N. Belgrade 11070, Serbia and Montenegro.

STEIJN Klaas, Unit Animal Health Department, Animal Diseases and Animal Health, VWA/RVV, P.O.B. 19506, NL-2500 CM Den Haag, The Netherlands.

SÜLI Judit, University of Veterinary Medicine, Department of Infectious Diseases, Komenskeho 73, Košice 04181, Slovak Republic.

SVRCEK Stefan, University of Veterinary Medicine, Department of Infectious Diseases, Komenskeho 73, Košice 04181, Slovak Republic.

TESORO Emiliano, Unidad de Investigación Médica en Inmunología, Hospital de Pediatría, CMN-Siglo XXI, IMSS, Av. Cuauhtemoc 330, Col. Doctores, México D.F. 06725, Mexico.

TORDO Noël, Virology Department, Unit Antiviral Strategies, Institut Pasteur, 25, rue du Dr. Roux, FR-75724 Paris, Cedex 15, France.

TREIBERG BERNDTSSON Louise, National Veterinary Institute, SVA, Ulls väg 2B, SE-751 89 Uppsala, Sweden.

VALTCHOUSER R., Pencho Slaveikov, 15 BG, BG-1606 Sofia, Bulgaria.

VERBITSKIY Petro I., State Department of Veterinary Medicine, Ministry of Agricultural Policy of Ukraine, 24, Khreshchatik str., Kyiv-01001, Ukraine.

VERMEERSCH Jean-Pierre, European Commission, Rue Froissard 101 3/84, BE-1049 Bruxelles, Bruxelles.

VERZHIKHOVSKIY Olexandr M., State Department of Veterinary Medicine, Ministry of Agricultural Policy of Ukraine, 24, Khreshchatik str., Kyiv-01001, Ukraine.

VITALIY Nodosekov, St. Kotelnikova 31 op 4, Kyiv, Ukraine.

VLASOV Nikolay, All-Russian Center for Control and Standartization of Medical Means for Animals, Zvenigorodsky avn. 5, RU-123122 Moscow, Russia.

VOS Ad, Viral Vaccines, IDT GmbH, Hemelseberg 3, NL-6862 BN Oosterbeek, The Netherlands.

VOUGIOUKAS George, 27 Popoflesse Str., GR-16673 Voula, Greece.

VRZAL Vladimir, Bioveta a. s., Komenského 212, CZ-683 23 Ivanovice na Hané, Czech Republic.

WANDELER Alexander, Center of Expertise for Rabies CFIA/ACIA, Ottawa Laboratory Fallowfield, 3851 Fallowfield Road, Ottawa ON K2H 8P9, Canada.

WARRELL Mary, The Centre for Tropical Medicine, Level 7, John Radcliffe Hospital, Headington, Oxford, OX3 9, U.K.

YAKOBSON Boris, Kimron Veterinary Institute, Bet Dagan P.O.B. 12, IL-50250 Bet Dagan, Israel.

YEHYA Ghazi, Kfarchima, Office de la Soie, B.P. 268 Hazmieh, Lebanon.

ZAKHAROV Valery, FGI Federal Centre for Animal Health, RU-600901 Vladimir, Yur'evets, Russia.

ZAKIEVA Samira, The National Laboratory of Azerbaijan Republic, The State Veterinary Service, Nadjaf Narimanova 7a, 1106 Baku, Azerbaijan.

ZGONNYK Nataliya, State Department of Veterinary Medicine, Ministry of Agricultural Policy of Ukraine, 24, Khreshchatik str. Kyiv-01001, Ukraine.

ZIETARA Magdalena, General Veterinary Inspectorate, 30 Wspolna Str., PL-00930 Warsaw, Poland.

ZMUDZINSKI Jan F., National Veterinary Research Institute, Al. Partyzantow 57, PL-24-100 Pulawy, Poland.

Index of Authors

Developments in Biological Standardization

Vol. 23: Madrid 1973	Sterilization and sterility testing of biological substances
Vol. 24: San Francisco 1973	Preservatives in biological products
Vol. 25: Lyon 1973	Requirements for poultry virus vaccines
Vol. 26: Budapest 1973	Selected veterinary vaccines
Vol. 27: Budapest 1973	Purity of human plasma proteins
Vol. 28: London 1974	Immunity to infections of the respiratory system in man and animals
46th Symp., London 1974	Breeding of simians and their uses in developmental biology. Ed. Lab. Animals Ltd. (6)
Vol. 29: Geneva 1974 (WHO/IABS)	Standardization and control of allergens administered to man
Vol. 30: Milan 1974	Viral hepatitis
Vol. 31: Rabat 1975	Brucellosis (II)
Vol. 32: Paris 1975 (OIE/IABS)	Colstridial sera and vaccines for veterinary use
Vol. 33: Douglas 1975	Vaccination by the non-parenteral route
Vol. 34: Budapest 1976	Pyrogenicity, innocuity and toxicity test systems for biological products
Vol. 35: Lyon 1976	Foot-and-mouth disease vaccines
Vol. 36: Lyon Washington D.C. 1976	Freeze-drying of biological products
Vol. 37: Geneva 1976	Standardization of cell substrates for the production of virus vaccines
Vol. 38: London 1977	Biological preparations in the treatment of cancer
Vol. 39: Geneva 1977	Influenza immunization (II)
Vol. 40: Marburg 1977	Standardization of rabies vaccines (III) (WHO/IABS)
Vol. 41: Guadeloupe 1978	Vaccinations in the developing countries
Vol. 42: Paris 1978	Second General Meeting of European Society of Animal Cell Technology
Vol. 43: Brussels 1978	Immunization: Benefit versus risk factors
Vol. 44: Villars 1979	Test methods for the quality control of plasma proteins
Vol. 45: San Antonio 1979	The Standardization of animals to improve biomedical research, production and control
Vol. 46: Oxford 1979	Third General Meeting of European Society of Animal Cell Technology
Vol. 47: Bilthoven 1980	Reassessment of inactivated poliomyelitis vaccine
Vol. 48: Geneva 1980	Standardization of albumin, plasma substitutes and plasmapheresis
Vol. 49: Leetown 1981	Fish biologics: Serodiagnostics and vaccines
Vol. 50: Heidelberg 1981	Joint ESACT-IABS Meeting on the use of heteroploid and other cell substrates for the production of biologicals
Vol. 51: Lyon 1981	Immunization of adult birds with inactivated oil adjuvant vaccines
Vol. 52: Lyon 1981	Herpes virus of man and animal: Standardization of immunological procedures
Vol. 53: Dublin 1982	Enteric infections in man and animals: Standardization of immunological procedures

Vol. 54: Athens 1982	Viral hepatitis: Standardization in immunoprophylaxis of infections by hepatitis viruses
Vol. 55: Copenhagen 1982	Fifth General Meeting of European Society of Animal Cell Technology
Vol. 56: Algeria 1983	IIIrd International Symposium on Brucellosis
Vol. 57: Paris 1983	Monoclonal antibodies: Standardization of their characterization and use
Vol. 58: Budapest 1983	BCG vaccines and tuberculins
Vol. 59: Geneva 1983	Standardization and control of biologicals produced by recombinant DNA technology
Vol. 60: Gardone Riviera 1983	Production and exploitation of existing and new animal cell substrates
Vol. 61: Geneva 1984	Proceedings of the Fourth International Symposium on pertussis
Vol. 62: Stockholm 1985	Diagnostics and vaccines for parasitic diseases
Vol. 63: San Francisco 1985	Use and standardization of chemically defined antigens
Vol. 64: London 1985	Reduction of animal usage in the development and control of biological products
Vol. 65: Amsterdam 1985	Use and standardization of combined vaccines
Vol. 66: Baden 1985	Advances in animal cell technology: cell engineering, evaluation and exploitation
Vol. 67: Melbourne 1986	Standardization in blood fractionation including coagulation factors
Vol. 68: Geneva, 1986	Cells – Products – Safety
Vol. 69: London, 1987	Cytokines Laboratory and Clinical Evaluation
Vol. 70:Arlington, VA, 1988	Continuous Cell Lines as Substrates for Biologicals
Vol. 71:Utrecht, 1989	Monoclonal Antibodies for Therapy, Prevention and In vivo Diagnosis of Human Disease
Vol. 72: Annecy, 1989	Progress in Animal Retroviruses
Vol. 73: Shizuoka, 1990	Pertussis: Evaluation and Research on Acellular Pertussis Vaccines
Vol. 74: Bethesda, MD, 1990	Biological Product Freeze-Drying and Formulation
Vol. 75: London, 1990	Virological Aspects of the Safety of Biological Products
Vol. 76: Bethesda, MD, 1991	Continuous Cell Lines - An International Workshop on Current Issues
Vol. 77: Annecy, 1991	Standardization of the Immunopharmacology of Natural and Synthetic Immunomodulators
Vol. 78: Bethesda, MD, 1991	Poliovirus Attenuation: Molecular Mechanisms and Practical Aspects
Vol. 79: Ploufragan, 1992	The First Steps Towards an International Harmonization of Veterinary Biologicals: 1993 and Free Circulation of Vaccines within the EEC
Vol. 80: Heidelberg, 1992	Transmissible Spongiform Encephalopathies - Impact on Animal and Human Health
Vol. 81: Cannes, 1992	Virological Safety Aspects of Plasma Derivatives
Vol. 82: Albany NY, 1993	Recombinant Vectors in Vaccine Development
Vol. 83: Annecy, 1993	Genetic Stability and Recombinant Product Consistency
Vol. 84: Langen, 1993	Non-Target Effects of Live Vaccines
Vol. 85: Santa Fé, NM, 1994	Genetics of Streptococci, Enterococci and Lactococci
Vol. 86: Langen, 1994	Replacement, Reduction and Refinement of Animal Experiments in the Development and Control of Biological Products
Vol. 87: Geneva, 1995	New Approaches to Stabilisation of Vaccines Potency
Vol. 88: Bethesda, MD, 1995	Viral Safety and Evaluation of Viral Clearance from Biopharmaceutical Products
Vol. 89: Rome, 1995	Pertussis Vaccine Trials
Vol. 90: Oslo, 1996	Fish Vaccinology
Vol. 91: San Francisco, CA, 1996	Development of Specifications for Biotechnology Pharmaceuticals Products
Vol. 92: Bergen, 1996	Modulation of the Immune Response to Vaccine Antigens
Vol. 93: Annecy, 1996	Safety of Biological Products Prepared from Mammalian Cell Culture
Vol. 94: Bethesda, MD, 1997	Simian Virus 40 (SV40): A Possible Human Polyomavirus
Vol. 95: Paris, 1997	Preclinical and Clinical Development of New Vaccines
Vol. 96: Washington, DC, 1995	Characterization of Biotechnology Pharmaceutical Products
Vol. 97: London, 1997	Biological Characterization and Assay of Cytokines and Growth Factors

Vol. 98: London, 1997	Inactivated Influenza Vaccines Prepared in Cell Culture
Vol. 99: Strasbourg, 1998	Animal Sera, Animal Sera Derivatives and Substitutes Used in the Manufacture of Pharmaceuticals: Viral Safety and Regulatory Aspects
Vol. 100: Geneva, 1998	A Celebration of 50 Years of Progress in Biological Standardization and Control at WHO
Vol. 101: London, 1998	Alternatives to Animals in the Development and Control of Biological Products for Human and Veterinary Use

Developments in Biologicals

Vol. 102: San Francisco, CA, 1999	Advances in Transfusion Safety
Vol. 103: Annecy, 1999	Physico-Chemical Procedures for the Characterization of Vaccines
Vol. 104: Langen, 1999	Development and Clinical Progress of DNA Vaccines
Vol. 105: Paris, 2000	Progress in Polio Eradication: Vaccine Strategies for the End Game
Vol. 106: Rockville, MD, 2000	Evolving Scientific and Regulatory Perspectives on Cell Substrates for Vaccine Development
Vol. 107: London, 2000	The Design and Analysis of Potency Assays for Biotechnology Products
Vol. 108: Langen, 2001	Advances in Transfusion Safety
Vol. 109: Washington, DC, 2000	Biologics 2000 – Comparability of Biotechnology Products
Vol. 110: Palm Cove, 2001	Orphan Vaccines – Bridging the Gap
Vol. 111: Utrecht, 2001	Advancing Science and Elimination of the Use of Laboratory Animals for Development and Control of Vaccines and Hormones
Vol. 112: Bethesda, MD, 2001	Immunogenicity of Therapeutic Biological Products
Vol. 113: Berlin, 2001	Process Validation for Manufacturing of Biologics and Biotechnology Products
Vol. 114: Ames, IA, 2002	Vaccines for OIE List A and Emerging Animal Diseases
Vol. 115: Bergen, 2002	Laboratory Correlates of Immunity to Influenza – A Reassessment
Vol. 116: Los Angeles, CA, 2003	Development of Therapeutic Cancer Vaccines
Vol. 117: Langen, 2003	Consideration of Alternative Licensing Procedures for Vaccines for Minor Species, Minor Indications and Autogenous/Autologous Products
Vol. 118: Langen, 2003	PDA/EMEA European Virus Safety Forum
Vol. 119: Buenos Aires, 2004	Control of Infectious Animal Diseases by Vaccination
Vol. 120: Bethesda, MD, 2003	Advances in Transfusion Safety
Vol. 121: Bergen, 2003	Progress in Fish Vaccinology
Vol. 122: Bethesda, MD, 2003	State of the Art Analytical Methods for Characterization of Biological Products and Assessment of Comparability
Vol. 123: Rockville, MD, 2004	Vaccine Cell Substrates 2004
Vol. 124: Paris, 2005	OIE/FAO International Scientific Conference on Avian Influenza

IMPRIMERIE MEDECINE HYGIENE GENEVE SUISSE

mai - 2006